Mammographic Image Analysis

Computational Imaging and Vision

Managing Editor

MAX A. VIERGEVER
Utrecht University, Utrecht, The Netherlands

Editorial Board

Mammographic Image Analysis

by

Ralph Highnam
Department of Engineering Science,
Oxford University, Oxford,
United Kingdom

and

Michael Brady
Department of Engineering Science,
Oxford University, Oxford,
United Kingdom

SPRINGER-SCIENCE+BUSINESS MEDIA, B.V.

A C.I.P. Catalogue record for this book is available from the Library of Congress.

ISBN 978-94-010-5949-7   ISBN 978-94-011-4613-5 (eBook)
DOI 10.1007/978-94-011-4613-5

Printed on acid-free paper

TABLE OF CONTENTS

PART III: FURTHER BREAST IMAGE ANALYSIS

PREFACE

Breast cancer is a major health problem in the Western world, where it is the most common cancer among women. Approximately 1 in 12 women will develop breast cancer during the course of their lives. Over the past twenty years there have been a series of major advances in the management of women with breast cancer, ranging from novel chemotherapy and radiotherapy treatments to conservative surgery. The next twenty years are likely to see computerized image analysis playing an increasingly important role in patient management.

As applications of image analysis go, medical applications are tough in general, and breast cancer image analysis is one of the toughest. There are many reasons for this: highly variable and irregular shapes of the objects of interest, changing imaging conditions, and the densely textured nature of the images. Add to this the increasing need for quantitative information, precision, and reliability (very few false positives), and the image processing challenge becomes quite daunting, in fact it pushes image analysis techniques right to their limits.

There are many stakeholders in the search for better ways to detect tumours and manage patient care. Most important are the teams of clinicians, typically comprising a radiologist, a surgeon, and a pathologist. They, in turn, rely on medical technicians and radiographers, medical physicists, and, increasingly, medical image analysts. Future developments mostly come from researchers and students (who first have to learn the basics of the subject effectively). Finally, women act as subjects and volunteers, and more and more want to be informed about the nature of their disease and the decision making process that concerns their well-being. Though we are image analysts, we have tried to write this monograph so that the ideas can be accessed by the widest possible range of stakeholders. To this end, we have tried to keep mathematical detail in boxes independent of the text and put in plenty of examples. So, if the going gets tough occasionally, please don't give up!

Many of the ideas described in the monograph originally appeared in journal articles written over a period of nine years, though we have discovered a lot of new material during the course of writing this monograph. We embarked on the roller-coaster ride that is writing a monograph because we wanted to promote two themes that underpin all of our work and which can only be described episodically in any single article. First, we believe that the high levels of reliability demanded of mammographic image analysis inevitably imply the development of techniques that are specific to mammography, irrespective of whether it is based on x-ray, magnetic resonance imagery (MRI), ultrasound, nuclear medicine, or any other imaging modality. We interpret this as meaning that it is necessary to base our algorithms on a set of detailed, explicit models: of image formation, of contrast agent take-up, of anatomy, and of pathology. Part I of the monograph develops such a model-based approach to x-ray mammography, Part II shows how it can be exploited, while Part III develops a model and exploits it for contrast-enhanced MRI mammography.

Second, the key contribution of our approach to x-ray mammographic image analysis is the development of a representation of the non-fatty compressed breast tissue that we show can be derived from a single mammogram. The importance of the representation, which we call h_{int}, is that it removes all those those changes in the image that are due only to the particular imaging conditions (for example, the film speed or exposure time), leaving just the non-fatty "interesting" tissue. Normalising images in this way enables us to enhance them, match them, and classify regions in them more reliably, because unnecessary, distracting variations have been eliminated. We show how the h_{int} representation can be developed in Part I, then put it to work on a range of clinically-important tasks in Part II.

This monograph has had a long gestation period, partly because we have made numerous discoveries while writing it, and partly because the subject is in a period of rapid development. One of the more pleasant tasks for the authors is to thank publicly the many people who have helped us realise this monograph and the ideas that it promotes. First, the UK Engineering and Physical Sciences Research Council funded RPH as a doctoral student and subsequently as a post-doctoral researcher, and awarded JMB a Senior Research Fellowship for five years and funded his major project on mammography. Max Viergever encouraged us to write the monograph and remained patient long after our estimated finish date. RPH thanks Philips Laboratories for the six month sabbatical he spent there, and in particular Charles Carman. JMB thanks Nicholas Ayache, the members of Project Epidaure and INRIA for hosting two stays on the Côte d'Azur that changed his life in many ways. We thank the staff of the Breast Care Unit at the Churchill Hospital, Oxford for their continuing support over many years, particularly Basil Shepstone, Ruth English, Yvonne Swainston, Wendy Hills, Hazel Bailey, Sue McDougal, June Pickvance, Coral James, Jane Cobb, Janet Green, Liz Robinson, Lorriane Tucker, Christine Cherry, Jan Lougher, Betty Harvey, Lettice Bowen, Geraldine Ashworth,

Jane Clarke and Ann Dickson-Brown. Special thanks go to Donald Peach for many informative talks. Similarly, the work reported in Chapter 15 could never have been possible without the enthusiastic support of the staff of the MRI Centre at the John Radcliffe Hospital, Oxford, particularly Niall Moore, Pieter Pretorius, and Dermot Dobson. We thank our colleagues and students for their many contributions to the research programme that we set out, particularly Alison Noble, Nick Cerneaz, Siew-Li Kok-Wiles, Margaret Yam, Paul Hayton, Maud Poissonnier, Christian Behrenbruch, Sebastien Gilles, Regis Guillemaud, Kostas Marias, and Yasuyo Kita (and ETL for making her visit to Oxford possible). It is impossible to thank individually the many professional colleagues who commented on our ideas, but we do wish to acknowledge David Dance, Ela Claridge, Nico Karssemeijer, and Paul Taylor. Finally, we thank the many volunteers who willingly participated in the clinical trials that we undertook to validate our ideas.

Finally, JMB dedicates this monograph to the memory of his wonderful mother-in-law, Dr. Irene Friedlander, whose untimely death from breast cancer was the spur for his research in mammography.

CHAPTER 1

INTRODUCTION

1.1. Introduction

Breast cancer is a major problem for public health in the Western world, where it is the most common cancer among women. In the European Community, for example, breast cancer represents 19% of cancer deaths and fully 24% of all cancer cases. It is diagnosed in a total of 348,000 cases annually in the USA and EC [68] and kills almost 115,000 annually. Approximately 10% of women will develop breast cancer during the course of their lives.

In almost every field of medical imaging other than mammography, clinicians and technicians increasingly rely on computer processing of images as a key part of their decision making. This can involve framing a diagnosis or deciding when to call for further investigation such as a repeat image, an image of a different type, or a biopsy. Images are also used to monitor therapy. This monograph brings together the work we and our colleagues have done over the past few years on attempting to bring the benefits of image processing into mammography.

For the most part, our work to date has been concerned with mammography, which is currently the most frequently performed breast imaging technique done in the clinic. Mammography implies x-ray imaging of the breast. There is an increasing array of breast imaging techniques, including magnetic resonance imaging (MRI), nuclear medicine, and 2- and 3-dimensional ultrasound, and some of these have begun to be referred to as mammography, for example MR mammography. However, we retain the strict usage and so whenever we do not further qualify the term, mammography will mean x-ray breast imaging.

There has been a huge amount of work over the past 30 years developing image processing for mammograms and it has become clear that mammography poses an extremely tough image processing challenge because the images are intrinsically complex and they have poor signal-to-noise ratio. The images are complex because, as we shall see, the breast anatomy is intrinsically complex as is the interaction with it of x-rays, MRI, and the other modalities used in medical imaging. Also, in clinical practice there is always a compromise between patient risk (for example, radiation dose or the amount of contrast agent injected in certain MRI examinations) and image quality. Worse, abnormalities appear as quite subtle, irregular, often non-local differences in intensity. Moreover, the images are inevitably cluttered due to superimposition, the background normal breast structure varies greatly between different breasts, and, despite the careful quality assurance that is enforced for taking mammograms, image acquisition is weakly controlled relative to industrial applications of image processing. In short, mammographic images strain techniques of image processing to their current limits, and beyond. The challenge is made doubly difficult by the need for levels of performance that are orders of magnitude more demanding than are the norm in computer vision. Millions of mammograms are taken annually in the USA and in Europe; consequently, even one image-processing related mistake per ten thousand mammograms can have serious consequences for many hundreds or thousands of women.

The viewpoint that we promote in this monograph is that, in order to be reliable and predictable, mammographic image processing must be based on a model of how the image is formed. In the case of x-ray mammography, this means that we must model the way that x-rays pass through breast tissue of different types and are absorbed and scattered before exposing the film. We need to model non-linearities in image formation due to the anti-scatter grid and intensifying screen glare . Our modelling is based on the work of a number of medical physicists, most notably Dance[51], Johns[137], Yaffe[137], Carlson[32], Day[50, 56], and Haus[103]. Throughout the project, we have worked very closely with radiographers and radiologists, at the Churchill and John Radcliffe Hospitals in Oxford.

A key component of our approach to x-ray mammography is the automatic construction from a given image of a quantitative measure of the breast tissue at each image location. The measure we use is h_{int}, which represents the thickness of "interesting" (non-fat) tissue between the image location and the x-ray source. The variation of this measure over the image constitutes what we call the h_{int} representation, and it can most usefully be regarded as a surface that conveys information about the anatomy of the breast. For example, masses which have high non-fat content appear as "hills" on the surrounding "undulating terrain". We will show that the h_{int} representation factors out of a mammogram information that is related to the imaging process, for example the exposure time or tube characteristics, leaving just the intrinsic "interesting" information about the breast anatomy. This is the fundamental reason why it is the basis of our approach to image normalisation: all effects in the image due to variations in the imaging conditions have been removed, leaving just the breast tissue. We normalise images in order to enhance them in some way, for example to remove the effects of degrading factors such as photon scatter. Furthermore, the h_{int} representation gives us a basis upon which to build object models and to reason about breast anatomy. We use this ability to choose features that are robust to breast compression and variations in breast composition. In a similar way, a key component of our approach to contrast-enhanced breast MR is the development of a pharmacokinetic model of the take-up of contrast agent by tissues of different types.

In the remaining sections of this introductory chapter, we first outline the current situation with respect to breast cancer screening, a policy that has been instituted to varying extents in many countries. Then we introduce those aspects of the anatomy, physiology, and pathology of the breast needed to make the book self-contained. We show why the h_{int} representation is necessary. Finally, we outline the organisation of the book.

We have tried to make the text accessible both to scientists interested in image processing and to clinicians and technicians. Throughout, we have first given a textual description of a problem and technique for solving it. Only then, and only when appropriate, have we added a mathematical account which we have "boxed" to isolate it from the text. The text is self-contained even if the mathematics is ignored. We have attempted to make the figures tell a lot of the story, and we have kept the figure captions non-technical. So, even if a "quick flick" through the book suggests that it is going to be a mathematical grind, we assure the reader that such is not the case! Don't give up!

1.2. Breast cancer screening

During the past sixty years, female death rates in the USA from breast cancer stayed remarkably constant while those from almost all other causes declined. The sole exception is lung cancer death rates, which increased sharply from 5 to 26 per 100,000. It is interesting to compare the figures for breast cancer with those from cervical cancer, for which mortality rates declined by 70% after the cervical smear gained widespread acceptance. In the UK, the current screening programme invites women between the ages of 50 and 65 for breast screening. If a mammogram displays any suspicious signs the woman is invited back to an assessment clinic where other views and other imaging modalities are utilized. If the results are still suspicious a biopsy is performed. It is hoped, and generally believed, that screening with mammography will have the same beneficial effect on breast cancer death rates as the Pap smear on cervical cancer. In his excellent "Overview of Breast Cancer Screening" [57], Peter B. Dean states that: "breast cancer screening has been introduced only recently, and only to certain specified age groups in a few chosen populations. The effect it will have on breast cancer mortality in large populations has yet to be demonstrated, but the success of well-designed trials gives us good reason to be optimistic."

Age Group	Incidence per 100,000	Age Group	Incidence per 100,000
15-19	0.2	55-59	228.9
20-24	1.1	60-64	251.2
25-29	8.3	65-69	282.9
30-34	26.7	70-74	302.2
35-39	57.2	75-79	338.0
40-44	106.2	80-84	350.0
45-49	173.8	85+	376.3
50-54	195.9		

TABLE 1.1. Average annual age-specific rates of incidence of breast cancer (per 100,000 females). From [266].

Since life expectancy has increased during the past sixty years, there has been a steady increase in the incidence of breast cancer in industrialised societies. Table 1.1 shows the average annual age-specific rates of incidence of breast cancer (per 100,000 females) in the USA between 1973 and 1977. It can be seen that the incidence is practically negligible before the age of 30, but then increases sharply until the age of 50 from which point it continues to increase but less sharply. The incidence practically doubles between the ages of 40 and 50. This fact, coupled with the sharply reduced utility of mammography for young women, has led to the lower age limit for breast cancer screening programmes being set at between 40 and 50.

One way in which younger women can check their breasts is through self-examination. Before breast screening was introduced, over 90% of breast tumours were detected by the woman herself[11]. This strongly suggests that regular and systematic examination by a woman of her breasts would improve her chance of detecting a breast cancer at the earliest possible palpable stage. The aim of breast self examination is to encourage a woman to learn how her breasts feel normally, so that she is in a good position to detect quite small abnormal changes. Generally, although people are not very good at describing how something as complex as a breast, arm, or knee feel, they are good at detecting localised *changes*. Since there is a wide variation in the size, shape and constitution of breasts, and since, in particular, some women have rather lumpy breasts, or breasts that change considerably during the normal menstrual cycle, they may be better placed to detect abnormalities by palpation than would a doctor.

There has been an ongoing programme in the UK to make women aware of the need for breast self examination, and schemes to teach them what to take notice of. There is some evidence that it can lead to earlier detection

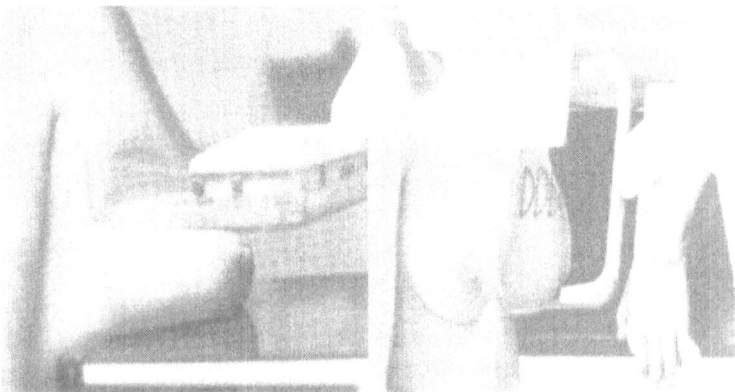

Figure 1.1. This picture shows the two views most commonly performed in mammography. The left picture shows the cranio-caudal view of the breast, in which the x-rays pass through the breast in a direction from the head towards the feet. The right picture shows the medio-lateral oblique view, which is taken diagonally across the body in a direction from the shoulder towards the opposite hip. The medio-lateral oblique view enables the radiologist to judge whether there has been metastatic spread of cancer to the axillae. Taking two views from different angles in principle enables the radiologist to discriminate between clinically significant areas and those that are not but which might appear so in a single image. This picture originally appeared in [34] and is reprinted by permission of Butterworth Heinemann Publishers, a division of Reed Educational & Professional Publishing Ltd.

of disease; but there is no proof of any impact on breast cancer death rates. One possible explanation for this is that 70% of women with breast lumps intentionally delay reporting their symptoms[11], largely through denial stemming from a fear of a diagnosis of cancer. Nearly half the cancers seen for the first time in a UK hospital clinic are already at an incurable stage. A second explanation could be that the difference in stage between tumours detected by breast self-examination and those found in the normal course of events is so small that it makes little difference to survival rates. Nevertheless, regular self-examination is seen as an important adjunct to mammographic screening.

Dean [57] reviews the development of national screening programmes, beginning with the much criticised but highly influential HIP study in New York during the 1960s, and the randomised, controlled, population-based trials in Sweden beginning in the late 1970s. Mammography screening expanded in Sweden to cover the whole country by 1994. Finland was the first country to begin nationwide screening of women in 1986, shortly followed by the UK which began its national programme in 1987. In contrast, most mammograms currently performed in the USA are on symptomatic women[57]. The UK programme resulted from the Government's acceptance of the report of the committee chaired by Sir Patrick Forrest [79]. It was quite bullish about the effects of a screening programme:

> "by the year 2000 the screening programme is expected to prevent about 25% of deaths from breast cancer in the population of women invited for screening ... On average each of the women in whom breast cancer is prevented will live about 20 years more. Thus by the year 2000 the screening programme is expected to result in about 25,000 extra years of life gained annually in the UK".

Dean notes that the parameters proposed by the Forrest Report, and subsequently established in the UK screening programme, were based on those chosen at the beginning of the Swedish trial in 1977, but significantly revised by the Swedes by the time the Forrest Committee started to deliberate. Most importantly, the Forrest Committee call for a single view of each breast and an interval between screening examinations of three years. This despite the fact that the Swedish authorities had in 1984 revised the parameters to the two views of each breast as shown in Figure 1.1, an independent reading by two radiologists, and a screening interval of at most two years (18 months for women aged 40-55). A recent study [260] has been published suggesting that the rate of presentation of tumours that arise in the UK within the three year screening interval (*"interval cancers"*) is much larger than expected. If these early results on interval cancers hold up to further study, this is likely to lead *inter alia* to pressure for a reduction in the screening interval and to two-view screening (cranio-caudal and medio-lateral oblique), with the consequent increased need to match reliably the views at a screening, and from successive examinations. The resource implications of such an increase in screening are considerable.

Dean notes that measuring the success of breast cancer screening programmes is fraught with difficulty, not least because it is difficult to isolate an effective control group that participates in a trial yet does not independently seek a mammogram. He concludes that "historical controls, i.e. whether or not the mortality from breast cancer begins to decline in the population screened, is likely to be the best method for evaluating screening". More recently, quotations such as the following have begun to appear: [1] "breast cancer mortality rates fell by more than 5% between 1989 and 1993, most markedly in women younger than 65 and in whites. The decline appears to stem from a combination of early detection and, probably, improvements in treatment". Indeed, despite the current lack of a quantitative evaluation of the effectiveness of screening, Dean suggests that "women offered screening should be told that their participation in the programme will more than double their chances of surviving breast cancer".

---

[1] Quotation from the *Scientific American* special issue on Cancer, 1996.

1.3. Basic breast anatomy, physiology and pathology

It is neither possible nor appropriate to present in this monograph a comprehensive account of the remarkably complex anatomy, physiology, and pathology of the breast. Rather, we introduce just those aspects that are needed to make the book self-contained. The reader who wants a more detailed account is referred to [97, 233]. Readers with little background in medical imaging may find some of the medical terms unfamiliar. A detailed understanding is not required to follow the developments here or in the body of the book.

Milk production and calcifications

The female breast is highly specialised for its primary function, the production of milk to nourish infants. The preponderance of milk-producing tissue in the breast of a female of child bearing age is typically converted to fat during the involution process that precedes the menopause. Minor involution processes also occur following the end of milk production and as part of the menstrual cycle. Milk contains a great deal of calcium, and calcium absorbs (more technically, attenuates) tens of times more x-ray photons than does other breast tissue[2]. In short, just like bone in a familiar x-ray, fragments of calcium are practically radio-opaque and appear bright white in a x-ray mammogram. Most other normal, non-fat breast tissue is water dense and also appears light, though less bright than calcium. Conversely, fatty tissue is practically radio-transparent and appears very dark in a mammogram. The practical consequence of these observations is that a mammogram such as that shown in Figure 1.2 of a typical woman of child bearing age appears predominantly white, making it difficult to detect the often localised structures characteristic of breast disease. It is usually far easier to detect similar localised structures in the predominantly dark mammograms also shown in Figure 1.2, of a post-menopausal woman whose breasts tend to have a far higher fat content. This is one of the major reasons that screening programmes, which are all currently based on x-rays, have excluded women below a certain age (typically 50 years of age). This is reinforced by the need to reduce as far as possible health risks due to radiation.

---

[2]We will give precise figures for x-ray attenuation by breast tissue in Chapter 2.

DENSE AND FATTY BREASTS

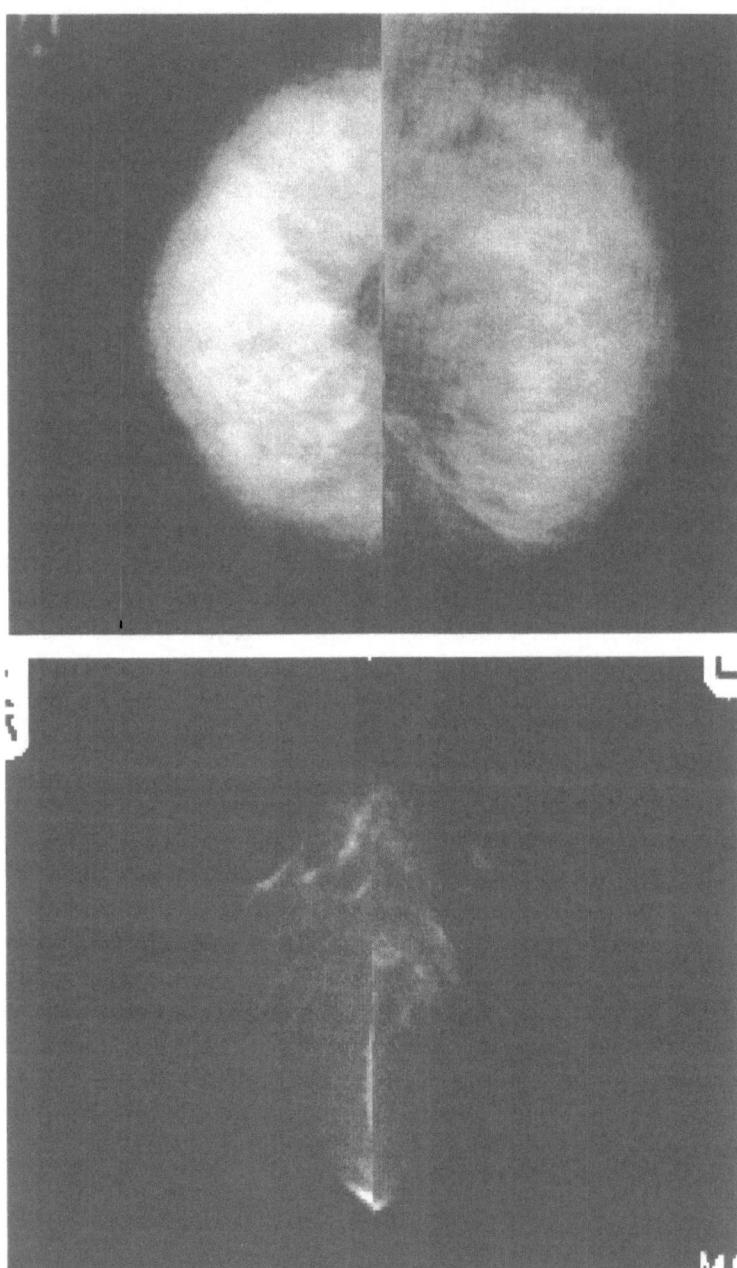

Figure 1.2. The top mammograms are from a younger woman with dense breasts, whilst the bottom ones are from an older woman with predominantly fatty breasts. It is much more difficult to find localised abnormal "bright" structures in the dense mammograms.

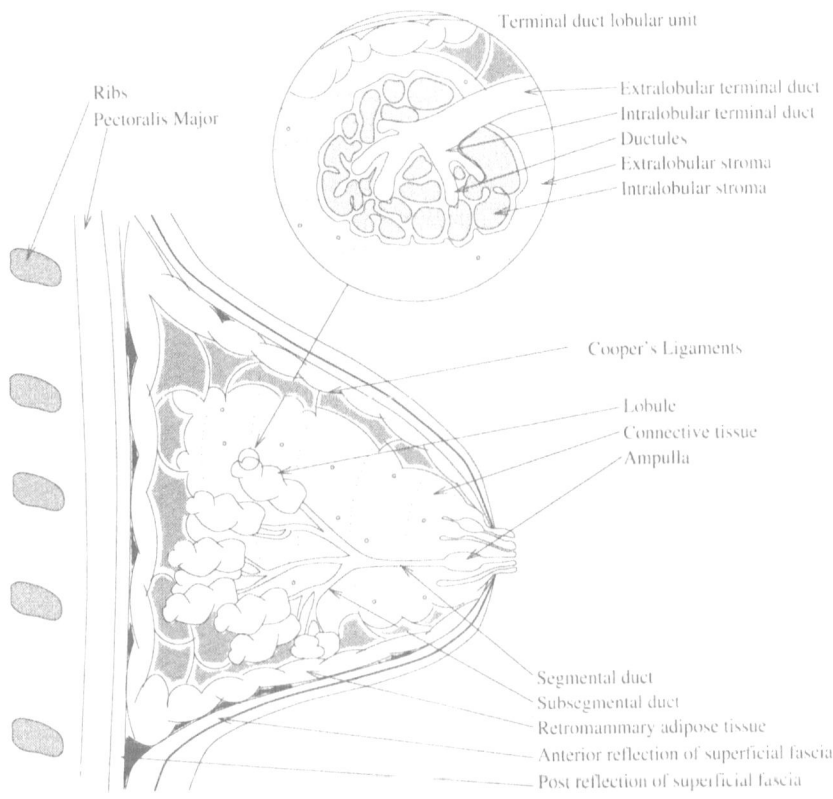

Figure 1.3. A simplified sketch of the hugely complex anatomy of the breast, showing the structures that are most relevant for breast cancer. See the text for details.

Figure 1.3 is a sketch of the main features of the anatomy of the breast. Milk production arises in the breast lobes. Generally, there are 15-20 lobes that converge on the nipple each of which spreads out radially from it in the form of a tree-like pattern of ductal structures. Working backwards from the nipple, the lobe begins with a collecting duct that transfers the milk from the lactiferous duct to the suckling infant. The collecting duct immediately widens into a pouch-like structure called the ampulla that narrows and forms the segmental duct that is the trunk of the ductal tree. This duct branches several times, forming subsegmental ducts with correspondingly smaller diameters, before they enter a complex and important structure called the lobule. Inside the lobule, each of the subsegmental ducts further divides into 10 to 100 intralobular terminal ducts each of which ends in a terminal ductule, where, finally, the milk is produced in sac-like units called acini, and from where it begins its voyage to the nipple. The structure surrounding the lobule is called a terminal duct lobular unit (TDLU) and it plays a key role in the pathology of breast cancer since it is there that many diseases arise. We turn to that now.

In situ (as opposed to invasive) carcinomas arise commonly in two forms: ductal and lobular. Ductal carcinoma *in situ* (DCIS) can involve a variable number of ducts and ductal structures, may be solid, and often involves central necrosis, but is always contained within the ducts. Occasionally the carcinoma cells of a deep DCIS can migrate towards the nipple pushing the skin layers ahead of it, resulting in an eczematous rash involving the nipple and areola. This condition, known as Paget's disease, may be indicative of DCIS. Lobular carcinoma *in situ* (LCIS) describes a proliferation of cancer cells within the lobule acini. In LCIS, the acini cavities are completely filled and swell to accommodate the growth, effectively reducing the intralobular connective tissue (stroma). However, the membranes remain intact containing the growth.

Localised cancers in the ducts or lobules often are associated with secretions that thicken or become necrotic. These are called calcifications, or microcalcifications if they are smaller. The identification of calcifications is a major goal of screening programmes, though benign calcifications are common (for example they often occur in blood vessels), and so the distinction between ductal and vascular microcalcifications needs to be made if the number of false positives is to be sufficiently low. This is not a problem for radiologists interpreting mammograms against the background of their knowledge of breast anatomy. It is, however, a challenge for image analysis programs. Not surprisingly, the development of algorithms to identify microcalcifications has been the subject of intensive (ongoing) effort in mammographic image processing, as we discuss in detail in Chapter 11. Some appreciation of the difficulty faced by the radiologist detecting microcalcifications, and by the developer of computer programs that aim to do the same, is shown in Figure 1.4. Attempts continue to detect cancers earlier and earlier, that is to detect smaller and smaller clinical significant signs. This in turn demands ever higher image resolution, and there is a perpetual debate over the image resolution that is necessary to reliably detect microcalcifications.

Curvilinear structures

Ductal structures in a mammogram take the form of curvilinear structures that are slightly brighter than their surroundings. An algorithm for their detection and removal is the subject of Chapter 12. Figure 1.5 shows the curvilinear structures detected by the algorithm for one breast. However, it

MICROCALCIFICATIONS AND NOISE

Figure 1.4.   Microcalcifications are localised secretions that have thickened and dried or that have become necrotic. They are primarily composed of Calcium salts. Generally, they are difficult to detect in mammograms because they are small and although they tend to be brighter than the surrounding tissue, the contrast can be both variable and small. It is often hard to distinguish between real microcalcifications and image noise that has no clinical significance. In this image, the bright spots at the top are, in fact, noise; while the duller bright spots at the bottom are microcalcifications.

is almost always the case that ductal curvilinear structures are confounded with other curvilinear structures, most notably blood vessels and supporting tissues called Cooper's ligaments. A technical name for the functioning tissue of the breast is the parenchyma, and it corresponds to the majority of the bright (water dense) patches of a mammogram. The parenchyma is held in place by the Cooper's ligaments, though of course the whole structure can move non-rigidly as the breast is compressed. We return to breast compression later in this section.

Masses

Other bright structures may appear in the midst of the parenchyma and blood vessels, assuming that they can be distinguished as such, and they may correspond to pathologies or, in some views, to lymph nodes. Left

CURVILINEAR STRUCTURES

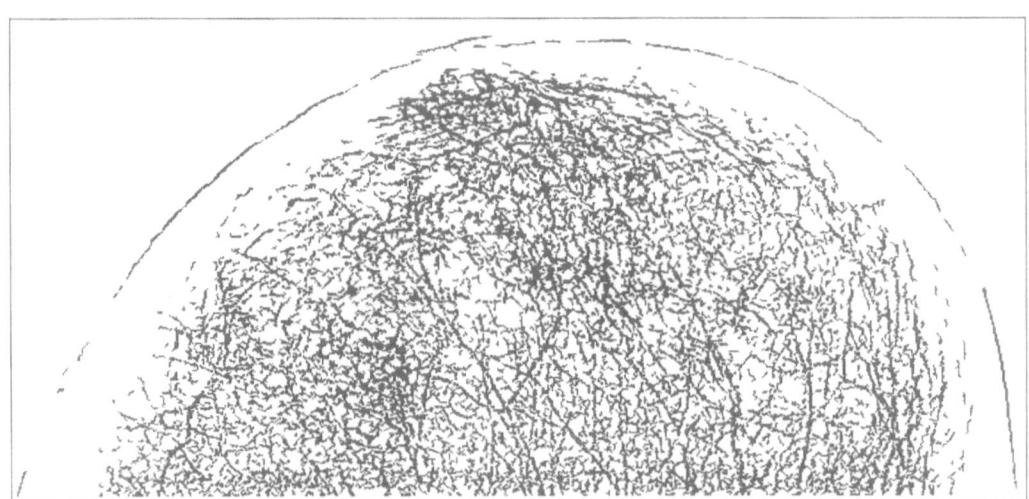

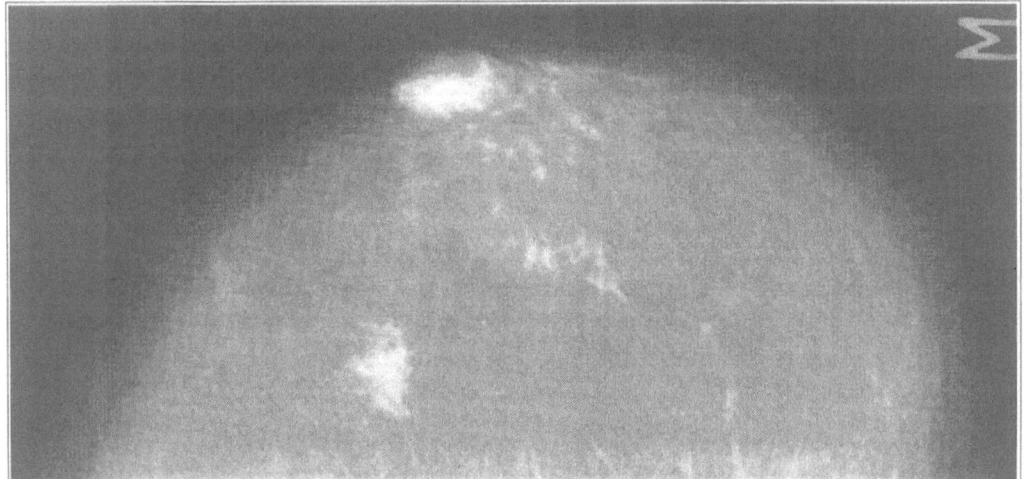

Figure 1.5.   Curvilinear structures is the name given to the ducts, blood vessels, and ligaments that appear as locally brighter and linear structures in mammograms. The right hand figure shows the curvilinear structures detected in the mammogram shown on the left. More details about curvilinear structures, and about the algorithm developed to detect them, is given in Chapter 12.

unchecked, *in situ* cancers eventually develop into invasive carcinomas by compromising their containing membranes, in which case the likelihood of metastasis increases sharply. Invasive carcinomas commonly present as either ductal in situ (more than 50% of cases), infiltrating lobular (about 10%), tubular, medullary, mucoid or papillary (< 1%). The blood vessels and lymphatic channels are thought to be the principal mechanism by which cancer cells metastasise to involve other parts of the body. An important goal of breast screening is to detect and eliminate cancers before they metastasise. The medio-lateral oblique image view (see Figure 1.1) was proposed because it provided the most comprehensive single view of the breast. Often, the axillae and lymph nodes are visible. Combining the information from the medio-lateral oblique and cranio-caudal mammograms is a difficult open problem in mammographic image processing and is a tough problem even for experienced radiologists. In Chapter 9 we describe a technique that we have developed to determine correspondences between features in a cranio-caudal mammogram and those taken medio-lateral obliquely. A key feature of the algorithm is that it simulates (un)compression.

Many kinds of benign abnormalities can appear in a mammogram. For example, cysts can occur in the TDLUs when the terminal duct becomes blocked and the normal secretions begin to accumulate. Cysts are not at all uncommon, and are normally quite easy to distinguish from other kinds of mass. Various types of fibrosis (formation of new scar tissue) or adenosis (development and/or enlargement of new glandular units) occur as "normal" changes, not least during pregnancy. The teaching atlas [233] developed by Tabar and Dean describes the many other kinds of benign and malignant masses that occur in mammograms. Locating and diagnosing correctly all the masses in a mammogram remains an open problem for mammographic image processing. It is likely to remain so for some time to come. An example of a cancer is in Figure 1.6 which shows a malignant mass.

It is often stated in handbooks for radiologists that "The breasts are mirror images; therefore, mammographically the distribution of the glandular tissue should appear the same, with only slight variation from one breast to the other ... Asymmetry is the radiologist's greatest aid in determining abnormalities both benign and malignant" [4]. Figure 1.7 shows a left-right pair of normal mammograms from one of our databases. Note that while overall structure and distribution of the parenchyma is roughly the same in the two breasts, the use of the word "symmetry" here is more qualitative than mathematical. In Chapter 13 we develop an algorithm for matching left-right pairs of mammograms, so that mis-matches correspond to possible pathologies. In a similar way, we referred earlier to "the branching, radial pattern of the ductal structures", though we noted also that it

MALIGNANT MASS

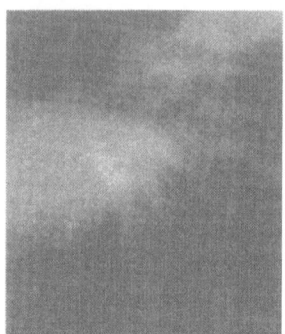

Figure 1.6. The detection of masses and their subsequent classification as either malignant or benign is a problem that is difficult for radiologists and for which the development of useful image processing algorithms remains essentially open. This is a fragment of a mammogram that corresponds to a malignant mass. The spicules that radiate from the central area have very variable size and contrast, though this is not a particularly difficult example to detect!

"SYMMETRICAL" MAMMOGRAMS

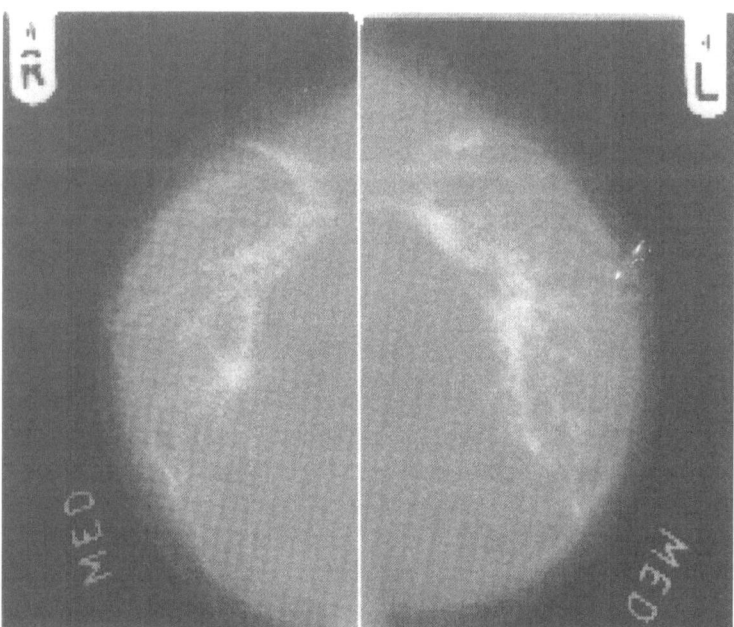

Figure 1.7. The approximate symmetry of the structures in a left-right mammogram pair is regarded by radiologists as extremely useful in detecting abnormalities that may indicate disease. Simplistically, such an abnormality disturbs the symmetry. The difficulty is to make precise the intuitive idea of symmetry, since it is considerably more general than the usual strict mathematical definition.

is typically confounded with curvilinear structures corresponding to blood vessels and stroma. Interruption of the radial ductal pattern is called "architectural distortion" or "radial scar", though it is quite qualitative, subtle, and can occur with both benign and malignant processes. There has been little work to date on algorithms for detecting and diagnosing architectural distortion or radial scar.

Fascial anatomy

So far in this section we have concentrated on the internal anatomy of the breast. We conclude with a different perspective, the so-called *fascial anatomy* of the breast. This regards the breast as a skin structure and is important because it provides a set of (albeit qualitative) constraints on breast compression. This proves to be very useful in developing algorithms for matching two images of the same breast over time, matching images of a left-right breast pair (see Chapter 13), and, what is much more important and difficult, matching a cranio-caudal view to a medio-lateral oblique view of the same breast (see Chapter 9). In this perspective, the breast is regarded as a "specially modified cutaneous apocrine gland" [187], that is, it is a gland that is contained within the woman's skin. The skin has many layers, of which, for present purposes we can distinguish three at increasing depths: the dermis (informally, the skin), the superficial fascia, and the deep fascia. The superficial fascia is bounded above by its superficial layer, and below by its deep layer. The breast is situated between the superficial and deep layers of the superficial fascia. The superficial layer is attached firmly to the dermis of the breast. The deep layer of the superficial fascia is separated from the deep fascia below it by the retromammary space, and is loosely coupled to it by ligaments. The deep fascia covers the pectoral muscle that is visible on many mammograms. An important consequence is that the breast moves on the thoracic wall during compression. Novak [187] reports a series of careful investigations in which he made markings on the breast surface and studied the resultant deformation of those markings after breast compression typical of mammography. In effect, these enable predictions to be made about the non-rigid deformations of tissue inside the breast, and as we describe in detail in subsequent chapters, this has enabled us to develop algorithms to match pairs of breast images, in three cases: a left-right pair of images taken with the same view, the same view taken at two different times, and, most challenging of all, a pair consisting of a cranio-caudal and a medio-lateral oblique view.

1.4. The image processing challenge

Current attempts at mammographic image analysis involve standard, general-purpose algorithms, but this is a highly questionable approach given the very demanding levels of performance that we hinted at in the opening section of this chapter. For convenience, we repeat what we wrote there:

"Millions of mammograms are taken annually in the USA and in Europe; consequently, even one image-processing related mistake per ten thousand mammograms can have serious consequences for many hundreds or thousands of women."

As an application of image processing, mammographic images pose a tough challenge because they have poor signal-to-noise ratio. This is largely because the images exhibit complex textures, because they are blurred by scattered x-ray photon radiation and by intensifying screen glare, and because there is a compromise between radiation dose and image quality. Being a two-dimensional projection of a three-dimensional anatomical structure, an x-ray mammogram inevitably superimposes tissue regions that are in fact not connected. As Figure 1.2 illustrate, mammograms vary enormously in contrast and brightness. Furthermore, there is relatively weak control of imaging acquisition.

Unfortunately, while there has been a great deal of research aimed at applying image processing to mammography, the vast majority of it has been of limited scope and incorporates only general *non-mammography specific* image processing considerations. The dangers are obvious; here are two clinically important examples:

– *Image smoothing* may appear to make large cancers easier to locate, but it can remove smaller signs such as calcifications and spiculations.
– *Edge sharpening* may appear to improve an image from the image analyst's perspective; but can transform a malignant lesion into one that appears to a radiologist to be benign.

Figure 1.8 shows an example. In addition to these possibilities of creating errors in diagnosis, currently available image processing systems use terms that are familiar to engineers but which are totally unfamiliar to clinicians. This inevitably leads to unreliability, a lack of confidence on the part of users (typically radiographers), and disuse.

The approach developed in this monograph is very different, and leads to very different algorithms. The basic principle is that in order to be reliable and predictable, image processing must be based on a model of how the image is formed. We develop this idea in Part I primarily for (x-ray) mammography then set it to work in Part II: our image analysis algorithms are rooted in a model of the way that x-rays pass through breast tissue, are absorbed and scattered before exposing the film. For instance, returning to the two examples *image smoothing* and *edge sharpening* mentioned above:

EXAMPLE OF IMAGE SMOOTHING

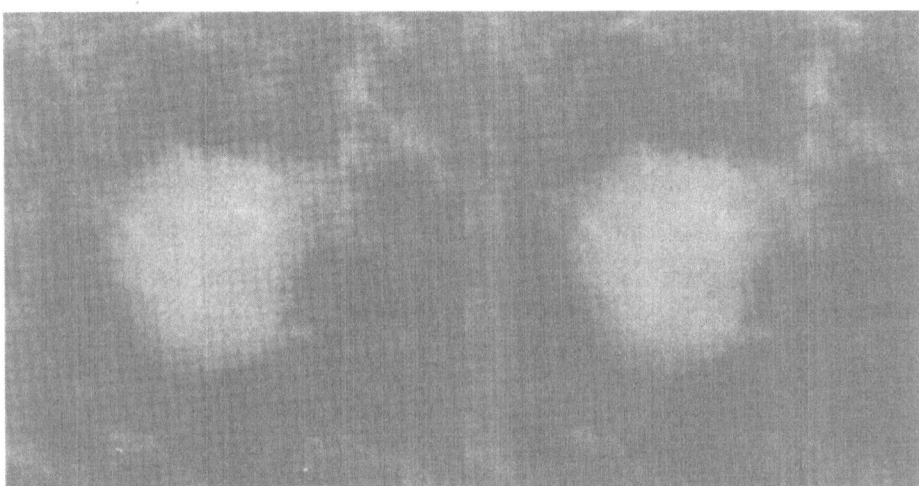

Figure 1.8. Image smoothing can remove noise, as in this example, but it can also remove real calcifications and make benign masses look more malignant by making them blend into the background.

- In Chapter 12 we develop a technique to estimate the curvilinear structures (CLS), the blood vessels, ducts, and fibrous tissue, that together give a mammogram its wispy textured appearance. We show how they can be removed from the image to facilitate the detection and analysis of abnormal masses. The CLS algorithm is based firmly on the representation h_{int} that we develop in Part I of the interesting, non-fatty tissue in the tiny column through the breast above each pixel. The h_{int} representation enables us to estimate the tissue surrounding any detected region, and this enables the image to be smoothed without removing calcifications and spiculations.
- In Chapter 2 we develop a technique to estimate the glare at each point in the image, then remove it: this further sharpens the image and facilitates more reliable extraction of microcalcifications. Again, in Chapter 3 we develop a method to estimate image blur due to the scattering of x-ray photons as they pass through the breast tissue. We are then able to remove this scatter-induced blur, to generate an image that is considerably less blurred but which retains all the clinically significant details of the image. Removing blur should aid measurements of, for example, lesion edge blur[44].

Many of the mammographic image processing algorithms described in this book have been incorporated into a software system **Xmammo** that is available under license from Oxford University and which is currently being evaluated clinically. A typical window display of **Xmammo** is shown in Figure 1.9. The interface and screen layout result from substantial and continuing interactions with radiographers at the Breast Care Unit in the Churchill Hospital, Oxford. Consider a typical case of a mammogram that has poor contrast. A general purpose image analysis package invites the radiographer to apply a standard technique such as histogram equalisation; but the radiographer cannot be expected to understand what that might mean! **Xmammo** encourages the radiographer to enhance the contrast in a way that corresponds to changing the tube voltage (there is usually a small knob on the machine to do this). This is a parameter with which the radiographer is very familiar, and, more importantly, is familiar with the kind of changes that are likely to result. We return to **Xmammo** in Chapter 7.

Throughout the monograph we will repeatedly emphasise that modelling the imaging process, and understanding breast anatomy, enables us to perform effective removal of the imaging parameters and thus image normalisation. This is a fundamental prerequisite of any form of population analysis, not least clinical trials, since without effective normalisation, populations statistics confound clinically insignificant image formation variations (exposure time, x-ray tube characteristics, film type) with those that are clinically significant. The following example aims to convince the reader that this is important and pervasive in mammographic image analysis.

Most reported mammographic image processing is performed on images that, once digitised, have pixel value linearly related to the film density of the corresponding position on the x-ray film. Such images are used for a variety of reasons, including their suitability for digital storage without losing too much information due to discretization and the absence of variations due to varying illumination conditions in the digitisation process.

To illustrate the susceptibility of features computed conventionally in image analysis to changes in the imaging conditions consider "contrast" in a film density image. We noted above that contrast can either be improved using a general tool such as histogram equalisation or by an application-specific approach such as is used in **Xmammo**. Contrast is normally estimated in a local region of an image, and a standard measure is the difference between the maximum and minimum value in the region, scaled, for example by the average or median value in the region, or at least by the sum of the maximum and minimum value. Box 1.1 shows that this so-called "normalised" measure depends on the digitiser transform.

XMAMMO

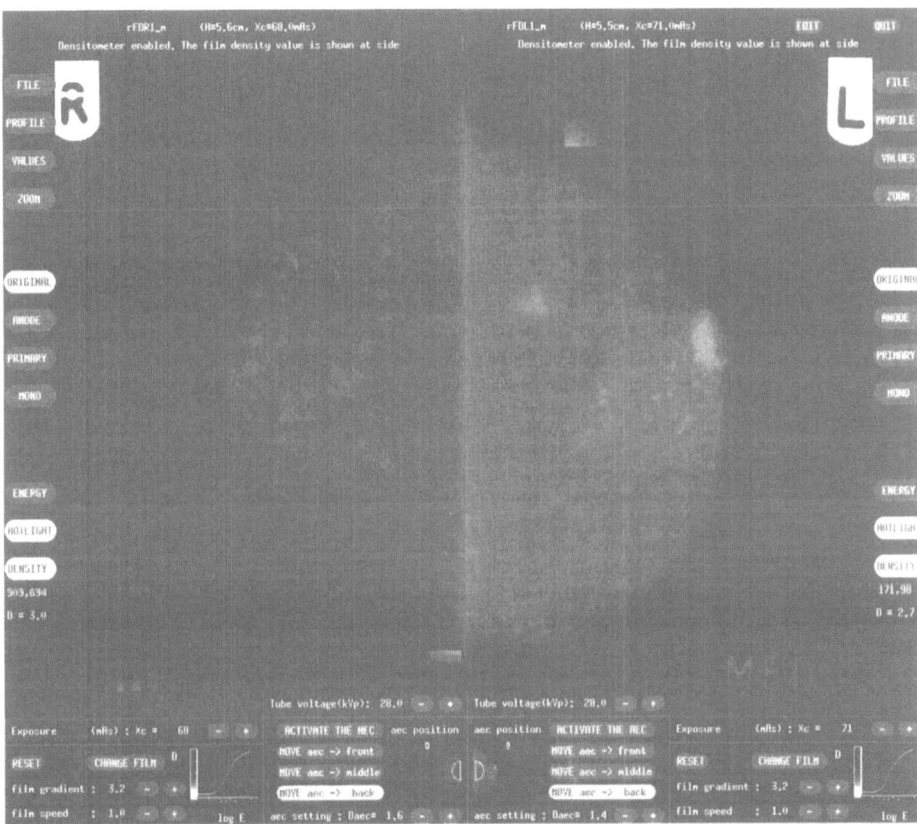

Figure 1.9. The **Xmammo** interface. A left- right breast pair is shown. The buttons on the left enable the user to select the original image, the primaries (scatter removal), to simulate the familiar hot-light, etc. A hot-light is shown as the bright square and allows close examination of the densities within the light, radiologists use it in practice to view the breast edge. The buttons are repeated on the right side. At the bottom, there are simple ways to change the time of exposure, the film and tube types, and to reposition the AEC.

BOX 1.1: Estimating contrast on a digitised mammogram

Let $P(x,y) = \alpha D(x,y) + \eta$ be the pixel value corresponding to the film density D within the film area corresponding to spatial position (x,y). This linear relationship is typical for laser film scanners. The constants α and η depend on the particular imaging device. Image contrast in a region can be estimated by:

$$
\begin{aligned}
C &= \frac{P_{max} - P_{min}}{P_{max} + P_{min}} \\
&= \frac{\alpha D_{max} + \eta - \alpha D_{min} - \eta}{\alpha D_{max} + \alpha D_{min} + 2\eta} \\
&= \frac{D_{max} - D_{min}}{D_{max} + D_{min} + \frac{2\eta}{\alpha}}
\end{aligned}
$$

Clearly, the contrast measure C depends not just on the image but also on the digitising device since $2\eta/\alpha$ is present in the equation. A typical 8-bit digitiser mapping a film density of 4.0 to a pixel value of 0 and a film density of 0.2 to 255 would have values of $\alpha = -91.07$ and $\eta = 273.21$, which makes $2\eta/\alpha = -6.0$ and means that the digitiser term is very significant.

BOX 1.2: Contrast in energy imparted

Assuming a linear film-screen curve gives the following relation between film density D and energy imparted to the intensifying screen E^{imp}:

$$
D = \gamma \log_{10}(\beta E^{imp})
$$

where γ is the film-screen gradient and β is related to the speed of the film-screen system. We can then expand the contrast definition of Box 1.1 to investigate the effects of the film processing conditions on the feature:

$$
\begin{aligned}
C &= \frac{\gamma \log \beta E^{imp}_{max} - \gamma \log \beta E^{imp}_{min}}{\gamma \log \beta E^{imp}_{max} + \gamma \log \beta E^{imp}_{min} + \frac{2\eta}{\alpha}} \\
&= \frac{\log E^{imp}_{max} - \log E^{imp}_{min}}{\log E^{imp}_{max} + \log E^{imp}_{min} + 2\log \beta + \frac{2\eta}{\gamma\alpha}}
\end{aligned}
$$

Clearly, the contrast measure depends heavily on the film-screen system, as well as on the digitiser.

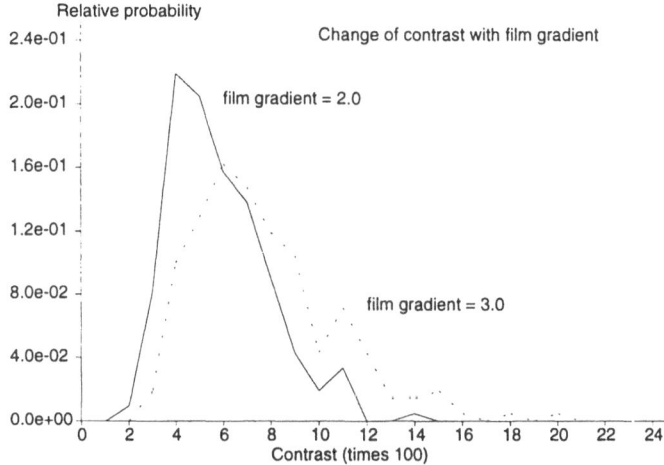

Figure 1.10. This shows the relative distribution of contrast values from small windows over a mammographic image using a simple contrast measure, 100 samples, and a film density image of a volume of fibroglandular tissue within the breast. The curves are for different film-screen characteristic curves with different gradients as marked.

But we can take the argument one step further. As we will show in Chapter 2, film density is usually assumed to be linearly related to the logarithm of the energy imparted to the intensifying screen. Energy, in turn, is related to the breast tissue whose analysis is the focus of the image analysis exercise, confounded by the characteristics of the x-ray beam. Box 1.2 adds this complication. The details are relatively unimportant; but the take-home message is clear: this familiar contrast measure is highly susceptible not only to the digitisation process, but also to changes in the other imaging conditions. To drive the point home further, Figure 1.10 shows the relative distribution of contrast measures for some normal fibroglandular tissue when the film gradient changes by simulation from 2.0 to 3.0.

In Chapter 2 we develop the h_{int} representation that enables mammograms to be normalised prior to image analysis, by separating out the effects due to imaging and x-ray beam characteristics from those due to the breast anatomy. As we will see, this leads to more reliable algorithms for estimating and using measures such as contrast.

1.5. Snapshot description of the contents

The book concentrates primarily on x-ray mammography, and is organised into three parts. Briefly, Part I, comprising Chapters 2 through 6, develops a model of the formation of an x-ray mammogram image, specifically a model of the passage of x-ray photons through compressed breast tissue and their subsequent interaction with an intensifying screen. Part II, comprising Chapters 7-13, applies the model developed in Part I to a variety of image analysis tasks. Finally, Part III, discusses work we have done with other breast imaging modalities; in particular in Chapter 14 we discuss work with our colleague Paul Hayton on breast MRI. Chapter 15 concludes the monograph with an overview of other imaging modalities including nuclear medicine and 2D and 3D ultrasound. Chapter 15 also provides a perspective for future research in a number of important problems related to mammographic image analysis that are tangential to the image analysis presented in this monograph.

The reader who wants either to avoid the mathematical details (at least, at first reading) or who wants to get straight to the image analysis, may proceed directly to Part II. We now end this introductory chapter by giving a slightly elaborated summary of Parts I, II and III.

Part I: Generating h_{int}

Chapter 2 explains how a digital mammographic image is generated and we develop a mathematical model of the mammographic imaging process and explain how we calibrate it. Our modelling is centred on conventional systems, but can be adapted to directly digital systems which are discussed in Chapter 15. We note that the projective nature of mammographic imaging inevitably loses the three-dimensional structure of the breast. A key contribution of Part I is to demonstrate that we can go some way to overcoming this limitation, by developing a $2\frac{1}{2}$ dimensional representation of the compressed breast tissue that we call the h_{int} representation of "interesting" (non-fatty) tissue, an example of which is shown as Figure 1.11. If we denote the thickness of interesting tissue at a pixel by h_{int} and that of fat by h_{fat}, then, assuming that we know the compressed breast thickness H, we have $h_{int} + h_{fat} = H$, so that we only need to store one variable, h_{int}, to accurately describe each cone of breast tissue. It turns out that, with sufficient calibration, we can generate an estimate of h_{int} at each pixel as long as we have an estimate of scattered and extra-focal radiation; Chapters 3 and 4 provide the details about how we can do that.

AN h_{int} SURFACE

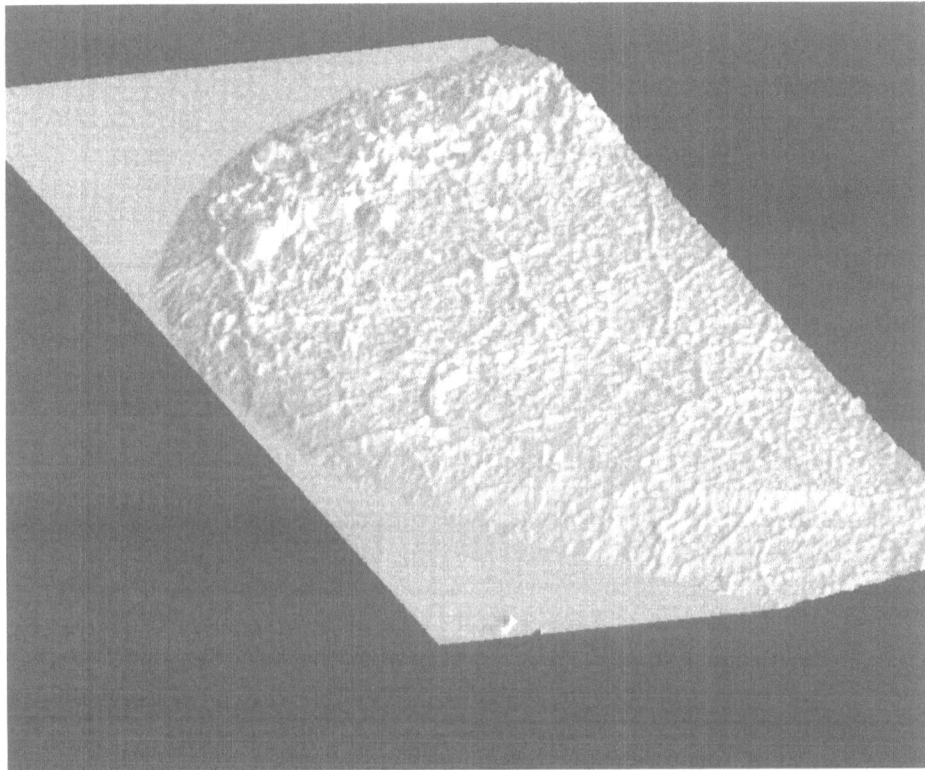

Figure 1.11.   Depiction of the h_{int} surface of a breast. The height corresponds to the amount of non-fatty tissue. In this way, anatomical features correspond to topographic features of h_{int} surfaces. Towards the nipple there is an obvious cyst which is represented here as a hill.

One important parameter that we need to know in order to compute h_{int} is the compressed breast thickness H. Unfortunately, only the newest machines record this. Chapter 5 provides the details of a technique we have developed for estimating H automatically from an image. Finally, Chapter 6 has a mathematical analysis that demonstrates that the models that we develop are not sensitive to slight errors in the calibration data.

Part II: Exploiting The h_{int} model

Part II begins in Chapter 7 with a set of image enhancement techniques that are based on the h_{int} representation and which together comprise the **Xmammo** software system for assisting radiologists. Each image enhancement routine adheres to the following schema:

$$D_{given}(x,y) \longrightarrow h_{int}(x,y) \longrightarrow D_{enhanced}(x,y),$$

in which $D_{given}(x,y)$ is the original image and $D_{enhanced}(x,y)$ is the enhanced result. Crucially, the image analysis processes described in Chapter 7 are expressed in terms that radiologists are familiar with: simulate a different exposure time or x-ray source, simulate moving the automatic exposure control, etc.

Chapter 8 then presents results that show how the h_{int} surface can be transformed prior to re-display, in order to simulate change in anatomical structure or breast tissue. In particular, we show how to simulate: the appearance of masses of various types in various contexts; microcalcifications; macrocalcifications; and curvilinear structures. These simulations can be represented in a similar manner to the above, by:

$$D_{original}(x,y) \rightarrow h_{int}(x,y) \rightarrow h'_{int}(x,y) \rightarrow D_{simulated}(x,y).$$

Note how in this case the h_{int} computed from the original image $D_{original}(x,y)$ is modified. In fact, precisely because h_{int} *normalises* the image by keeping a representation of the anatomical structure of the compressed breast, and by removing information that pertains to a particular image of it, it is easier, more precise, and more reliable to modify the h_{int} that corresponds to $D_{original}$ than to modify $D_{original}$ directly. Figure 1.12 shows a simulation example.

Chapter 9 discusses the fundamental problem of breast compression, and introduces two novel techniques. The first of these is called differential compression mammography , and exploits image changes when the breast is imaged at two slightly different compression thicknesses. We show how this can give important information about tissue movement and hardness. The second technique aims to relate a cranio-caudal image to one taken with a different compression thickness in a medio-lateral oblique view.

The differential compression mammography technique that we introduce in Chapter 9 seems, on the face of things, impractical because it requires that two images be taken, doubling the radiation exposure to the breast. In current practice, it is normal to fit an anti-scatter grid to the x-ray machine, in order, as the name implies, to cut down on x-ray photon

MASS SIMULATION

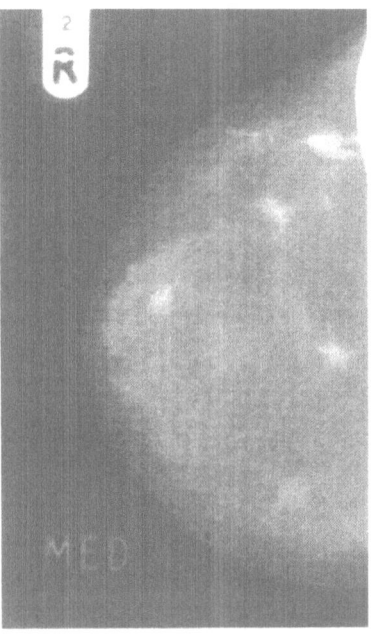

Figure 1.12.   This fatty breast has had two spherical volumes implanted into it to simulate cysts, and two irregular shaped volumes to simulate malignant lesions. The cysts volumes are "filled" with tissue which has a lower x-ray attenuating tissue than for the two irregular malignant volumes. The circular shape near the nipple, is a genuine cyst. The irregular shaped masses have the shape of a malignant lesion from a different mammogram.

scatter and so improve the appearance of the image. Unfortunately, using an anti-scatter grid increases the radiation dose to the patient, in fact it approximately doubles the dose. We are able to show in Chapter 10 that one can enhance a mammogram taken *without* an anti-scatter grid using image analysis techniques, so that it appears indistinguishable from one taken with a grid. This holds out the prospect that one can dispense with the anti-scatter grid. In this way, the differential compression mammography technique becomes practically and ethically feasible.

Chapter 11 summarises our recent work aimed at applying the h_{int} representation to improve the sensitivity and specificity with which micro-calcifications can be detected in mammograms. We present a novel technique for estimating different sources of image noise and for estimating the thicknesses of calcifications. In the original presentation in Chapter 2, the algorithm to generate the h_{int} representation assumes that there is no calcium in the breast. Chapter 11 revisits that assumption and shows that the calcification thicknesses are, in fact, recorded in the h_{int} representation.

In Chapter 12, we develop a technique to identify and remove curvilinear structures (CLS), a process that is important in its own right for distinguishing ductal and vascular calcifications. It turns out that matching or interpreting breast images is made difficult by the presence of CLS that correspond to ducts, blood vessels, and fibrous tissue, and so the algorithms to locate and remove the CLS are an important pre-cursor to matching, which is the focus of Chapter 13.

For matching, we consider three important cases:

- *Temporal pairs*: "Salient" regions are extracted independently in two mammograms of the same breast, the same view at two different times. The salient regions in the first mammogram are then matched with those in the second, and those that have either appeared in the later mammogram but not in the earlier one, or which have changed significantly between the two mammograms are drawn to the attention of the radiologist.
- *Bilateral pairs*: In a similar fashion, salient regions are extracted from the same-view left and right breast mammograms of the same patient, taken at approximately the same time. They are matched by an algorithm that draws the radiologist's attention to those that appear in one breast but not in the other.
- *Locating abnormal regions*: Salient regions are extracted from a breast image and for each a number of features are computed. These features are used to assess the "normality" of the region, as defined by a probabilistic model that is learned automatically. If a salient region is determined to be in the tails of the probabilistic model, it is declared to be "abnormal" and is drawn to the attention of the radiologist.

Part III: Further Breast Image Analysis

Although the monograph is primarily concerned with x-ray mammography images, in Chapter 14 we describe work carried out over the past two years with our colleague Paul Hayton that has resulted in a system **xmri** for processing contrast-enhanced MRI breast images. MRI is showing promise in aiding breast cancer diagnosis in young women and in women with scar tissue from previous surgery. Finally, in Chapter 15 we briefly introduce the developing use of both nuclear medicine and ultrasound in mammography, and we discuss a number of issues that are increasingly involved in clinical decision aids based on image analysis.

1.6. Concluding introductory remarks

We have written this monograph partly to present a set of what we believe to be novel and clinically useful image analysis techniques and partly to illustrate a particular model-based approach to image analysis that is firmly rooted in the physics of mammographic image formation. In related work we have adopted a similar approach to analysing infrared images [115], aerial images, and MRI brain images. Nevertheless, the reader is asked always to bear in mind that this monograph represents an initial attack on some very difficult image analysis problems in an application area that is of immense importance.

The output of Part I of the monograph is the h_{int} representation of "interesting tissue". It is based on conventional x-ray film technology. The details of the approach will inevitably change when, for example, digital mammography becomes the norm; but it seems that the h_{int} representation will be invariant to such changes. Because of this, the image analysis techniques based on h_{int} presented in Part II should stay broadly unchanged, though improved techniques will inevitably be invented, and novel computer architectures may require their implementations to be revisited.

We contend that the essential interface between Parts I and II, namely the h_{int} representation, should stand the test of time.

PART I

Generating h_{int}

CHAPTER 2

A MODEL OF MAMMOGRAM IMAGE FORMATION

2.1. Introduction

In this chapter we explain how a digital mammographic image is generated and we develop a mathematical model of the entire imaging process and explain how we calibrate it and generate the h_{int} representation. Our modelling is centred on conventional systems, but could be adapted to directly digital systems. Our aim in this chapter is to show that with sufficient calibration we can generate an estimate of h_{int} at each pixel as long as we have an estimate of scattered and extra-focal radiation; Chapters 3 and 4 explain how we attain those.

2.2. Mammographic imaging process model

Overview

Figure 2.1 shows a schematic representation of the mammographic imaging system. There are several books which explain the mammographic process in great detail [197, 206, 208] and substantial modelling of the mammographic process has taken place previously. This previous work has been inspired by the need to keep the radiation dose to the breast as low as possible, whilst giving an optimal signal-to-noise ratio [134, 150, 185, 220, 230, 261]. Because of the orientation of such work, the modelling has been used to optimise the radiographic equipment involved in mammography. Notably, this has included choice of anode material and x-ray tube voltage. The model developed in this chapter is similar in spirit to those referenced. However, in the related work the authors usually predict the appearance of a mammogram performed on a "standard breast" and then optimize some contrast measure with respect to radiation dose to the breast; our model works backwards from the mammogram itself to find some measure of the object being imaged. This means that we are able to ignore radiation dose to the breast, but have to take account of degrading factors, as well as variations in breast size and composition, rather than assuming idealised imaging conditions and a standard breast.

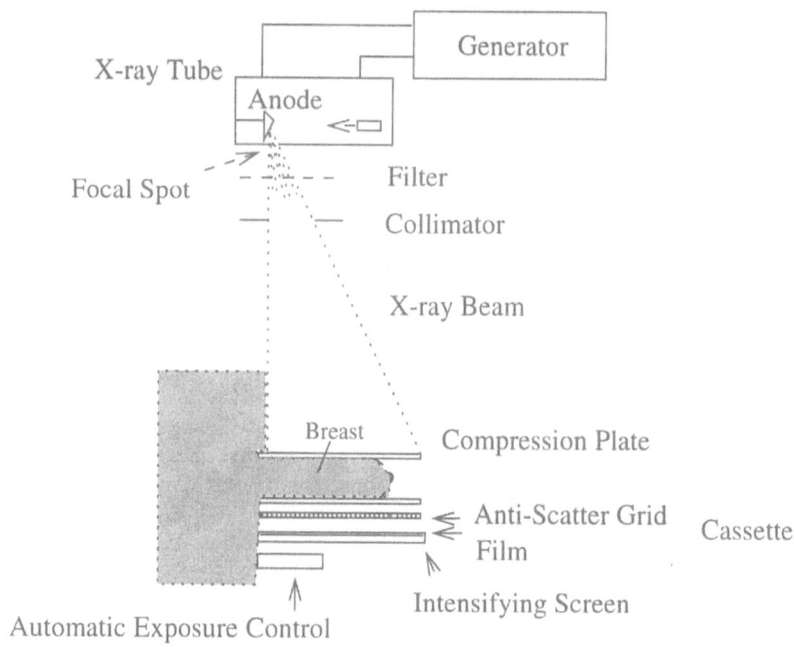

X-ray Tube

Generator

Anode

Focal Spot

Filter

Collimator

X-ray Beam

Breast

Compression Plate

Anti-Scatter Grid

Film

Cassette

Intensifying Screen

Automatic Exposure Control

Figure 2.1. This shows a schematic representation of the components of a conventional screen-film mammographic system. When a mammogram is performed, a beam of x-ray photons is directed towards a compressed breast. This beam is filtered to remove low energy photons and collimated to the area of interest. The beam has a spectrum of energies that is characteristic of the tube voltage and, in particular, the anode material. The spectrum is independent of the woman being scanned and the view taken. The intensity of the beam exiting the breast is related to the thickness and type of tissue in the breast. The x-ray photons leaving the breast have to pass through an anti-scatter grid before they reach a phosphorous intensifying screen. If an x-ray photon is absorbed in the screen, light photons are emitted by the phosphor and these light photons expose a film which is processed to produce a mammogram. The exposure to the breast is stopped once an automatic exposure control, positioned under a section of the breast, has received a set exposure. There are several effects which lead to degradation of the image, including scattered radiation, beam hardening and possible poor exposure. To generate a digital image the x-ray film is typically digitised using a laser scanner system.

The mathematical model proposed in this chapter is developed by following the path of the x-ray photons from production to exposure to the film. The initial discussion is of the incident x-ray beam and how it is polyenergetic and varies across the breast. Then the x-ray photon path through the breast is discussed and a breast model based on the x-ray attenuation properties of breast tissue is proposed. The next step is discussion of the photons leaving the breast, their origin, and how they have to pass through an anti-scatter grid before reaching the film-screen combination. The final part of the model discusses film digitisation.

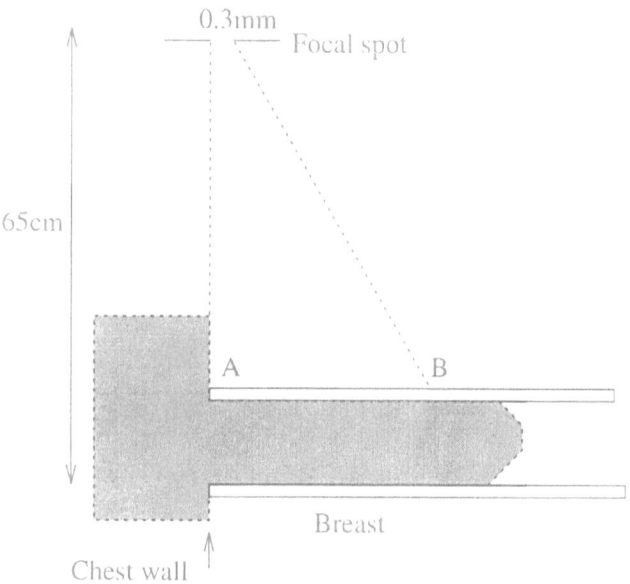

Figure 2.2.   The x-rays form a divergent beam from the source whose focal spot and anode are situated above the chest wall of the woman currently being examined. The distance from the focal spot to the film is typically 65cm, and although the specified focal spot size is typically 0.3mm by 0.3mm, the effective focal spot size can be nearer 0.5mm by 0.5mm [59]. There is a compromise between focal spot size, x-ray tube output and overall image blur [160]. The small focal spot size and large distance from source to breast, mean that a model of the source as an infinitesimal spot is reasonable. Using simple geometry it is possible to show that the volume of tissue is constant above any pixel, and that the path length only varies marginally over the image. The incident radiation intensity varies spatially due to the "anode heel effect" and diverging beam to the extent that the intensity at point A can be 25% greater than that at point B.

Incident radiation to breast

The x-rays form a divergent beam from the source, whose focal spot and anode are situated above the chest wall of the woman currently being examined, Figure 2.2 shows the geometry. The small focal spot size and large distance from x-ray source to breast, mean that it is reasonable to model the source as an infinitesimal spot.

Many manufacturers make x-ray tubes specifically for mammography,

kVp	Photon output $(photons/mAs/mm^2)$	Average photon energy (keV)
25	0.2438×10^6	16.036
28	0.3660×10^6	16.610
30	0.4604×10^6	16.954

TABLE 2.1. This shows the photon output and average incident photon energy at a distance of 75cm for three tube voltages for a typical x-ray tube as reported in [13]. These values show that as the tube voltage is increased the x-ray tube becomes more efficient in terms of photon production. The table also shows that, as one would expect, the average exiting photon energy from the tube rises with tube voltage.

BOX 2.1: Computing incident photon flux

Let $\phi(V_t, x, y)$ be the photon flux over the area corresponding to spatial position (x, y) when the tube voltage is V_t kVp. The units of flux are photons per unit area per unit time:

$$\phi(V_t, x, y) = f(V_t) \times I_t(V_t)$$

where $f(V_t)$ is the photon output given in Table 2.1 and I_t is the tube current.

---

but their characteristics are usually quite similar. X-ray tubes are more efficient at higher tube voltages. Table 2.1 shows the total photon output for a typical x-ray tube at different tube voltages. The tube current varies with tube voltage on some machines to compensate for the tube efficiency. For example, the Philips Diagnost U-M has a current of 120mA at 25kVp, 107mA at 28kVp and 100mA at 30kVp. When a mammogram is performed an exposure value measured in mAs (milli-Ampere seconds) is usually read-out and noted down by the radiographers. Typically, the exposure value varies between 30mAs and 500mAs depending on how large and dense the breast is; the actual value is determined by the automatic exposure control (AEC). Figure 2.3 shows a mammogram under simulated variation of the AEC position value, Chapter 7 contains the details of how the simulation was performed. Armed with knowledge of the x-ray tube and tube voltage, the incident radiation can be quantified, as shown mathematically in Box 2.1.

The incident x-ray beam is polyenergetic, that is, it comprises x-ray photons of many different energies and has a spectrum which varies according to the x-ray tube anode material and subsequent filtering. The most

CHANGING AEC POSITION

Back   Front

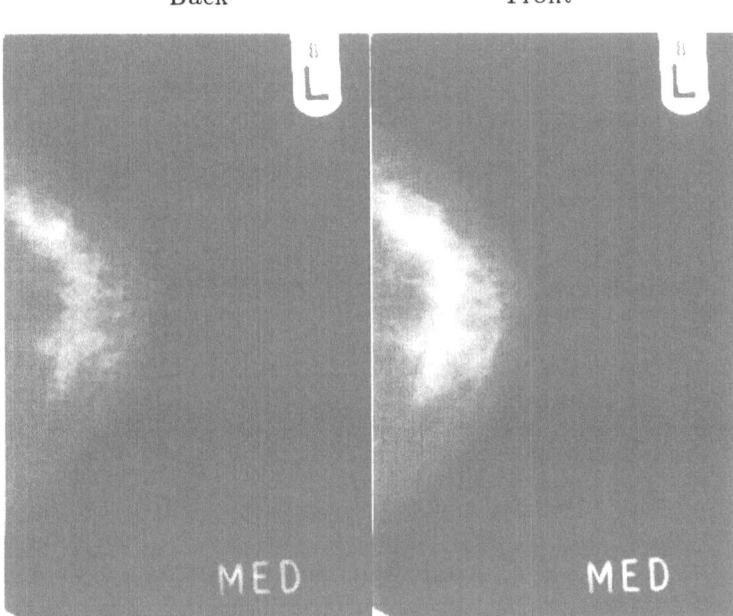

Figure 2.3. The mammogram on the left was taken with the automatic exposure control situated close to the chest wall. The control unit was set to give an average film density of 1.4 and the "exposure" was 45.1 mAs. The mammogram on the right shows a simulation of the effect of having the automatic exposure control beneath the middle of the breast. In this case the "exposure" was 36.9mAs. This kind of simulation is relatively simple using the computer, but care has to be taken to ensure that the information for the simulation is actually present within the original image.

common anode material is Molybdenum and this has strong characteristic radiation contributions at 17.4keV and 19.6keV. Typical incident spectra for tube voltages of 25kVp and 28kVp are given in Figure 2.4 which, we assume, represents the number of incident photons at each energy relative to the maximum (i.e. the number at 17.4keV) *anywhere* across the x-ray field. Such figures are generated from theoretical models due to the expense and technical difficulties involved in measuring the spectrum [13]. The incident radiation to the breast is simply the integral over all the energies, see Box 2.2 for the mathematical details.

The energy of the x-ray photons is important because the difference between the attenuation coefficients of the breast tissues rises with lower energy and thus there is a greater difference in the x-ray signal exiting the breast when a lower energy beam is used. This, in turn, leads to more

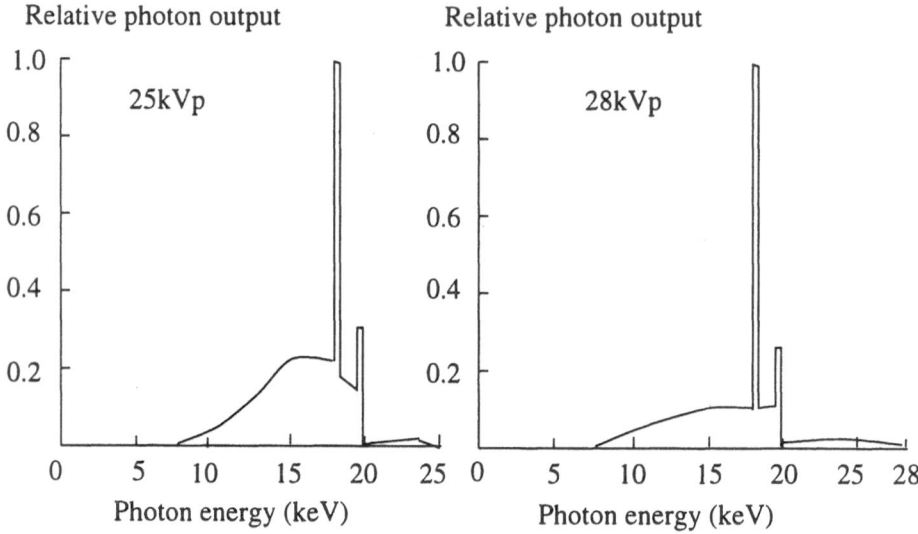

Figure 2.4.   X-ray spectra of a beam from a tube with a Molybdenum anode, filtered by 0.8mm of Beryllium, from the tube window, and 0.03mm of Molybdenum. The tube voltages are marked. The actual number of x-ray photons at 28kVp is far greater than at 25kVp, see Table 2.1.

contrast in the image. However, lower energy photons are more readily attenuated both in the breast tissue so that lower energy photons lead to a greater radiation dose. Thus there is a trade-off between contrast in the mammogram and radiation dose to the breast: low energy photon beams give better contrast, but the breast receives a higher radiation dose. This trade-off is the crux of most modelling which aims to optimise radiographic techniques, but can be ignored in our modelling because radiation dose to the breast is irrelevant.

The greater absorption of low energy photons can lead to unwanted variation of contrast across a mammogram, particularly in dense parts of the breast. Imagine a fatty (low x-ray attenuation) breast with a highly attenuating material (such as calcium) at the bottom and then the same thickness breast with the fat replaced by fibro-glandular tissue (higher attenuation than fat). By the time the x-ray beam reaches the calcium it has already been attenuated and the average x-ray photon energy is higher for the fibro-glandular breast than for the fatty breast. Since the energy is higher, the calcium has less effect on the x-ray beam in the fibro-glandular case than in the fatty case and thus the same object exhibits different con-

---

BOX 2.2: Incident radiation

Let $N_0^{rel}(V_t, \mathcal{E})$ be the number of photons at energy $\mathcal{E}$ relative to the total number of photons in the incident spectrum. We assume that the incident spectrum is uniform across the x-ray field, and so the incident energy on a small area (A_p) of the lucite compression plate at spatial position (x, y) is simply the integral over all energies:

$$E_0^{plate}(x, y) = \phi(V_t, x, y) A_p t_s \int_0^{\mathcal{E}_{max}} N_0^{rel}(V_t, \mathcal{E}) \, \mathcal{E} d\mathcal{E}$$

As the x-ray photons pass through the lucite compression plate some are absorbed. The probability of absorption depends on the energy of the photon, the material and the thickness of the material. Beer's law [9, 254] relates the number of incident photons to a material to the number of exiting photons:

Number of exiting photons = Number of incident photons $\times e^{-h\mu(\mathcal{E})}$

where h is the material thickness and $\mu(\mathcal{E})$ is the linear attenuation coefficient of the material at energy $\mathcal{E}$. Using Beer's law we can estimate the number of photons exiting the plate at spatial position (x, y) and hence the total incident energy to the breast:

$$E_0(x, y) = \phi(V_t, x, y) A_p t_s \int_0^{\mathcal{E}_{max}} N_0^{rel}(V_t, \mathcal{E}) \, \mathcal{E} e^{-\mu_{luc}(\mathcal{E}) h_{plate}} d\mathcal{E}$$

where $\mathcal{E}_{max}$ is the maximum photon energy which depends on the tube voltage; h_{plate} is the thickness of the lucite compression plate, and μ_{luc} is the relevant linear attenuation coefficient; and t_s is the time of exposure.

---

trast depending upon the material that the x-ray beam has passed through. This effect is termed "beam hardening" and is caused by the average energy of the x-ray beam rising as the beam is attenuated. As well as loss of contrast, beam hardening can also cause the automatic exposure control to terminate the exposure early. Figure 2.5 shows an example of beam hardening.

The incident radiation intensity varies spatially for several reasons the most significant of which is the "anode heel effect" (Figures 2.2 and 2.6). An x-ray tube produces x-rays by firing an electron beam at an anode. As the electron beam penetrates the anode the electrons are absorbed at varying depths and the x-ray photons that are produced have to travel through varying thicknesses of anode material before leaving the anode. This leads to varying attenuation of the emergent x-ray beam thus giving spatial variations in the incident x-ray spectrum, this is termed the anode heel effect [13] and is quite substantial. Another source of spatial variation

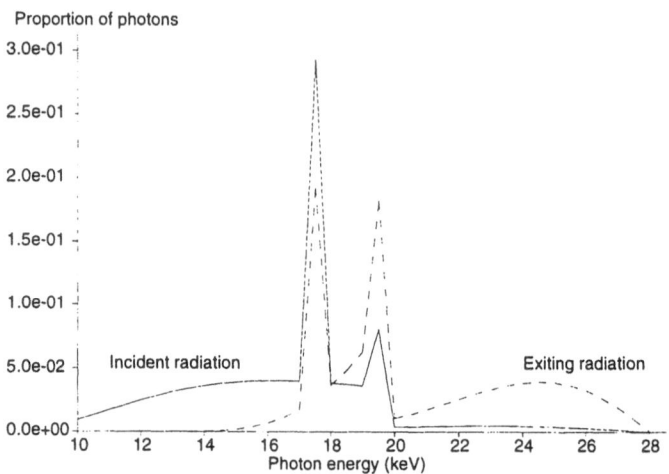

Figure 2.5. The solid line represents the relative incident radiation spectrum to a volume of breast tissue of thickness 6cm which is 50% fat. The dashed line shows the simulated relative exiting radiation spectrum. The lower energy photons are readily absorbed by the breast (thus giving radiation dose and no image) whilst the higher energy photons pass through relatively easily. This can be seen in the average energies: the exiting radiation has an average energy of 20.798keV whereas the incident radiation has an average energy of 16.610keV. This effect is termed "beam hardening".

is due to the diverging nature of the beam. This means that the further away from the source the more spread out the x-ray beam is. However, this effect is small given that the distance from the source to the breast is large relative to the breast size.

It is assumed in our work that the spatial intensity variation is due to the number of incident photons varying across the image rather than the relative incident energy spectrum changing. The main variation is a smooth intensity reduction from the back of the film out towards the nipple, and this can be as great as 25% of the maximum value. The variation along the back of the film is much smaller, Figure 2.6. The spatial variations can be measured by performing an exposure with no object present. Using that data, we show on Page 54 in Box 2.9 how to compensate a mammographic image for the spatial variations. After the mammogram has been compensated, it appears as it would with a uniform incident radiation intensity and pencil beam geometry.

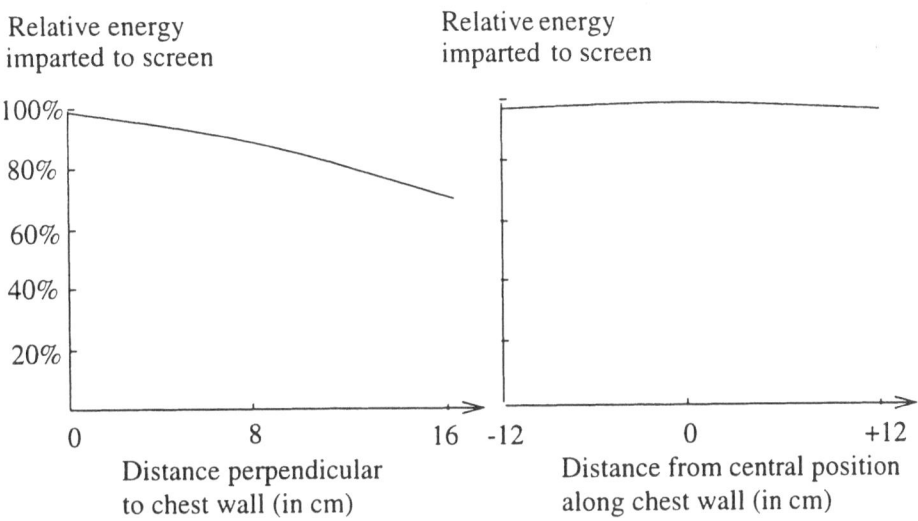

Figure 2.6. The incident radiation intensity varies spatially due to the anode heel effect and diverging beam. These graphs show the spatial variation along the chest wall and from the chest wall out to the nipple. They were found by performing an exposure with no object present and calculating the energy which must have been imparted to the intensifying screen to give the measured film density. On the left is the effect outward from the chest wall, and on the right is the effect along the chest wall.

X-ray photon path through the breast

As the x-ray photons travel through the breast they are attenuated by both scattering and absorption processes. The probability of attenuation is related to the type of tissue through which the photons have to pass. As we noted in Chapter 1, the normal breast consists of fibrous, glandular and adipose tissue, and sometimes calcification. Adipose tissue is fibrous connective tissue packed with fat cells. The tissues are poorly recognisable on macroscopic examination [157]. In order to estimate the absorbed radiation dose to the breast, Hammerstein et al. [98] determined the elemental compositions and densities of fat, adipose tissue, skin and glandular tissue. They found that skin and fat yielded consistent results, but that the carbon and oxygen components varied greatly in adipose and glandular tissue. They ascribe this variation to difficulty in removing fibrous stroma from the adipose tissue, and from removing fatty material from the glandular tissue. Johns and Yaffe [137] do not report such difficulties, and include neoplastic tissue in their study.

Tissue type	No. patients		μ (cm^{-1}) at energy (keV)		
			18	20	25
Fat	7	Minimum	0.538	0.441	0.314
		Mean	0.558	0.456	0.322
		Maximum	0.585	0.476	0.333
Fibrous	8	Minimum	1.014	0.791	0.499
(Glandular)		Mean	1.028	0.802	0.506
(Parenchymal)		Maximum	1.045	0.816	0.516
Infiltrating	6	Minimum	1.061	0.826	0.519
duct		Mean	1.085	0.844	0.529
carcinoma		Maximum	1.137	0.884	0.552

TABLE 2.2. The linear attenuation coefficients for various breast tissue types reported by Johns and Yaffe [137]

Table 2.2 gives the linear attenuation coefficients reported by Johns and Yaffe. Clearly, the attenuation coefficients for fibrous, glandular and cancerous tissue overlap at all energies so that it is impossible to distinguish them on grounds of attenuation alone. In fact, their attenuation coefficients are comparable to water which is a term that radiologists sometime use to describe them. Fat has much lower x-ray attenuation than the other tissues and is thus distinguishable based upon attenuation. We refer to fibrous, glandular and cancerous tissue as "interesting tissue", as distinct from fat and calcium. We assume that skin and blood can also be classified as interesting tissue from the point of view of x-ray attenuation.

Typical linear attenuation coefficients for calcifications are 26.1 at 18keV, 19.3 at 20keV, and 10.8 at 25keV. These relatively large values are why they appear bright and indicate the high attenuation of calcification, but since calcification occurs only in small quantities, the total attenuation is often more comparable to larger thicknesses of other breast tissues. For example, 0.1mm of calcification has a similar attenuation to 2.6mm of fibroglandular tissue and thus may not be obvious.

In our model, it is assumed either that calcification is not present or that it can be detected prior to further processing; in Chapter 11 we explain how that might be achieved. In any case, we can show that our algorithms do not remove any sign of calcifications. With this assumption the remaining breast tissues can be classified according to their linear attenuation coefficients into interesting tissue or fat. This assumption is necessary to reduce the number

---

BOX 2.3: Analytical formula for attenuation coefficients

The linear attenuation coefficients of Johns and Yaffe cover the energy range from 18keV upwards, but the mammographic energy range starts at 10keV. In the mammographic energy range, the photoelectric absorption component (μ_a) of the linear attenuation coefficient (μ) varies with the cube of the photon energy, whilst the scatter component (μ_s) is near constant [9]:

$$\mu(\mathcal{E}) \approx \frac{\lambda}{\mathcal{E}^3} + \mu_s$$

where λ is a constant related to the atomic numbers and densities of the materials being considered. Using this equation and the values in Table 2.2, the linear attenuation coefficients for the different tissues can be interpolated and extrapolated to cover the entire mammographic energy range.

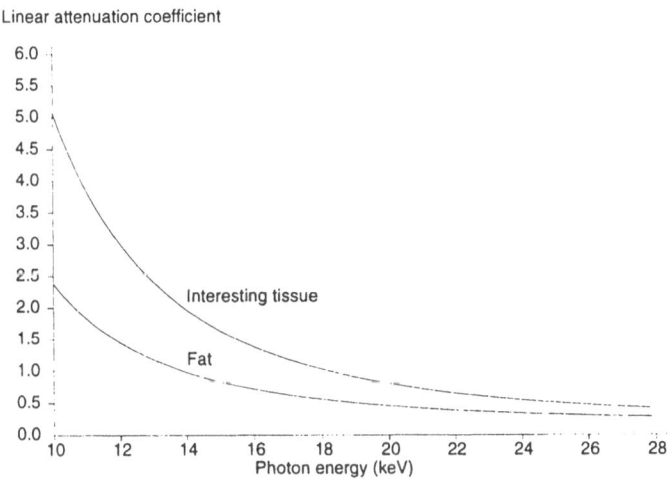

Figure 2.7.   Values of the linear attenuation coefficients used for fat and interesting tissue. These are the averages of the values reported by Johns and Yaffe [137], with suitable interpolation and extrapolation to cover the entire mammographic energy range.

of unknowns in the system and to allow correction for beam hardening. We require the linear attenuation coefficients over a range of energy values so we interpolate and extrapolate from the values of Johns and Yaffe, see Figure 2.7 and Box 2.3.

When a mammogram is performed, the breast is firmly compressed in order to: reduce motion artifacts by immobilizing the breast; reduce geometric

blur by having objects nearer the film-screen; reduce the film density range
through having a more uniform breast thickness; reduce scattered radiation;
improve separation of tissue structures through increased projected area;
reduce radiation dose to the breast. However, the word compression, taken
in an engineering sense, is misleading as the breast tissues do not compress
but deform and displace with no loss of volume [215]. This is important
because no change of volume implies no change in density and thus the
linear attenuation coefficients of the tissues remain constant.

Let the distance between the compression plates be H cm and let h_{int}
be the thickness of interesting tissue on any x-ray path and h_{fat} be the
thickness of fat on the same path:

$$H = h_{int} + h_{fat} \qquad\qquad (2.1)$$

The top compression plate is sometimes at an angle to the bottom compression plate rather than being parallel, but this is easily measured and
corrected for. Equation 2.1 is incorrect at the breast edge with the film
where the total thickness of tissue is reduced. In Chapters 4 and 5 we model
the breast edge as consisting of pure fat and use detection of the reduced
thickness as a verification test of the model and as a way of estimating
compressed breast thickness H.

X-ray beam reaching the film-screen

The x-ray signal exiting from the breast has components due to photons passing straight through the breast (primary radiation), photons that
have been scattered, and photons that come from other than the focal-
spot (extra-focal radiation). It is the primary radiation that contains the
most useful information for diagnosis because there is a direct relationship
between the primary intensity and h_{int}. In order to reduce the other two
components there is an anti-scatter grid positioned between the breast and
the film-screen combination. The mathematics in Box 2.4 deals in detail
with the primary radiation and shows how the primary radiation can be
computed knowing the thickness of just the interesting tissue, h_{int}. The
scattered and extra-focal radiation components are dealt with mathematically in Chapters 3 and 4.

Of the total x-ray signal exiting the breast, about 40% is scattered radiation! The spatial variation of the scatter component depends mainly on the
local tissue composition and local tissue placement. The incident radiation
intensity determines the intensity of the scatter. Our scatter model works
by noting that even in the presence of scatter and extra-focal radiation the
x-ray beam contains useful information about the local tissue composition.
Extra-focal radiation is a significant proportion of the total radiation and

---

BOX 2.4: Primary and total x-ray radiation exiting breast

There are three components making up the signal exiting the breast, primary, scatter and extra-focal:

$$E^{exit}(x,y) = E_p^{exit}(x,y) + E_s^{exit}(x,y) + E_e^{exit}(x,y)$$

We now derive an equation for the primary component. The total attenuation of photons at energy E passing through h_{int} centimetres of interesting tissue and h_{fat} centimetres of fat is simply:

$$\begin{aligned} h\mu(\mathcal{E}) &= h_{int}\mu_{int}(\mathcal{E}) + h_{fat}\mu_{fat}(\mathcal{E}) \\ &= h_{int}(\mu_{int}(\mathcal{E}) - \mu_{fat}(\mathcal{E})) + H\mu_{fat}(\mathcal{E}) \end{aligned} \quad (2.2)$$

So that the number of primary photons N_p at energy $\mathcal{E}$ after the incident beam has passed through h_{int} centimetres of interesting tissue and h_{fat} centimetres of fat can be determined by applying Beer's law:

$$N_p(\mathcal{E}) = N_0(\mathcal{E})e^{-h\mu(\mathcal{E})}$$

where N_0 is the number of incident photons and $\mu_{int}(\mathcal{E})$ and $\mu_{fat}(\mathcal{E})$ are the linear attenuation coefficients of interesting tissue and fat respectively. This leads to an equation giving the intensity of the primary beam after traversal of the breast. This has just one unknown, namely h_{int} contained within $h\mu(\mathcal{E})$:

$$E_p^{exit}(x,y) = \phi(V_t, x, y)A_p t_s \int_0^{\mathcal{E}_{max}} N_0^{rel}(V_t, \mathcal{E})\, \mathcal{E}e^{-\mu_{luc}(\mathcal{E})h_{plate}}\, e^{-h\mu(\mathcal{E})}d\mathcal{E}$$

$$(2.3)$$

---

is reported to be up to 15% of the total [13, 27]. As the x-ray photons pass through the anti-scatter grid, the total proportion of scatter falls to near 13%, but this is at a cost of almost halving the number of primary photons.

Image formation: conventional film-screen system

X-ray photons passing through the breast and anti-scatter grid also have to pass through the film before being absorbed by an intensifying screen which produces visible light. The energy imparted due to primary radiation is explained mathematically in Box 2.5. The light given off by the intensifying screen exposes the film and creates the image, although a small percentage of the x-ray photons are absorbed as they pass through the film. We assume that the exposure to the film is directly proportional to the energy imparted to the intensifying screen. The greater the exposure to the film, the darker it becomes and this darkness is usually measured in terms of

---

BOX 2.5: Primary energy imparted to screen

Knowing the values for screen absorption and grid transmission allows us to write down an equation for the primary energy imparted to the screen:
$E_p^{imp}(x,y) =$

$$\phi(V_t, x, y) A_p t_s \int_0^{\mathcal{E}_{max}} N_0^{rel}(V_t, \mathcal{E}) \mathcal{E} S(\mathcal{E}) G(\mathcal{E}) e^{-\mu_{luc}(\mathcal{E}) h_{plate}} e^{-h\mu(\mathcal{E})} d\mathcal{E} \quad (2.4)$$

where $S(\mathcal{E})$ is the screen absorption ratio, shown in Figure 2.8, $G(\mathcal{E})$ is the anti-scatter grid transmission ratio shown in Figure 3.3 and:

$$h\mu(\mathcal{E}) = h_{int}(\mu_{int}(\mathcal{E}) - \mu_{fat}(\mathcal{E})) + H\mu_{fat}(\mathcal{E})$$

With the exception of the tissue thicknesses, all these values are known. However, glare from the intensifying screen causes the energies to be blurred so that some kind of compensation is required.

---

film density, D:

$$D = \log_{10}\left(\frac{I_l}{T_l}\right)$$

where I_l is the intensity of the illuminating light and T_l is the intensity of the light transmitted through the film. So, a film density of 1.0 indicates that only one-tenth of the illuminating light passes through the film, whilst a film density of 2.0 indicates that only one-hundreth of the illuminating light passes through. Of the film density range stored on a mammogram, only a certain range of film densities can be seen on a standard light box (without the use of a "hot" light).

There are three main sources of noise in film/screen mammography: film granularity, the limited number of x-ray quanta, and random inhomogeneities in or on the intensifying screen. The statistical noise in film-screen mammograms has been studied extensively elsewhere [7, 9, 144, 141] and in Chapter 11 we show how to detect the "shot noise" which occurs due to dust and dirt on the intensifying screen and discuss statistical noise in more depth.

An intensifying screen is used in mammography because it acts as a signal amplifier. Figure 2.8 gives the relative absorption of the different energy photons by the intensifying screen, as reported by Dance and Day [50]. Although use of an intensifying screen dramatically reduces x-ray dose to the breast, it also increases image blur, sometimes (unfortunately) called unsharpness. The intensifying screen increases blur because when the x-ray photons are absorbed in the phosphor, light photons are emitted isotropically. The greatest exposure to the film is near where the x-ray photon was

Energy absorption efficiency (S)

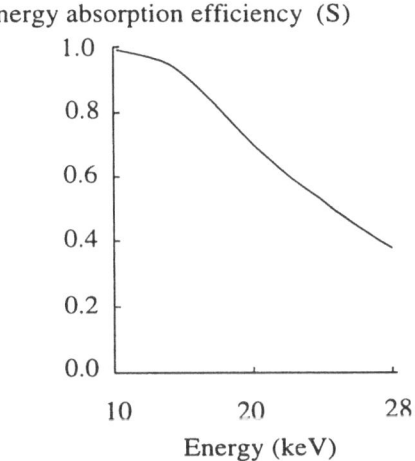

Figure 2.8.   Relative absorption of primary photons by the intensifying screen, as reported by Dance and Day [50].

absorbed, but the overall effect is a blur rather than a precise point. Figure 2.9 shows a schematic of this "glare" process. Giakoumakis and Miliotis [87] and more recently Maidment and Yaffe [169] present analytical models and practical measurements of the performance of intensifying screens. Giakoumakis's model is of a phosphor screen divided into thin layers with the angular distribution of light being Lambertian. They include attenuation of light between the point of x-ray absorption and exposure to the film. Maidement and Yaffe extend the model by including the overcoat layer that protects the phosphor material. The results from these papers show that the spectral distribution of the x-rays and the angle of x-ray incidence are not important but that the grain size, screen thickness and refraction in any coupling media are. The modulation transfer function of various intensifying screens has been measured and presented by various other researchers [3, 49, 59, 102]. In Box 2.8 on Page 53 we describe in detail how we correct an image to appear as if there had been no glare and Figures 2.13 and 7.7 show examples. In Chapter 11 we show how to use knowledge of the blur expected due to glare to detect film-screen "shot" noise.

The film-screen response to energy imparted to the intensifying screen is given by a characteristic curve (Figure 2.10). The characteristic curve changes with the film processing conditions and must therefore be checked regularly if quantitative measures are required. Ideally, the energy imparted to the intensifying screen would be measured and simply plotted against

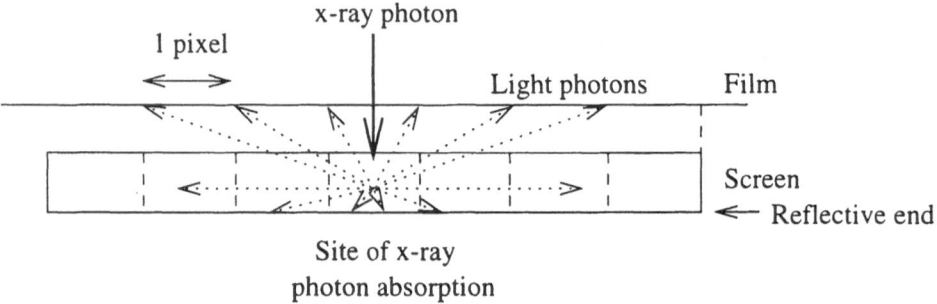

Figure 2.9. When an x-ray photon is absorbed in the intensifying screen, light photons are emitted isotropically (the dotted lines) which results in a blurred image. We seek a way of removing this effect and we do so using a model of the intensifying screen. We assume that the x-ray photons are absorbed equally across each part of the intensifying screen corresponding to one pixel and at different depths within that small volume. Knowing the pixel size, the solid angles between each potential absorption site and the neighbouring pixels can be computed. These solid angles define the proportion of light photons that the neighbouring pixels receive. The solid angles are weighted by distance from absorption site to the pixel (representing light absorption by the screen) and by the actual x-ray energy reaching that site. Using these values glare can be estimated and removed from an image as explained in full detail in Box 2.8.

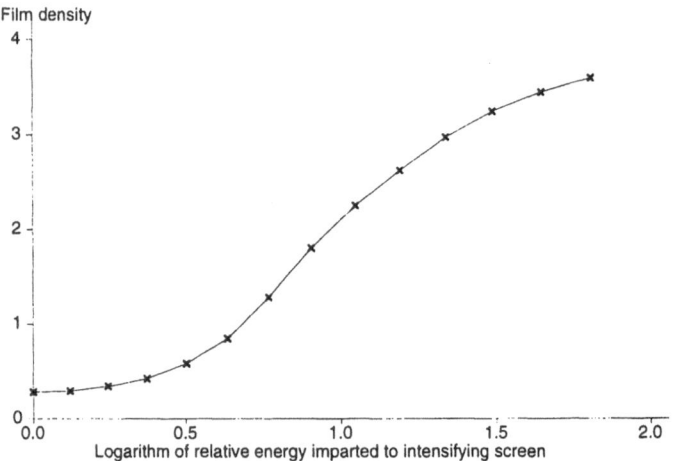

Figure 2.10. Film-screen characteristic curve found by exposing a lucite step wedge, measuring the film densities with a densitometer and plotting them against the results of a simulation to determine the energy imparted to the intensifying screen.

film density. However, determining the energy imparted to the intensifying screen accurately is difficult. We approximate the characteristic curve by using a lucite step wedge and simulating the attenuation of the x-ray beam by the different thicknesses of lucite. Lucite is chosen because of its similar absorption and scattering properties to a breast consisting of half fat, half interesting tissue. A small correction for scattered radiation is made, and the logarithm of the calculated relative energy imparted is plotted against film density, which is measured with a densitometer. Using the step wedge is a simple, cheap technique which can be used over many sites, it also allows us to calibrate every film-screen cassette.

The minimum film density is in the range 0.15 - 0.17 (called the base-fog), and the characteristic curve is approximately linear between film densities of 0.6 and 3.0; Box 2.6 presents the mathematical equations. The automatic exposure control aims to keep the mean film density at about 1.6 but is adjusted according to the tastes of the particular radiologist. The linear approximation is adequate for exploring the system character-istics, but a more realistic approximation is needed for quantitative work. For our work the linear approximation is used to derive analytical expres-sions, whilst a piecewise linear approximation is used to find the energy imparted to give any particular film density. Figure 2.11 shows an original mammographic image next to an image showing the energy imparted to the intensifying screen.

One further effect needs to be considered when dealing with film-screen systems and that is reciprocal law failure. The reciprocity law states that the density produced on a film depends only on the total amount of light energy employed. This law has been found to fail in mammographic films when a screen is used: greater exposures are needed to produce the same film density as the time of exposure rises. Stanton [230] quotes Haus' as-sertion that to create the same film density Kodak Ortho-M film needs an increase in exposure (as measured in mAs) of 7%, 17% and 36% as the time of exposure is increased from 0.5 seconds to 1s, 2s and 4s respectively. Kimme-Smith et al. [150] found that reciprocal law failure occurred to sim-ilar degrees in all modern film-screen combinations, including Fuji. Arnold [5] concluded that the main consequence of reciprocal law failure is on the speed of the film, thus we assume that the film-screen contrast does not change due to it. We also note that the delayed processing of films, such as happens when the mammograms are performed on a mobile van, leads to apparently slower film-screen systems [150]. We correct our film-screen cal-ibration data to be correct for the time-of-exposure for each mammogram.

ENERGY IMPARTED
Original Image   Energy Image

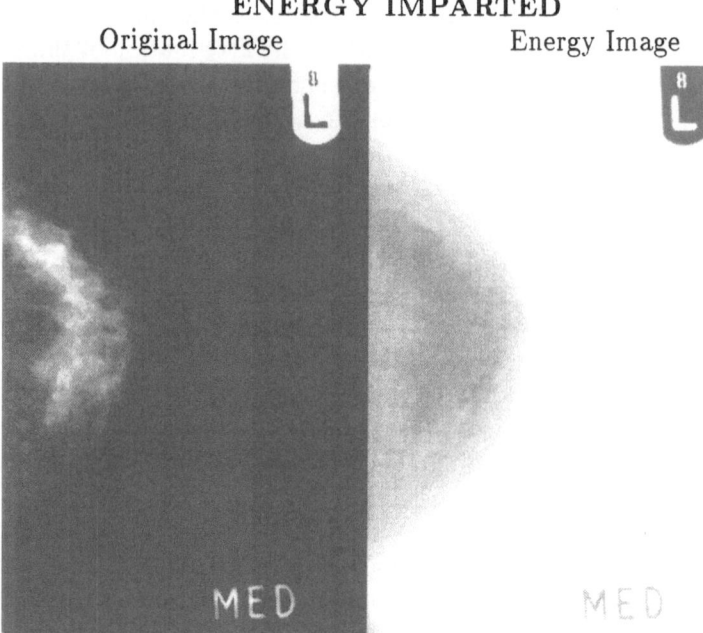

Figure 2.11.   On the left is the original mammogram, on the right is a representation of the energy imparted to the intensifying screen. The image on the right has luminance directly proportional to the logarithm of the energy imparted (this transform requires knowledge of the terminal display characteristics). The energy imparted is due to primary, scattered and extra-focal radiation.

BOX 2.6: Film-screen characteristic curve equations

With the linear assumption in the region of interest the following equation describes the relationship between film density and energy imparted:

$$
\begin{aligned}
D(x,y) &= \gamma \log_{10} E_{pse}^{imp}(x,y) + \beta' \\
\beta' &= \gamma \log_{10} \beta \\
D(x,y) &= \gamma \log_{10}(\beta E_{pse}^{imp}(x,y))
\end{aligned}
\tag{2.5}
$$

where γ is the film-screen gradient, and β is the other linear constant and is related to film-screen speed. The energy imparted has three components:

$$
E_{pse}^{imp}(x,y) = E_p^{imp}(x,y) + E_s^{imp}(x,y) + E_e^{imp}(x,y)
$$

The gradient γ can be found from the characteristic curve. Typically this has a value of just over 3.0. It's found by taking the minimum and maximum values of the linear part of the curve: $\gamma = \dfrac{D_{max} - D_{min}}{\log_{10} E_{max}^{imp} - \log_{10} E_{min}^{imp}}$

Digitizing films

Mammography is not as yet directly digital, although it promises to become so within the near future as discussed in Chapter 15. There are several reasons why it has not yet become directly digital, including the concern that the quality of the digital images is not yet good enough to satisfactorily image the smallest mammographic abnormalities. An alternative to directly digital systems is to digitise a mammographic film using some kind of scanning device. However, if digitising mammograms is seen to be a long-term option for digital mammography then it will be important that the x-ray film is seen as a recording device, and not a viewing device.

There are a variety of scanning devices that can be used, ranging from laser-scanning devices through to CCD cameras taking a picture of a lightbox. In all cases, it is essential that the relationship between pixel value (the output from the digitiser) and film density is known. Recording film density rather than the intensity of the light transmitted through the film is preferable because the film density is independent of the illuminating light intensity level. Calculation of film density can be made robust to spatial variations in the illuminating light intensity by measuring the illuminating light intensity at the same time as the transmitted light intensity, rather than measuring it once and assuming that it remains constant.

Some scanning devices, such as CCD cameras, tend to have hidden automatic gain controls which equalise image intensities - fine for viewing outdoor scenes but totally unsuitable when quantitative measurements are required. Fortunately, high quality, laser-scanning devices are becoming more common. These devices tend to have a linear relationship between film density and pixel value:

$$P(x, y) = mD(x, y) + c$$

Some of the most recent laser-scanners are capable of digitising films to a pixel resolution of under 50 microns, spanning the film density range from 0 to 4.0 with 12-bit resolution (i.e. using the pixel values of 0 to 4095 to represent the film densities from 0 to 4.0).

As well as quantisation error, any digitising equipment also introduces additional noise and blur into the system. Caldwell and Yaffe [31] restored their mammographic images in order to compensate for resolution degradation due not only to the digitising aperture, but also the finite size of the focal spot and glare in the intensifying screen. They did this by applying, in the frequency domain, an inverse filter based on the modulation transfer function (MTF). We also perform this restoration process and examples of the MTF of various digitising devices can be found in [54].

Naturally enough, the debate concerning the definition of 'sufficient res-olution' has been intense with the desire for greater resolution in the hope of achieving greater accuracy conflicting with technological and practical limitations. Karssemeijer et. al. [144] conclude that "100 μm resolution does not prohibit high-quality diagnostic performance in digital mammography" since "spherical calcifications with diameters smaller than 130 microns are not detectable with film-screen mammography". This issue is far from re-solved, however given that 50 micron resolution is commonly available to-day. Especially as it appears that the increased contrast in digital systems can overcome the loss of resolution [144].

The work in this book is directly applicable to directly digital systems as well as conventional systems. The only difference is in the modelling and calibration of the imaging device itself. With such modelling for a directly digital system it ought to be possible to map from pixel value to thickness of interesting tissue, h_{int}, and so algorithms which originally ran on h_{int} images from conventional systems should work on h_{int} images generated from directly-digital systems. However, some words of warning do need to be sounded, since modern machines offer more sophisticated hardware techniques which might prove extremely difficult to calibrate for. For example, an image taken with a machine that automatically varies the time of exposure across the breast will be extremely difficult to map to the h_{int} representation.

2.3. Summary and Results: Computing h_{int}

Having explained how we calibrate each step in the mammographic process and the assumptions that we make in our modelling the full algorithm for generating h_{int} is shown in Box 2.7. Figure 2.12 shows an example of an h_{int} image generated using our models. It is shown as a surface to underline the fact that the absolute jumps in the h_{int} values between pixels have a corresponding physical reason. The next two chapters provide the missing information for our modelling, namely estimates of scattered and extra-focal radiation.

BOX 2.7: Computing h_{int}

(1) Convert pixel value $P(x,y)$ to film density $D(x,y)$ using the digitiser calibration data including deblurring using the modulation transfer function.

(2) Convert film density $D(x,y)$ to energy imparted to intensifying screen $E_{pse}^{imp}(x,y)$ using film-screen calibration data.

(3) Compensate $E_{pse}^{imp}(x,y)$ for glare, see Box 2.8.

(4) Compensate $E_{pse}^{imp}(x,y)$ for the anode-heel effect and diverging x-ray beam, see Box 2.9.

(5) Estimate the scattered radiation $E_s^{imp}(x,y)$ using the model proposed in Chapter 3.

(6) Estimate the extra-focal radiation $E_e^{imp}(x,y)$ components using the model proposed in Chapter 4.

(7) Compute the primary radiation E_p^{imp}:

$$E_p^{imp}(x,y) = E^{imp}(x,y) - E_s^{imp}(x,y) - E_e^{imp}(x,y)$$

(8) $E_p^{imp}(x,y)$ is the measured primary energy. Equation 2.4 in Box 2.5 gives a theoretical primary energy for different values of $h_{int}(x,y)$. By equating the measured and theoretical values we can solve for $h_{int}(x,y)$ using a numerical approach.

AN h_{int} SURFACE

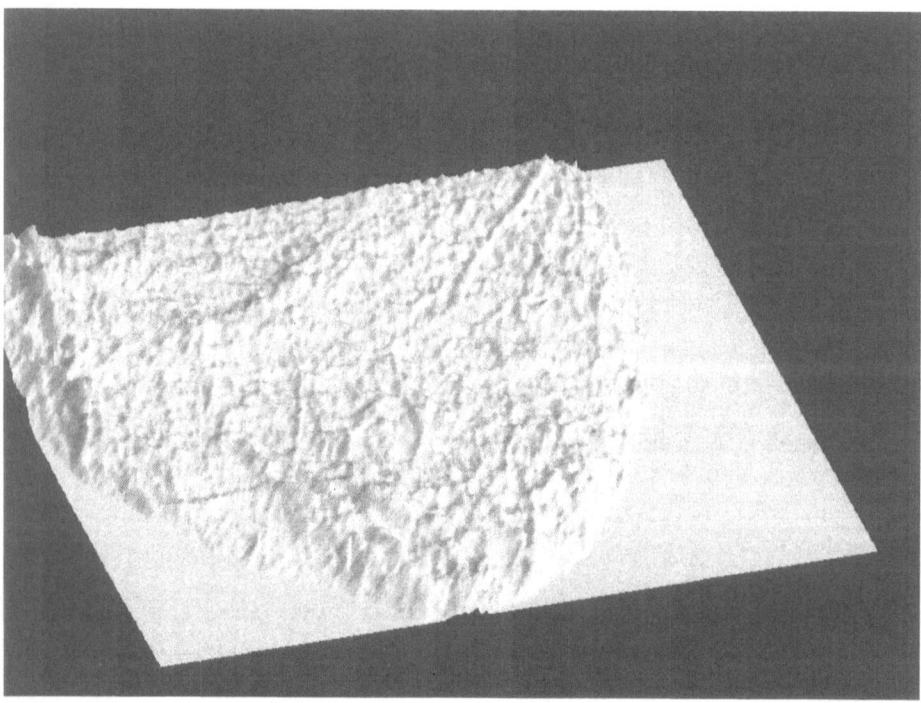

Figure 2.12. Depiction of the h_{int} surface of a breast. The height corresponds to the amount of non-fatty tissue. In this way, anatomical features correspond to topographic features of h_{int} surfaces. Towards the nipple there is an cyst which is represented here as a hill all around it is fibroglandular tissue making it quite hard to see on the mammogram.

BOX 2.8: Compensating for intensifying screen glare

We compensate for glare by using the point-spread function of the intensifying screen. To derive this function we consider the screen to be divided into layers and then each layer to be sub-divided into sub-pixel size units. Each of these units is considered to be a potential site of absorption of an x-ray. Let t_p cm be the thickness of the intensifying screen. We consider the screen to be in n layers so that each layer has a thickness of $dt_p = \frac{t_p}{n}$ cm. The layer is subdivided into pixels (whatever resolution is being used) and then each pixel is split into 100 smaller elements. We assume that the x-ray film lies directly on top of the intensifying screen separated only by a screen overcoat. For each layer we compute a weighting mask $w_z(x, y)$ (effectively the point spread function for that layer) which gives the percentage of light photons emitted at (x_c, y_c), depth z, that reach the film corresponding to the spatial position (x, y). The proportion of photons from (x_c, y_c) reaching (x, y) is related to the solid angle $d\theta$ from (x_c, y_c) depth z to (x, y). We assume symmetry round the azimuthal angle and just consider the 1D case. Some of the light photons that are emitted from (x_c, y_c, z) are absorbed by the phosphor so that we weight $d\theta$ using Beer's law:

$$\text{relative glare} = d\theta e^{-\mu_{phosphor}^{light} z / \cos\theta}$$

Where μ_{light} is an average linear attenuation value. Dividing the relative glare by the total relative glare gives a weighting mask for each layer. We now incorporate the x-ray energy being imparted to each layer. The energy into each layer is:

$$E_z^{imp}(x_c, y_c) = E^{in}(x_c, y_c)e^{-\mu_{phosphor}^{xray} z} - E^{in}(x_c, y_c)e^{-\mu_{phosphor}^{xray}(z + dt_p)}$$

where E_z^{imp} is the energy imparted and E^{in} is the incident energy. So that the relative glare now becomes:

$$\text{relative glare} = d\theta e^{-\mu_{phosphor}^{light} z / \cos\theta} E_z^{imp}(x_c, y_c)$$

We combine these values for each layer and for each sub-pixel to get the full weighting mask $w(x, y)$ and we scale the results so that $\sum_{(x,y)} w(x, y) = 1.0$. To properly compensate for glare it is necessary to know exactly where the edges of the mammographic film are since no glare comes from outside the film and those areas should be treated as zero in the convolution. Also, the energies imparted outside the breast area but on the film saturates the film so that to model the true effect of glare the energies on those regions have to be set to the expected incident energy as computed using the known time-of-exposure. The weighting mask w defines the point spread function for the intensifying screen so that the energy imparted image attained is simply the result of the energy imparted without glare convolved with w:

$$E^{\text{glare}} = E^{\text{no glare}} * w$$

This can be solved by deconvolution. Figure 2.13 shows an example of the effects of compensating for the glare.

BOX 2.9: Compensating for the anode heel effect

The primary component at (x, y) is directly proportional to the number of photons incident to the volume of tissue projected onto that pixel:

$$E_p^{imp}(x, y) = \phi(V_t, x, y) t_s A_p E_{p \ nd}^{imp}(x, y) \qquad (2.6)$$

where the last term is used to denote that part of Equation 2.3 which is independent of the total number of photons (nd stands for not-dependent). We assume that the x-ray energy spectrum stays the same but that the total number of photons $\phi(V_t, x, y)$ changes with (x, y) due to the anode heel effect and diverging beam. The scatter component at the pixel (x, y), mostly comes from the x-ray photons that are entering the breast tissue in the surrounding neighbourhood. This neighbourhood is small enough to allow us to ignore the anode heel effect over it so that the scatter component is also directly proportional to the incident radiation at (x, y):

$$E_s^{imp}(x, y) = \phi(V_t, x, y) t_s A_p E_{s \ nd}^{imp}(x, y) \qquad (2.7)$$

The total energy imparted is the sum of the primary and scatter components so that using Equations 2.6 and 2.7 gives:

$$E^{imp}(x, y) = \phi(V_t, x, y) t_s A_p (E_{p \ nd}^{imp}(x, y) + E_{s \ nd}^{imp}(x, y)) \qquad (2.8)$$

The incident photon flux is greatest underneath the anode, let the position on the film at this point be (x_a, y_a). We aim to change $E^{imp}(x, y)$ to be as if from that incident photon flux. By using Equation 2.8 we can reach:

$$E_{corrected}^{imp}(x, y) = \frac{\phi(V_t, x_a, y_a)}{\phi(V_t, x, y)} E^{imp}(x, y) \qquad (2.9)$$

We need to compute the ratio of the two photon fluxes. To determine the anode heel effect for a specific system and to thus compute the ratio we perform an x-ray exposure with no object present which gives us an apparently "blank film". The energy imparted to the screen comes mostly from the primary radiation since there is no scattering material:

$$E_{blank}^{imp}(x, y) = \phi(V_t, x, y) t_s A_p (E_{p \ nd}^{imp}(x, y) + E_{s \ nd}^{imp}(x, y))$$

$$E_{blank}^{imp}(x_a, y_a) = \phi(V_t, x_a, y_a) t_s A_p (E_{p \ nd}^{imp}(x_a, y_a) + E_{s \ nd}^{imp}(x_a, y_a))$$

We now note that since the parts of the signal not dependent on the number of photons are equivalent (there is no object) we have that:

$$\frac{\phi(V_t, x_a, y_a)}{\phi(V_t, x, y)} = \frac{E_{blank}^{imp}(x_a, y_a)}{E_{blank}^{imp}(x, y)}$$

Substituting this into Equation 2.9 allows us to compensate for the anode heel effect.

EXAMPLE OF GLARE REMOVAL

Original Energy Image Glare-Removed Energy Image

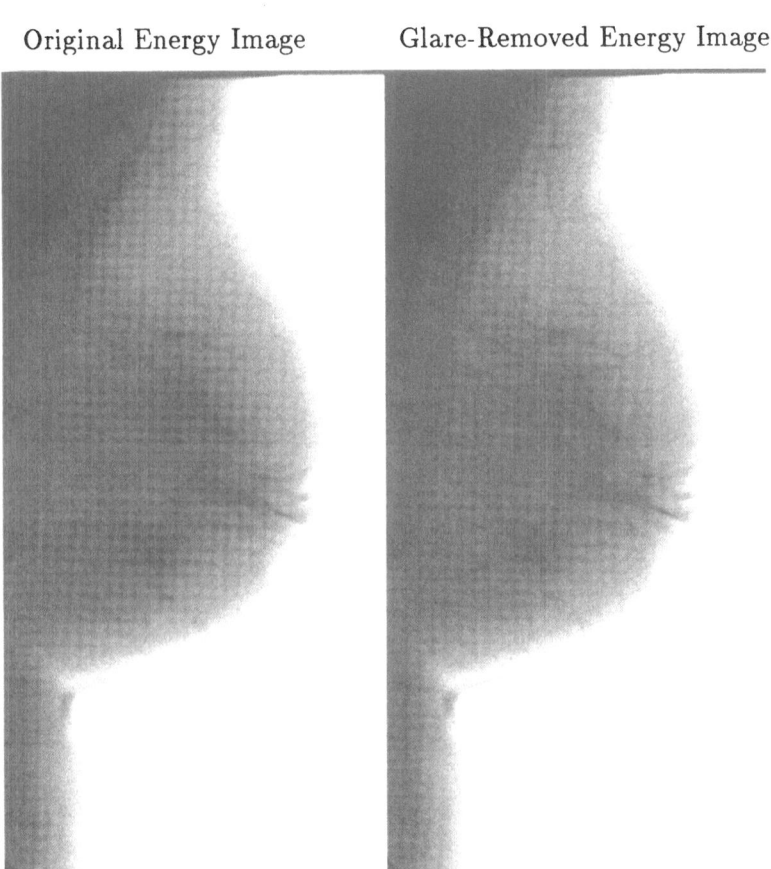

Figure 2.13. The image on the left shows the energy imparted with glare. The image on the right shows the energy imparted after compensation for glare. This is a sharpening operation which apparently makes the image far better. In Chapter 7 the results of performing this operation on a mammogram and then creating another mammogram are shown.

CHAPTER 3

A MODEL OF SCATTERED RADIATION

3.1. Introduction

Scatter is a major degrading factor in the appearance of mammographic images therefore removal of its effects improves perceived image quality. Scattered radiation degrades mammographic images by imparting a smoothly varying energy component to the intensifying screen. This component carries no information about the breast tissue on the specific x-ray path from x-ray source to pixel, although, as we show, scatter does contain information about the breast tissue in the immediately surrounding area. This chapter develops a method to model and remove scattered radiation[116]. The model is based on the conjecture that the amount of scattered radiation reaching a given pixel is related to the energies imparted in a neighbourhood surrounding the pixel. Of course, the exact relationship is highly complex, and we introduce a number of approximations. Still the proof of the pudding is in the eating, and the range of results we show later in the monograph demonstrates that the approximations are reasonable in practice. In essence, the energies imparted in a neighbourhood are used to estimate the composition of the local tissue and from this composition the scatter component is estimated from published data. However, tissues nearer to the central pixel affect the scatter component more than those tissues further away, and so the energy values need to be weighted to reflect this. Estimation of scatter plays a crucial role in allowing *quantitative measures* of the breast tissue to be found.

Other researchers have tackled the removal of the effects of scattered radiation from x-ray images, but not specifically for mammographic images. This specialisation enables us to make a number of mammography-specific approximations which allow us to develop more reliable algorithms. There have been two approaches to scatter removal: the first considers the scatter distribution as a blurred version of the original (similar to the method proposed here) and then subtracts it [180]. The other sharpens the original by deconvolving with an estimate of the point spread function for scattered radiation [218]. Both of the referenced papers consider glare, which comes from the emitted light photons of the intensifying screen, to be similar to scattered radiation, and correct for it in the same way. We have found it necessary and useful to treat the two separately. For general en-

hancement, Chan et al. [39] used the standard image-processing technique
called unsharp-mask filtering, which is similar to the technique used here,
but they set their parameters subjectively and work on the original image.
In our case, the original has been transformed to an energy imparted image first, and all the variables have been derived from published research
dealing with the physics of mammography.

Most of the work in this chapter is based on papers by physicists dealing
with scattered radiation in radiography. The papers on scatter in mammography have mostly been written with a view to estimating the quantity of
scatter, and to investigating the trade-off between the benefits of using an
anti-scatter grid and the increased radiation dose to the breast. This previous work has largely ignored what occurs around the breast edge where
the breast thickness is reduced and extra-focal radiation starts to have an
effect. That is the subject of the next chapter.

The chapter begins by discussing the anti-scatter grid, a device that
gives increased image quality but requires a doubling of the radiation dose
to the breast. We then start presenting our model of scattered radiation.
The first step requires definition of a "scatter volume" which indicates
where scatter reaching a central point actually comes from. This volume is
then refined using data about the anti-scatter grid allowing us to define a
weighting mask that holds at each "cell" the percentage of the total scatter
reaching the central pixel and coming from the column of tissue above that
cell. The final step is to use published data to compute a scatter function
that maps the convolution of the weighting mask with energy imparted to
an estimate of scatter. We discuss the implementation of the algorithm and
then show results of the scatter computation. In a later chapter we show the
results of scatter removal from images taken without an anti-scatter grid.
In the not too distant future mammography will become digital. When this
happens, the details of the model presented here will have to be changed,
but the basic idea underlying the scatter model will still be directly relevant.

3.2. Anti-scatter grid

Scatter was recognised as a problem in mammography when Barnes and
Brezovich [8] measured the number of scattered and primary photons reaching a detector having passed through a circular lucite phantom 14cm in diameter. They varied the thickness of the lucite phantom and the diameter
of the circular radiation field. The measurements were carried out without
a grid and were taken beneath the centre of the lucite phantom, Figure 3.1
shows some of their results. Shortly after this work, anti-scatter grids were
introduced into mammography with apparently dramatic effects [50, 51].
Figure 3.2 shows how an anti-scatter grid functions.

Scatter-to-primary ratio

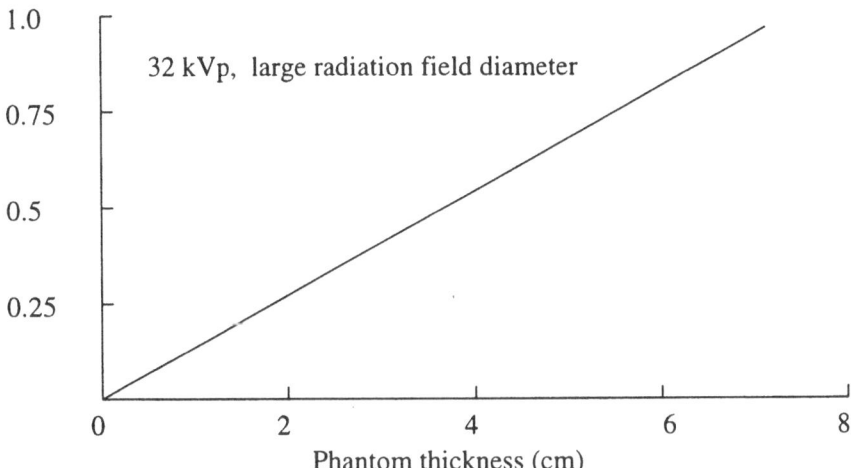

Scatter-to-primary ratio

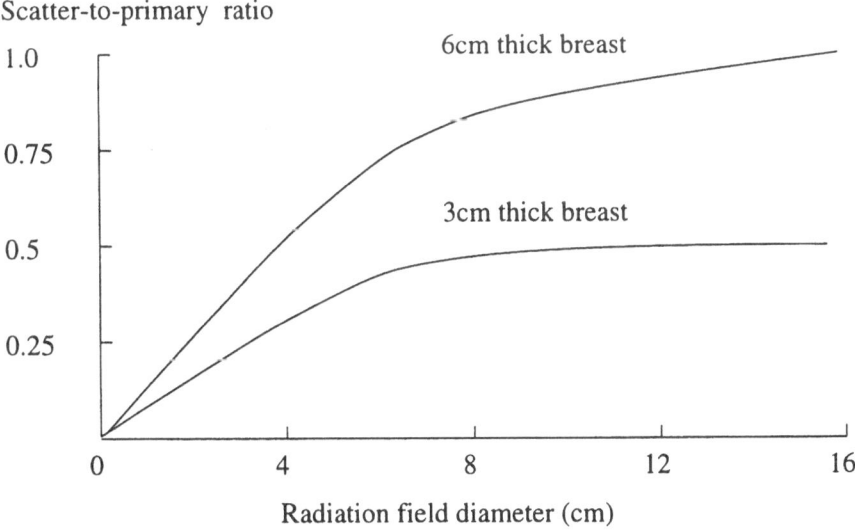

Figure 3.1.   These show the variation of scatter-to-primary ratio with lucite phantom thickness (top) and radiation field diameter (bottom) when no anti-scatter grid is
used, according to Barnes and Brezovich [8]. The top graph shows the benefit of firm
breast compression in reducing the scattered radiation component of the signal. The
rate-of-change of the bottom curves with radiation field diameter effectively tells us the
amount of scatter reaching a central point and coming from a certain distance away. We
use the rate-of-change to give us a weighting mask w that contains the percentage of
scatter coming from distances away from the central pixel.

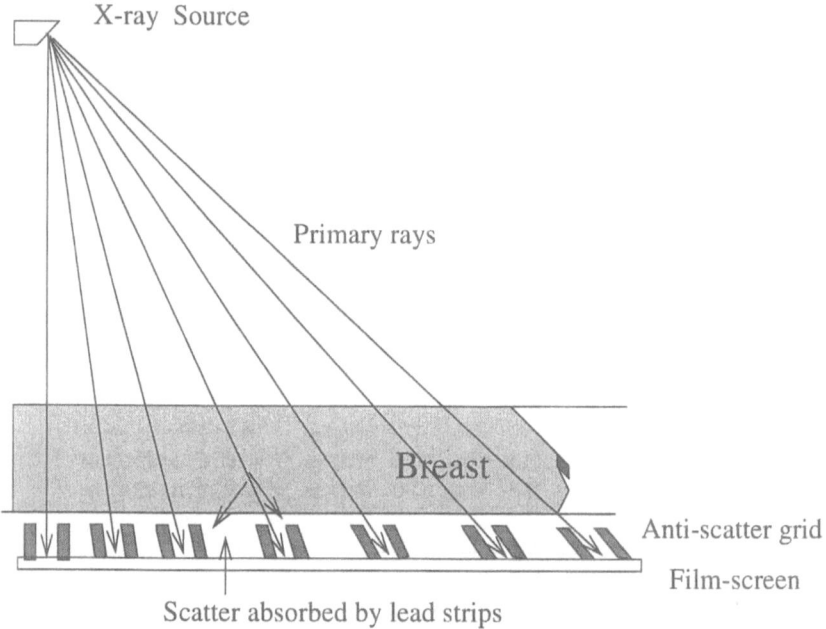

Figure 3.2. A typical anti-scatter grid consists of a series of angled lead strips separated by paper. The angle is set so that x-ray photons travelling directly from the source will pass through the grid without attenuation, whilst photons that are scattered, and therefore are travelling in unexpected directions, will be stopped. Although effective, a scatter-to-primary ratio of 0.15 with the grid is quite normal. Furthermore, to prevent the appearance of grid lines across the image it is necessary to move the grid rapidly back and forth. This causes attenuation of almost half the primary beam and therefore requires a near doubling of the radiation dose! In Chapter 10, we show how we can use the model of scattered radiation proposed in this chapter to perform software removal of scatter rather than using the grid, so we could, in principle, reduce the radiation dose required by half!

Although successful, grids also remove a significant amount of the primary beam necessitating an increase in dose to the breast in order that the film is satisfactorily exposed. The increase in radiation dose (the "Bucky factor") to the breast is often double. Scatter reduction can be obtained with no increase in dose to the breast by introducing an air gap between the breast and film, but this introduces unacceptable blurring through magnification. Due to the increased exposure using a grid, their use is likely to remain a subject of debate, especially for women with small breasts. Carlsson et al. [32] report that in Sweden, where grids haven't been used in screening, experience has shown that their use would reduce the number of healthy women recalled to the assessment clinic. Modelling of the mammographic process and of the effects of scattered radiation could provide an

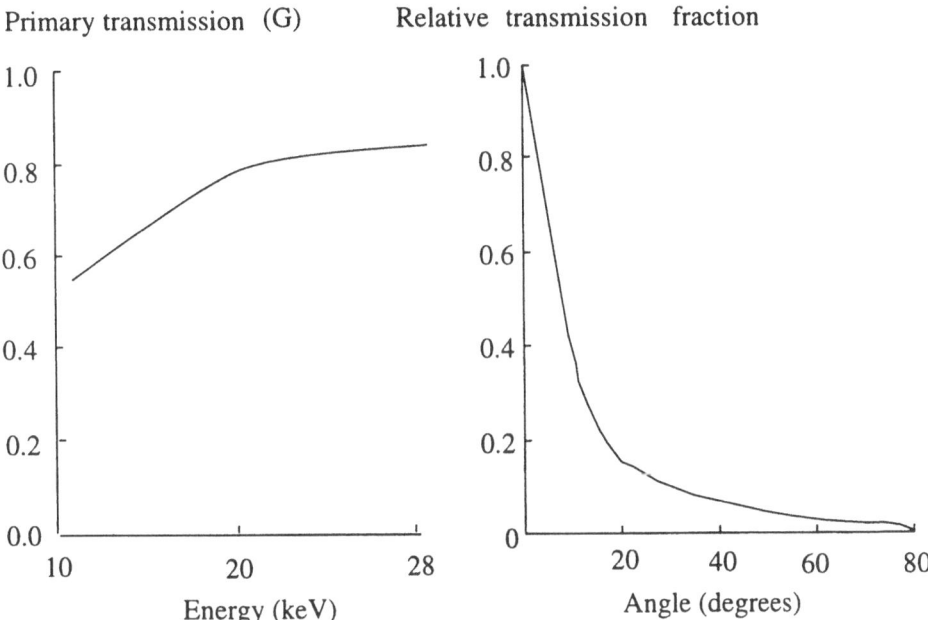

Figure 3.3. On the left are the transmission ratios (G) through a moving anti-scatter grid of primary photons at different energies. These are the values used in Equation 2.4. On the right are the relative transmission ratios through a moving anti-scatter grid of scattered photons with energies in the range 12.5 − 25keV. The values are relative to the transmission of primary photons and the angle shown is the elevation angle (i.e. the angle between the image plane and the photon). Both sets of data are as reported by Dance and Day [50].

alternative to using a grid, and hence could halve the radiation dose to the breast. We investigate removing the grid in Chapter 10.

Figure 3.3 shows the relative transmission of the anti-scatter grid to primary photons at different energies, and the relative transmission of scattered photons with different elevation angles (the values have been integrated over the azimuthal angle). Both graphs are as reported by Dance and Day [50]. Scatter-to-primary ratios, calculated with and without an anti-scatter grid, as reported by Carlsson et al. [32], are shown in Table 3.1. We use those values in Section 3.5 when we construct a "scatter function".

Phantom composition	Phantom thickness(cm)	Scatter-to-primary ratio	
		no grid	with grid
Fat	2	0.2340	0.0376
	5	0.4832	0.0899
	8	0.7578	0.1469
Half fat, half glandular	2	0.2527	0.0425
	5	0.5412	0.1041
	8	0.8244	0.1630
Glandular ("interesting")	2	0.2695	0.0481
	5	0.6018	0.1173
	8	0.9070	0.1868

TABLE 3.1. Scatter-to-primary ratios calculated with and without an anti-scatter grid, and for different breast compositions, as derived from Carlsson et al. [32] for a typical film-screen mammographic system. These ratios are averages over the phantom image, and do not include extra-focal radiation. The ratios are based upon energies imparted to the intensifying screen. Carlsson et al. report that the scatter-to-primary ratio in the centre of the breast is around 15% higher than the average, i.e. when breast edges effects and extra-focal radiation aren't considered the scatter component drops off considerably at the breast edge.

3.3. Defining the "scatter volume" when the grid is not used

The first step towards scatter removal is to define where the scattered photons reaching an image pixel come from without an anti-scatter grid. No data has been published for this, but it can be derived for lucite (which approximates 50% fat and 50% interesting tissue by mass) using the results published by Barnes and Brezovich [8]. We assume that the scattering locations for lucite are similar to that which would be found for fat and interesting tissue. This is only an approximation, as shown by the apparent forward-peaking of scattered radiation, and differences in the degree of this peaking for different materials and different photon energies [136, 152, 166, 179].

Although the exact circumstances under which Figure 3.1 was derived are different from those currently used in mammography, the results are appropriate here because we do not require the exact values of scatter-to-primary radiation, rather the percentage of the total scatter as a function of distance from the pixel. In the figure, the thickness of the phantom is fixed

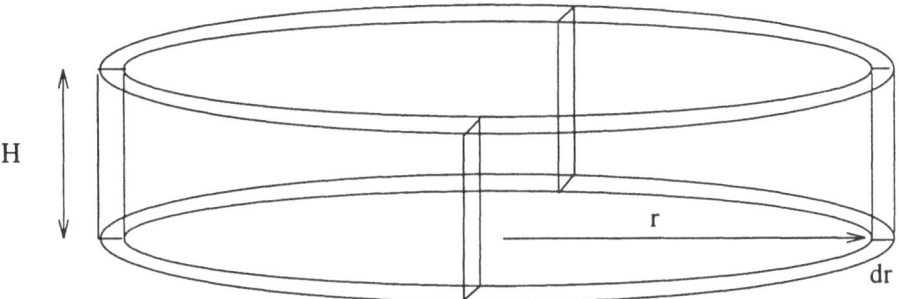

Figure 3.4. The data reported by Barnes and Brezovich [8] allows us to estimate the percentage of the total scattered photons coming from any chosen cylinder (inner radius r, outer radius $r + dr$, height H) and reaching the centre. The value of dr will later be made equal to the pixel size in an image.

for each curve, so the primary component is constant. That is, the rate of change of the curve gives the rate of change of the scatter component with increasing radiation field diameter, and so it is possible to determine the percentage of the total scatter reaching the detector from various distances.

In order to accommodate any breast thickness, a linear relationship between the scatter-to-primary ratio and phantom thickness is assumed for any fixed field diameter. This allows us to interpolate, or extrapolate, to find the scatter-to-primary ratios for phantom thicknesses other than 3 or 6 cm. This assumption is in agreement with the linear relationship Barnes and Brezovich found between scatter-to-primary ratio and phantom thickness for a large radiation field diameter.

Using this data enables the percentage of the total amount of scattered radiation coming from cylinders of lucite (Figure 3.4) with the width of a pixel and various radii to be estimated. This percentage forms the basis for deriving a weighting mask w which represents where in a neighbourhood of a pixel the scattered photons come from. The mathematics is shown in Box 3.1.

The underlying model here assumes that the mask derived for lucite is similar to that which would be found for fat and interesting tissue. Furthermore, we take no account of the differential absorption of the scattered photons, depending upon incident angle, by the intensifying screen. Also, the possibility of a photon reaching the centre pixel having been multiply scattered is not considered in the scatter model because the scattering loca-

---

BOX 3.1: The proportion of total scatter from each cylinder

Let $\frac{s}{p}(r)$ be the scatter-to-primary ratio for a phantom of thickness H and radiation field radius r, and let dr be a small increment in this radius (this will later be equal to the size of the pixels in the image). Let $E_s^{imp}(r)$ be the total energy imparted to the detector due to scattered radiation from a lucite phantom with radiation field radius r, and let $E_p^{imp}(r)$ be the primary signal. The amount of scattered radiation $dE_s^{imp}(r)$ coming from the cylinder of lucite defined by the inner radius r and outer radius $r + dr$ can be approximated as follows:

$$
\begin{aligned}
dE_s^{imp}(r) &= E_s^{imp}(r + dr) - E_s^{imp}(r) \\
&= E_p^{imp}(r + dr)\tfrac{s}{p}(r + dr) - E_p^{imp}(r)\tfrac{s}{p}(r) \\
&= E_p^{imp}(r)\left(\tfrac{s}{p}(r + dr) - \tfrac{s}{p}(r)\right)
\end{aligned}
$$

using the fact that the primary component E_p^{imp} is constant for any radius with a fixed phantom thickness H. In practice, the amount of scattered radiation reaching the detector stops increasing once the field radius is greater than some radius R. The stopping radius R increases with phantom thickness H. At this radius, the scatter-to-primary ratio is $\frac{s}{p}(R)$, and the total scatter can be written as follows:

$$
E_s^{imp}(R) = E_p^{imp}(r)\tfrac{s}{p}(R)
$$

Thus the proportion of the total scattered radiation which comes from the cylinder described above is:

$$
\frac{dE_s^{imp}(r)}{E_s^{imp}(R)} = \frac{\tfrac{s}{p}(r + dr) - \tfrac{s}{p}(r)}{\tfrac{s}{p}(R)}
$$

---

tion being found is the initial scattering site rather than the final scattering site. This has consequences when the grid data is applied because the angle from initial scattering site to pixel is used rather than the final angle. It is conjectured that this will not be significant especially since it is reported that single scatter contributes 60-85 percent of the total scatter depending upon breast thickness [166].

The scatter model does not, and cannot, differentiate between a block of fat with a layer of interesting tissue at the bottom and a block of fat with a layer of interesting tissue at the top. In both these cases the primary energy imparted will be the same, yet it is likely that the scattered radiation distribution will be different. However, initial investigations by [62] indicate that the scatter components will be similar.

3.4. Defining the scatter volume when a grid is used

In most countries, mammography is always performed with the aid of an anti-scatter grid. Such a grid prevents photons reaching the film from unexpected directions (with respect to the source and position on the film) and thus prevents loss of image contrast. Day and Dance [56] derived a formula expressing the transmission of photons through the grid as a function of varying directions, and their later paper [50] reproduced the results with the transmission values integrated over the azimuthal angle, Figure 3.3. This figure shows the values for transmission relative to that of primary photons (also in [50]). The values given are for photons between the energies of 12.5keV and 25keV. This does not quite cover the range of energies used in mammography; but suffices, since a massive proportion of the photons are within this range. Day and Dance's data is for a focused, moving Phillip's anti-scatter grid, with grid ratio 5:1, lead strips 0.02mm thick, 1.5mm high and separated by 0.3mm of cotton fibre. The grid is discussed in more depth in Chapter 10.

In order to find the scatter volume when a grid is used, grid data is applied to the scatter volume already derived under the assumption that no grid is used. To do this, some knowledge is needed of the angle at which the scattered photons arrive at the central pixel. This requires an assumption about the height of the scattering locations within each hollow cylinder. We assume that the initial scattering locations are distributed evenly over height. We make this assumption since there are two main factors affecting the number of scattered photons reaching the detector from a particular volume of the breast. One is the number of photons reaching the volume (which is related to the thickness of breast tissue between the source and the volume), the other is the distance of the volume to the detector. From the previous section we know that most of the scattered photons reaching the detector come from cylinders with relatively small radius. For volumes of tissue within such a cylinder, the two factors effecting total scatter tend to cancel out, thus the assumption of equal distribution, although obviously simplistic, is justified. Box 3.2 shows the mathematical detail.

Using the scatter volume derived from the paper of Barnes and Brezovich, the percentages of scatter from the various initial locations are redefined by application of Dance and Day's grid transmission values for the angle at which the photon would have arrived at the grid if scattered just once. Box 3.3 shows the mathematics and Figure 3.6 shows the results for phantoms 3cm and 6cm thick respectively. As expected, the scattered photons come from a lot closer when an anti-scatter grid is used. This effect is unavoidable if the primary signal is not to be attenuated greatly, but it does make digital scatter removal more difficult by making the scatter

---

BOX 3.2: The proportion of scatter from each tube of the cylinder

Consider a typical hollow cylinder, and divide this into n horizontal tubes (Figure 3.5). Let $x\%$ be the percentage of the total scattered photons reaching the central pixel from the cylinder. The percentage of the total scattered photons reaching the centre from each tube in the cylinder is $x/n\%$ with our assumption. In our work, each hollow cylinder is divided into 1mm high tubes, so that $n = 10H$, where H is the breast thickness in cm. Let $p(r, h)$ be the percentage of the total scattered photons coming from the tube with inner radius r, outer radius $r + dr$, lower height h and upper height $h + dh$, then:

$$p(r, h) = 100 \times \frac{dE_s^{imp}(r)}{E_s^{imp}(R)n}$$

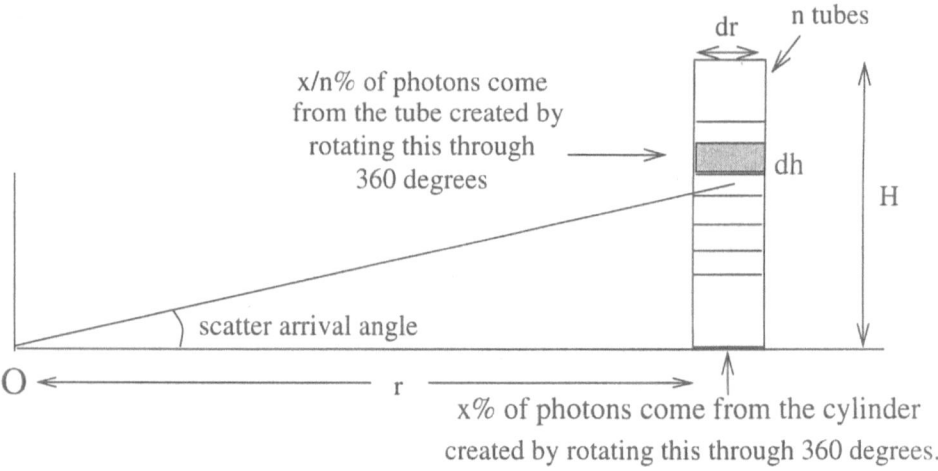

Figure 3.5. In order to use the grid data reported by Dance et al. [50], the scatter arrival angle needs to be known. For our work we divide the cylinder into n horizontal tubes and assume an equal percentage of the scattered photons comes from each tube.

component of a higher frequency through it becoming more reliant on the local tissue. Figure 3.7 illustrates this.

The percentages of scatter from the various initial locations are quantised into weighting masks w, where the value (or height) at each pixel is directly proportional to the percentage of the total scattered radiation coming from the column of tissue above that pixel and reaching the central pixel. The masks vary for each breast thickness, the thicker the breast the more likely that the scattered photons come from further away. Typically,

---

BOX 3.3: Calculating the proportion of scatter when a grid is used.

For simplicity, rotational symmetry is assumed and the data integrated over azimuthal angle. Let $p_g(r, h)$ be the percentage of the total scattered photons coming from the tube with inner radius r, outer radius $r + dr$, lower height h, upper height $h + dh$ when an anti-scatter grid is used and let $T(\theta)$ be the relative transmission through the grid for a photon with incident angle θ as shown in Figure 3.3:

$$\theta = \tan^{-1}\left(\frac{r}{h}\right)$$

$$p_g(r, h) = p(r, h)T(\theta)$$

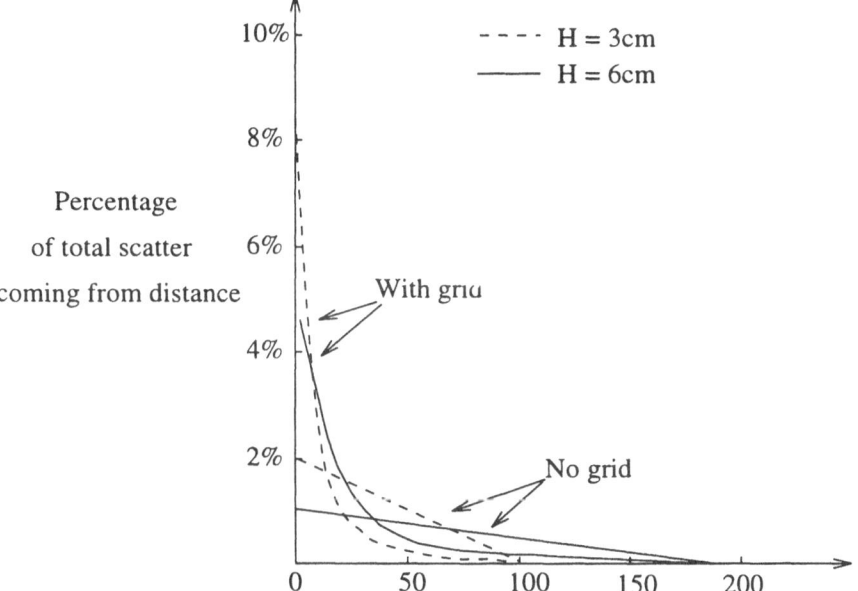

Figure 3.6. Percentage of total scatter coming from various distances away from the central pixel for lucite phantoms of thickness 3cm and 6cm. The curves for both with and without grid are marked. Notice how the grid makes the scatter much more local, and thus much more dependent on the tissue locally.

the mask will have diameter of about 1cm so that at 50 microns the mask will be 200 by 200 pixels and at 300 microns the mask will be 34 by 34 pixels.

The assumptions in this section appear to be supported by the reduction

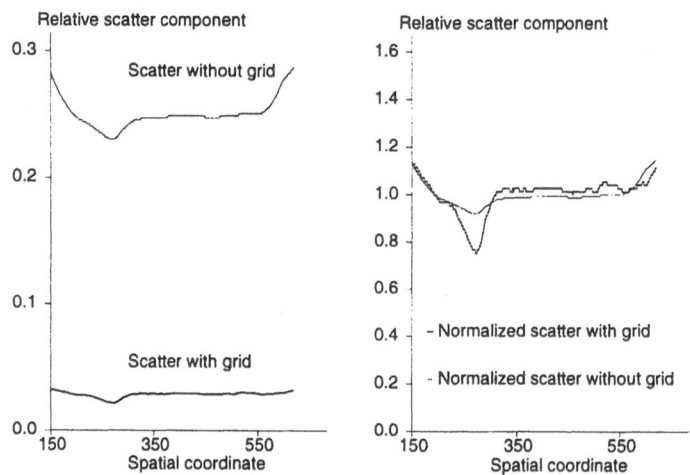

Figure 3.7. The figure on the left shows the relative scatter component along a profile across an actual image for the case when a grid is used and when not. The scatter without the grid is clearly massive compared to the scatter with the grid. However, when the grid is used the scatter component is more reliant on the local tissue and so is of a higher frequency, i.e. far more jagged. This can be seen by dividing the two curves by their averages. This is shown on the right.

that Carlsson et al. [32] predict in scatter-to-primary ratio with the grid. The results from our method are of the same order that they report, a reduction factor in both cases of between 5 and 6. The values are not directly comparable because Carlsson et al. use breast tissue rather than lucite, and photon energy has an important bearing on the result. As an example, our method predicts a reduction factor of 5.8 in the scatter-to-primary ratio when the primary transmission is considered at 20keV and the lucite phantom is 5cm thick, compared to the reduction by a factor of 5.2 which Carlsson et al. report for a 5cm thick breast consisting of 50% fat and 50% glandular tissue by mass. An improved model would consider non-isotropic absorption and use the formula proposed by Day and Dance [56].

3.5. Estimate "scatter function"

Let us review where we have reached: a weighting mask $w(x, y)$ has been calculated which represents the percentage of the total scatter reaching the central pixel and coming from the column of lucite above each pixel in a neighbourhood The aim now is to estimate the amount of scattered radiation at the central pixel by convolving the weighting mask with the energy imparted image $E_{pse}^{imp}(x, y)$, and using the resultant convolution sum as the input to a "scatter function", s. We propose to determine this function by consideration of three example cases: 100% fat, 100% interesting tissue, and 50% fat/50% interesting tissue by mass.

Carlsson et al. [32] have theoretically calculated the scatter-to-primary ratios for blocks of the three examples. Their results are shown in Table 3.1. (Note that in their report the authors refer to glandular rather than interesting tissue.) The scatter-to-primary ratios given by Carlsson et al. do not include the effects of extra-focal radiation and are averages over the breast shadow. They report that the scatter-to-primary ratio for a point in the centre of the breast is around 15% higher than the average.

Using calibration data, and the equations developed in the previous chapter, the energy imparted to the intensifying screen due to primary photons can be estimated for the three reference cases as shown mathematically in Box 3.4. The scatter component can then be found from Carlsson et al. from which we can calculate the expected total energy imparted. Convolving that value with the weighting mask provides us with a function mapping from the convolution of energy imparted and weighting mask to scatter. In fact, this function turns out to be linear as Figure 3.8 shows. Using this function it is proposed that the scatter component at any pixel in a heterogeneous breast can be determined by using the appropriate weighting mask convolved with the real energy imparted values to give the input.

A source of concern with this scatter model is that the results depend on the relationship between total energy imparted in the surrounding neighbourhood and scatter component at the central pixel. In fact, the total energy imparted in the surrounding neighbourhood itself depends on the scattered radiation coming from the tissue outside the neighbourhood. Again, it is difficult to judge the error, but one might consider a two-pass algorithm in which the second pass uses the predicted primary components to predict more accurately the scattered components, and then in turn update the primaries.

Note that when the weighting mask w is applied at the very edge of the breast, approximately half of the mask falls outside the breast image and half inside. Thus, without taking any account of the edge effects, the scatter component at the edge is already being partly estimated. In fact, the estimate is similar to what occurs at the chest wall where the convolution uses zero if the mask falls outside the breast image.

BOX 3.4: Derivation of the scatter function

Let $U(x_c, y_c)$ be the convolution sum at the pixel (x_c, y_c):

$$U(x_c, y_c) = \sum_{(x_c-x, y_c-y) \in \mathcal{N}} E_{pse}^{imp}(x_c - x, y_c - y)w(x, y),$$

where $\mathcal{N}$ is a neighbourhood around (x_c, y_c) assumed to lie within the breast image. The neighbourhood should contain most of the initial scatter locations and this can be determined when creating the weighting mask with the neighbourhood size increasing with breast thicknesses. Using the calibration data for the specific breast (i.e. time of exposure, breast thickness), the primary energy imparted to the intensifying screen can be estimated for three reference cases: 100% interesting tissue, 100% fat and 50% fat/50% interesting tissue. Once $E_p^{imp}(x, y)$ is known, the scatter-to-primary ratio can be used to find $E_{pse}^{imp}(x, y)$, assuming extra-focal minimal over most of the breast image:

$$E_{pse}^{imp}(x, y) = E_p^{imp}(x, y)(1 + \tfrac{E_s}{E_p}),$$

where the values for $\frac{E_s}{E_p}$ come from Table 3.1. Using this value the convolution sum $U(x_c, y_c)$ can be found for the three reference cases at the required breast thickness. For each of these blocks of tissue the energy imparted due to scatter is:

$$E_s^{imp}(x, y) = E_p^{imp}(x, y) \times \tfrac{E_s}{E_p}$$

The function s from convolution sum to scatter can be approximated using these three cases:

$$E_s^{imp}(x_c, y_c) = s(U(x_c, y_c))$$

In fact, this function turns out to be linear so that it could be combined with the weighting mask so that a convolution of E_{pse}^{imp} and the weighting mask gives E_s directly. Figure 3.8 shows an example scatter function.

3.6. Implementation

Our modelling is specific to particular regions of the mammographic image, so that the first stage in the implementation is to segment the breast and pectoral muscle area from the film area and parts of the image that are from off-the-film, see Figure 3.9. For our purposes, we do not need to segment pectoral muscle from the breast area itself since, for scatter, we can consider the pectoral muscle to consist of mostly interesting tissue (in fact, this later provides a very useful check on our modelling).

We segment the film from regions off-the-film by performing linear Hough transforms in those areas where the film edges are expected to be. Simple tests on the gradient of the determined film edges provides evidence

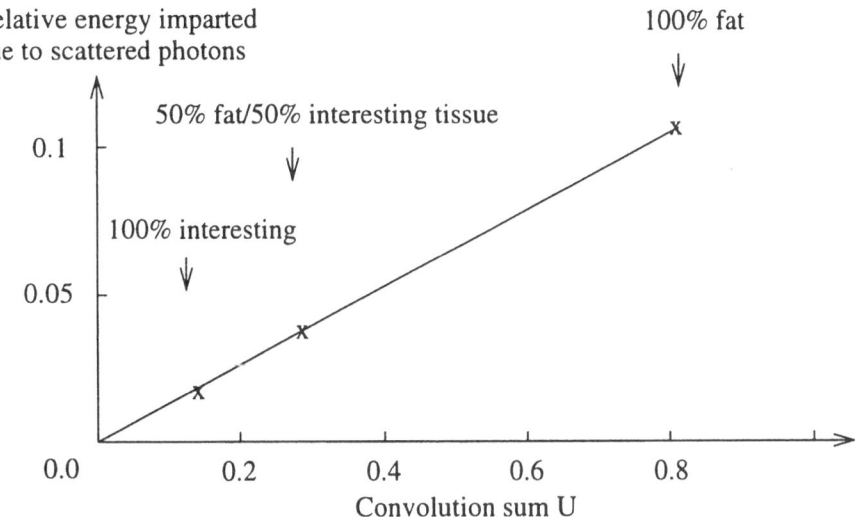

Figure 3.8. This shows a scatter function s for a breast 6.5cm thick. The convolution sum U is the result of convolving a weighting mask w, representing where scatter comes from, with the energies imparted to the intensifying screen. In this way, U is a measure of local tissue composition and tissue placement. The scatter function maps from U to an estimate of the scatter energy imparted. The function is worked out on the basis of three references cases as marked on the graph.

about whether the transform has worked or not. A linear Hough transform can also be used to remove the patient label from the image, thus ensuring patient confidentiality when the image is used for research.

The second stage of segmentation involves determining where the breast edge meets the film. The film image is obviously far darker than most of the breast image suggesting thresholding as a way to segment the breast region from the background. However, film labels, smear from the digitiser, the smooth intensity transform from breast to film, and noise makes thresholding unreliable. We use a technique based on image gradients and morphology that is simple, robust and can be implemented efficiently. Firstly, we note that the film area is the only area within the image where we can be certain of extremely low image gradients. Thus candidate pixels for being on the film rather than within the breast area can be attained by thresholding the image gradients. We compute the image gradients on the film density values rather than the pixel values thus making the process robust to variations in the actual digitisation process. The threshold value

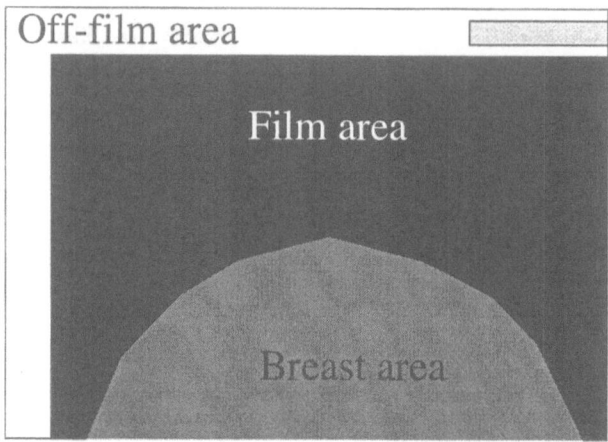

Figure 3.9. The scatter algorithm requires segmentation of the breast area from what we term the film area and the off-film area. The film area is that part of the film exposed directly to the x-rays. The off-film area arises from the digitiser over-scanning and part of the film being shielded from the x-rays by the film-screen cassette.

has been set at 0.001 and has been seen to be suitable for a whole range of mammographic images from 12-bit, 50 microns through to 8-bit, 300 microns. The thresholding does not have to be 100% accurate since the next step is post-processing to remove erroneously marked points. We take the film area candidates to be set to zero and the breast area to be set to one. We eliminate the few pixels wrongly marked in the film area by using a small mask to perform a binary morphological erosion. A binary closing operation (dilation followed by erosion) with a large mask makes the breast and film areas into coherent areas, although other small areas marked as being on the film can persist. If this happens, the actual film area is obvious through its size and position. Taking the area marked as on the film and extrapolating to the edges of the image ensures an enclosed area representing those pixels inside the breast area. Some post-processing might be required to remove labels that touch the breast area. Figure 3.10 illustrates the process on both a cranio-caudal and a medio-lateral oblique mammogram.

At 50 micron resolution, the scatter approximation requires a mask of size 200 by 200 to be convolved with an image of dimensions approaching 4800 by 2500, which is a very time consuming process. To speed up the convolution Fourier and parallel processing techniques can be used as can multi-scale techniques since the scatter component is smooth.

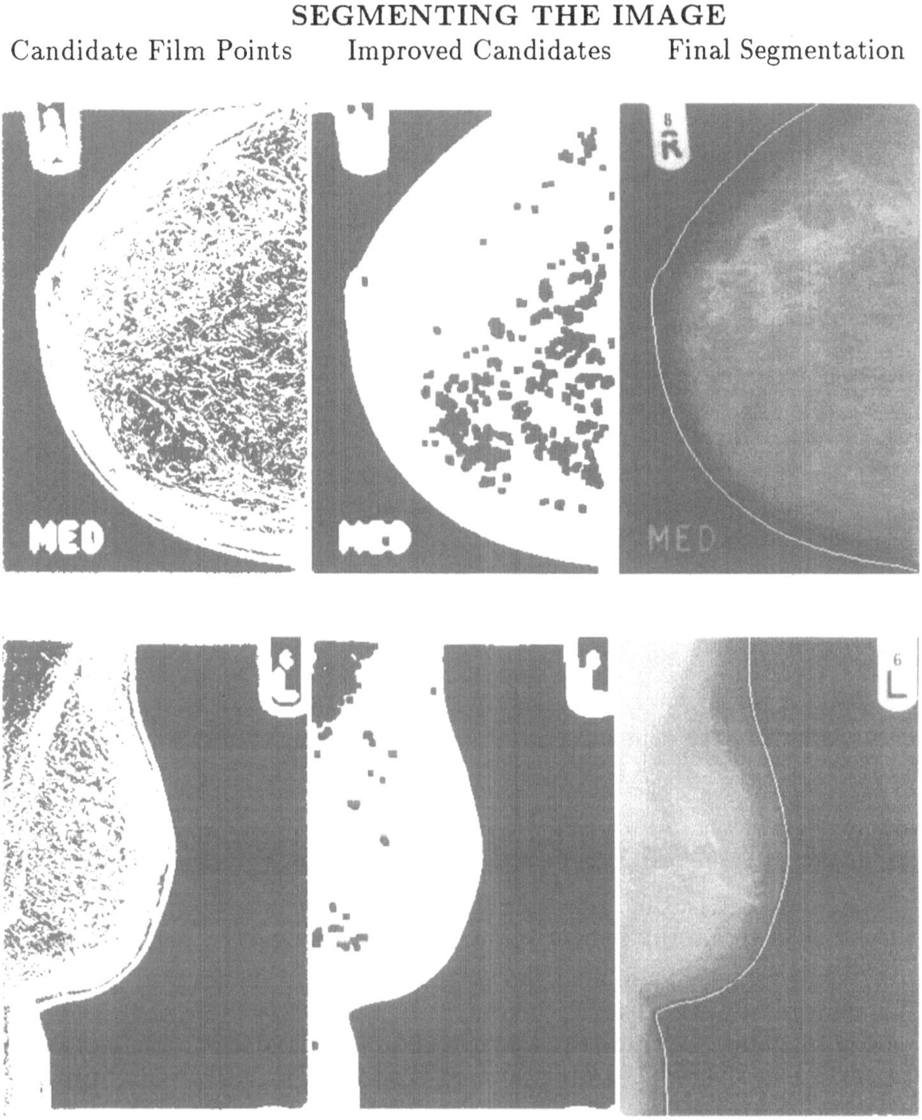

SEGMENTING THE IMAGE

Candidate Film Points   Improved Candidates   Final Segmentation

Figure 3.10. The left-hand pictures show in black the candidate pixels for being on-film. The candidates are selected on the basis of a low spatial gradient in the film density values. The middle picture shows the result of a morphological closing operation (dilation and then erosion) which merges together all the areas within the breast area by using a large mask. Most of the isolated candidate pixels disappear leaving only a few connected regions of candidate pixels, and only one of any real size - the film area. The right pictures shows the image with the breast/film boundary marked in white along with the original mammogram. The top example is of a cranio-caudal mammogram, and the bottom is a medio-lateral oblique. The algorithm is robust, having been tested on many images and being devised on simple, but well-founded principles.

BOX 3.5: Computing scatter

(1) Construct scatter weighting mask:
    (a) Determine the relative scatter reaching the central pixel and coming
        from a cylinder of thickness dr at a distance of r when a grid is not used
        and the breast thickness is H using the equations on Page 64.
    (b) Determine the relative scatter from each "tube" within the cylinder
        using the equations on Page 66.
    (c) Use the grid transmission formula to adapt the relative scatter to be
        as if a grid were used, Page 67.
    (d) Integrate the relative scatter at each location to construct a weighting
        mask w where the value at each pixel is directly proportional to the
        percentage of the total scatter coming from the column of tissue
        above that pixel and reaching the central pixel.

(2) Derive the scatter function s which maps from the convolution sum of
the energies $(E_{pse}^{imp} * w)$ to the scatter component E_s^{imp} using the approach
on Page 70.

(3) Convolve the energy imparted image E_{pse}^{imp} with the weighting mask w
and then apply the scatter function s to determine the scatter component
E_s^{imp}.

(4) Subtract the scatter from the total energy to obtain the energy imparted
due to primary and extra-focal: $E_{pe}^{imp}(x,y) = E_{pse}^{imp}(x,y) - E_s^{imp}(x,y)$

3.7. Summary and Results: Computing scatter

The scatter estimation algorithm is summarised in Box 3.5. Figure 3.11
shows examples of the scatter component computed for two mammograms.
As expected, the component is lowest towards the chest wall where scatter only reaches the image from one side whilst retaining a full thickness
of breast tissue. Towards the breast edge the component rises because although there is less scattering material there is also less attenuating material. The scatter model has been applied with success to hundreds of images.
It is difficult to verify the modelling but from practical results we've seen
that the values for scatter compare favourably with those expected, for
example the average scatter-to-primary computed over the breast area is
always very similar to the value expected from the work of Carlsson et al.
[32] (compare Table 3.1 to Figure 3.12).

    In later chapters, the results of removal of the scatter component for
image enhancement are shown (Figures 7.9 and 7.8) and we verify the
modelling by computing values of h_{int}. However, we first have to deal with
extra-focal radiation and that is the subject of the next chapter.

EXAMPLES OF SCATTER

Original Image   Energy Image   Scatter Component

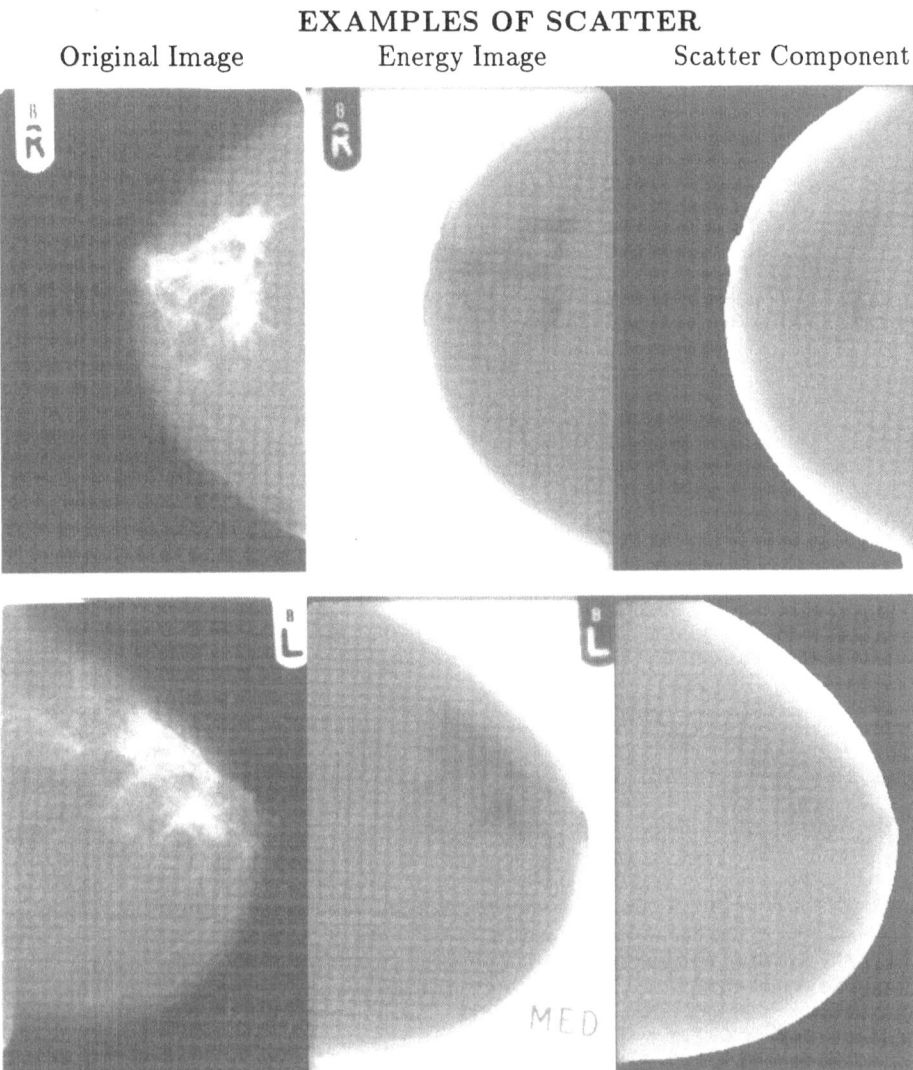

Figure 3.11. The images on the left represent original mammograms. The images in the middle show the energy imparted to the intensifying screen, and the images on the right show the scatter components of that energy, computed using our model. The scatter component rises near the breast edge due to the breast thickness reducing so that even though there is less scattering tissue there is also very little attenuation. The film area has been made artificially dark. Figure 7.9 shows results from removing the effects of scatter on mammographic images.

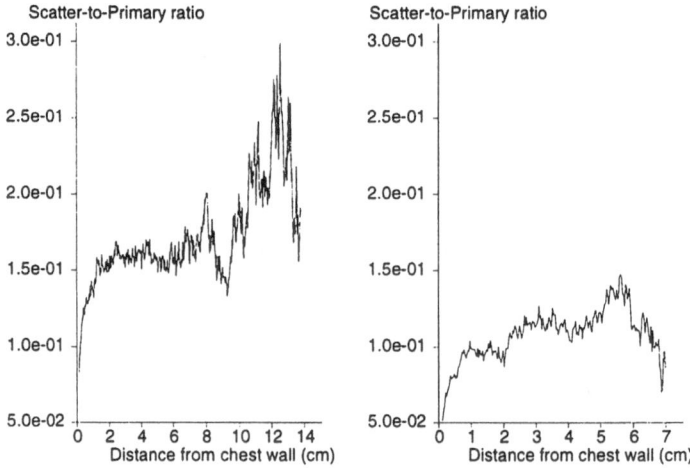

Figure 3.12.   These graphs show the scatter-to-primary ratio from the chest wall out to the nipple. The breast on the left is rather large with a compressed thickness of 7.6cm which suggests an expected average scatter-to-primary ratio of about 0.15 from the work of Carlsson et al.[32] if the breast is composed of half fat, half interesting tissue. The average ratio using our model of scatter on this particular mammogram is 0.17. On the right the breast is much smaller with a compressed thickness of 4.4cm. From Carlsson's data one would expect an average scatter-to-primary-ratio of about 0.10. In both cases, the scatter component drops off near the chest wall due to scatter only coming from one side.

CHAPTER 4

A MODEL OF EXTRA-FOCAL RADIATION

4.1. Introduction

Recall from Chapter 2 that the energy imparted to the intensifying screen has primary, scatter and extra-focal components:

$$E_{pse}^{imp} = E_p^{imp} + E_s^{imp} + E_e^{imp}$$

In order to generate h_{int} we need to find the primary component:

$$E_p^{imp} = E_{pse}^{imp} - E_s^{imp} - E_e^{imp}$$

Chapter 2 explained how we compute E_{pse}^{imp} and Chapter 3 explained how we can estimate the scatter component E_s^{imp}. In this chapter we show how to model and estimate the extra-focal component E_e^{imp}.

Figure 4.1 is a schematic diagram illustrating some of the concepts that we discuss in this chapter. Most of the x-ray photons that help create the mammogram leave the x-ray tube through the focal spot but a significant number leave the x-ray tube via other points of the x-ray tube; these photons constitute what is termed extra-focal radiation [50, 156]. The main effect of extra-focal radiation is to cause exposure of parts of the body which have been excluded by the collimation but it can also impart a significant amount of energy to the intensifying screen especially near the breast edge since the breast curves allowing easy access to the screen to x-ray photons arriving at low angles. It has been reported that up to 15% of the total radiation is extra-focal [13, 27]. Although the anti-scatter grid will remove much of the extra-focal radiation some of it will still reach the film-screen and, furthermore, we need an accurate model of extra-focal for our work in Chapter 10 when we consider mammograms performed without the anti-scatter grid.

Our model assumes that extra-focal radiation is travelling in random directions much the same as light from the sun on a cloudy day and is arriving at a point on the intensifying screen from all directions equally. We assume that we know the thickness and the composition of the breast along some curve C so that we are able to estimate the expected primary and scatter components along C. We know the total energy imparted so that

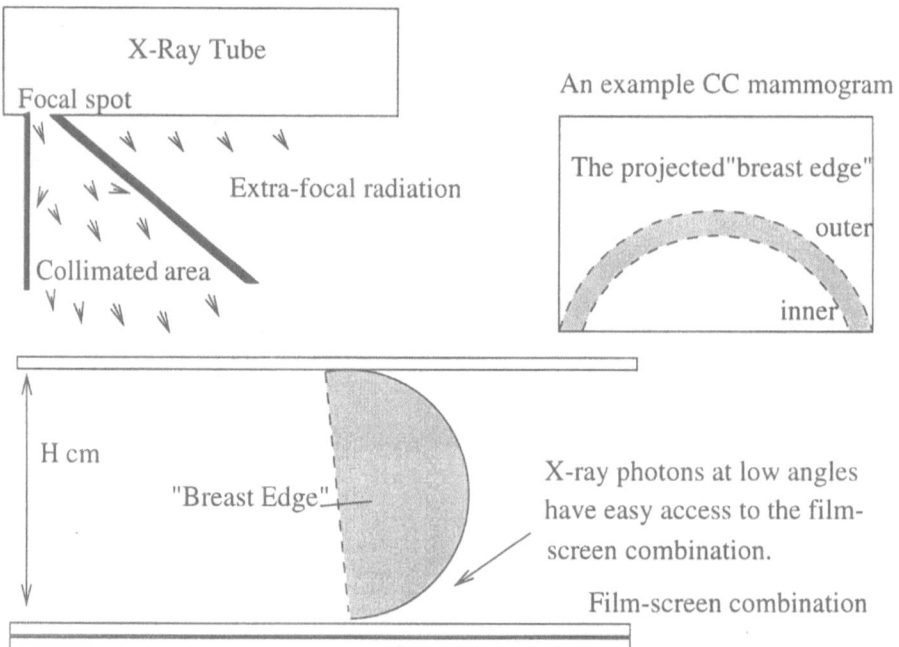

Figure 4.1. Most x-ray radiation comes from the focal spot. However, up to 15% of the total radiation has been reported as being extra-focal. Some of this is scattered so that it reaches the film-screen and contributes to the final image. Since the breast edge is curved, photons arriving at low angles have easy access to the film-screen and thus have a significant impact on the final image. Our model to compute extra-focal uses the shape and size of the breast edge. We define the breast edge to be that volume of the breast that is fat and is where the breast thickness descends from H towards zero. On a mammogram this area can be depicted by an inner and outer curve as shown in the top-right of this figure.

we can find the extra-focal component along C by straight subtraction:

$$E_e^{imp} = E_{pse}^{imp} - E_s^{imp} - E_p^{imp}$$

We then use our model of extra-focal radiation to extrapolate this value over the entire image.

The curve C that we use is the "inner projected breast edge": this is the breast tissue around the edge of the compressed breast which is fat and which is where the breast starts to curve, Figure 4.1 shows this pictorially. Chapter 5 discusses the breast edge in depth and develops a technique to determine the extent (the inner and outer curves in Figure 4.1) of the projected breast edge and we use the inner curve as our curve C. We model the breast edge as consisting entirely of fat and being semi-circular. Using this assumption, we can compute the thickness of tissue between any point and where the extra-focal is perceived to be coming from and then use this to adjust the extra-focal estimate accordingly.

When proposing any image processing routine, care must be taken not to create any artifacts, or remove any important signs. One sign to be especially aware of while dealing with the breast edge is skin thickening (a possible sign of cancer). This presents as a white edge to the breast image with an apparently fatty area inside, exactly what would be seen if the extra-focal or scatter component were over-estimated at the edge. It is therefore critical that the breast edge and extra-focal radiation are treated carefully.

The chapter starts with a summary of Lam and Chan's work [156] on scattered and extra-focal radiation. We use the results of that work to support our modelling. We then explain more fully our model of extra-focal radiation and our model of the breast edge. Our model requires that the extra-focal component be known along the curve C and we explain how we estimate that before showing results. An initial, simpler, model of extra-focal radiation, also proposed by us, can be found in [114, 116].

4.2. The work of Lam and Chan

Lam and Chan [156] published a paper about the improvement in quality of a mammogram which can be obtained when a balloon full of water is placed around the edge of a 4.5cm thick breast phantom. They concluded that one reason for this was the reduction of "scattered radiation"; they implicitly include extra-focal in their definition of scatter. The breast phantom had uniform thickness up to 8.5cm from the chest-wall. The left graph in Figure 4.2 shows the scatter-to-primary ratio found by Lam and Chan without an anti-scatter grid when the balloon was not used. The decrease at the "chest wall" is due to scattered radiation only coming from one side. The increase at the edge of the breast is due to breast edge effects and extra-focal radiation. The ratio dips close to the edge due to the breast phantom thickness decreasing rapidly and the consequent rise in the primary component, rather than the scatter component reducing. The right graph shows the relative scatter component calculated from the values reported by Lam and Chan. Notice that the scatter component (as defined by Lam and Chan) rises rapidly near the breast phantom edge with the film. This is in spite of the fact that the scattered radiation from the breast phantom itself is only coming from one side. Extra-focal radiation and the breast phantom edge shape are obviously having a large effect.

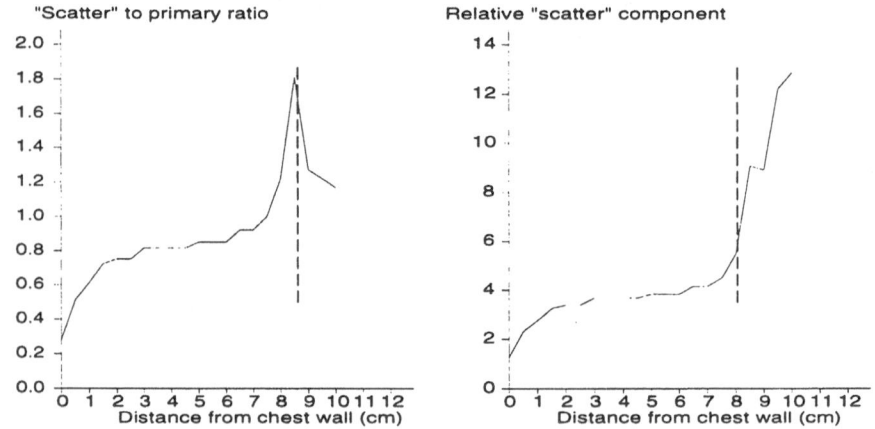

Figure 4.2.   These graphs show the change in the scatter-to-primary ratio out from the chest-wall towards the nipple. The left graph has values as reported by Lam and Chan [156]. Note that an anti-scatter grid was not used. The dashed lines show where the breast phantom thickness starts to decrease. See the text for comments and analysis of these graphs.

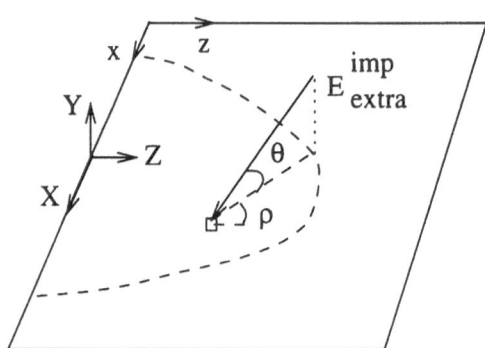

Figure 4.3.   We use (X, Y, Z) to be the 3D coordinates of a point, with the X axis along the chest wall, the Z axis perpendicular to the chest wall, and Y the vertical axis towards the x-ray source. We use (x, z) to be a point in the 2D image plane. When no breast is present we assume that the film-screen combination at (x, z) receives the same extra-focal radiation from all directions (θ, ρ). ρ is termed the azimuthal angle, θ the elevation angle and we use E_{extra}^{imp} to be the "extra-focal constant", that is, the energy incident on (x, z) from any direction.

4.3. A model of extra-focal radiation

Lacking a more precise account, we simply model extra-focal radiation as x-ray photons travelling in random directions, Figure 4.3 shows the coordinate system that we use. The energy imparted to the screen due to extra-focal can be assumed to be constant across the image if there were no breast present. With the breast present, the extra-focal radiation is attenuated by that quantity of breast tissue present along any particular path of travel. We aim to estimate that quantity of breast tissue using a model of the breast edge and to compute the constant E_{extra}^{imp} that would have been imparted had no breast been present. The equations in Box 4.1 give the mathematical details.

4.4. A model of the breast edge

We assume that the intensity of the extra-focal is sufficiently small that any significant tissue thickness will effectively annihilate it, so that the only tissue of importance is that around the breast edge - which we assume to consist entirely of fat. Thus, for extra-focal purposes we consider the breast to be entirely fat. We model the breast edge as being semi-circular and thus we can compute the thickness of fat from any point along any direction, Box 4.2 provides the details. Using those thicknesses we can now rewrite the basic extra-focal radiation equations in Box 4.1, as shown in Box 4.3.

We note that at the edge of the breast the amount of scatter produced in the breast and travelling towards the film-screen is reduced but this scatter has to pass through less tissue to reach the screen. This is taken into account by our estimation.

4.5. Estimating the extra-focal constant

In order to compute the extra-focal signal at each point we need to estimate the constant E_{extra}^{imp}. We assume we know where the projected breast edge is and since we assume it is all fat we know where there is a curve which has $h_{int} = 0$ and $h_{fat} = H$ (the inner curve in Figure 4.1). Thus we can estimate the primary and scatter components along the curve and by subtracting those values away from the total energy we can find the extra-focal component along the curve. Knowing just one value for the extra-focal allows us to compute the constant E_{extra}^{imp}, the mathematical details are in Box 4.4.

BOX 4.1: The basic extra-focal radiation equations

At each pixel (x, z), let θ be the incident elevation angle of the extra-focal radiation, let ρ be the azimuthal angle and let E_{extra}^{imp} be the (spatially constant) extra-focal energy that would be imparted if there was no grid or breast present from any one direction so that the energy imparted when a grid is used can be approximated by: $\forall \theta : 0 - \pi, \rho : 0 - 2\pi E_e^{imp}(x, z, \theta, \rho) = E_{extra}^{imp} T(\theta, \rho)$, where T is the transmission through the anti-scatter grid as shown in Figure 3.3, and we are assuming that the screen absorbs all the photons reaching it, regardless of angle. To simplify the analysis we deal with a monoenergetic case with photon energy $\mathcal{E}$. The total extra-focal radiation imparted to the intensifying screen at any point when no object is present is given by:

$$E_e^{imp}(x, z) = \int_0^{2\pi} \int_0^{\pi} E_e^{imp}(x, z, \theta, \rho) d\theta d\rho = E_{extra}^{imp} \int_0^{2\pi} \int_0^{\pi} T(\theta, \rho) d\theta d\rho$$

Let $\mu h(x, z, \theta, \rho)$ be the attenuation due to the breast along the path to point (x, z) from angles θ, ρ:

$$\mu h(x, z, \theta, \rho) = h_{int}(x, z, \theta, \rho)\mu_{int}(\mathcal{E}) + h_{fat}(x, z, \theta, \rho)\mu_{fat}(\mathcal{E}),$$

with $\mathcal{E}$ the relevant photon energy. The energy imparted due to extra-focal radiation can be estimated using Beer's Law, ignoring scatter, for when the breast is present:

$$E_e^{imp}(x, z) = E_{extra}^{imp} \int_0^{2\pi} \int_0^{\pi} e^{-\mu h(x, z, \theta, \rho)} T(\theta, \rho) d\theta d\rho$$

To study the problem analytically, we need to simplify this equation. We do this by first assuming symmetry around the azimuthal angle ρ so that the problem becomes essentially one dimensional:

$$E_e^{imp}(x, z) = 2\pi E_{extra}^{imp} \int_0^{\pi} e^{-\mu h(x, z, \theta)} T(\theta) d\theta$$

We aim to estimate E_{extra}^{imp} and the attenuation along each ray using a suitable model of the breast and breast shape. We can reduce the problem further since $\frac{\pi}{2} < \theta < \pi$ represents the angles of extra-focal radiation coming from the chest wall where we have a full thickness of breast and body, so we can assume that contribution is minimal. Furthermore, the most important part of the breast for extra-focal radiation is the breast edge and we can consider that to be just fat, so that the equation can be further simplified:

$$E_e^{imp}(x, z) = 2\pi E_{extra}^{imp} \int_0^{\frac{\pi}{2}} e^{-\mu_{fat} h_{fat}(x, z, \theta)} T(\theta) d\theta \qquad (4.1)$$

Box 4.2 shows how to compute $h_{fat}(x, z, \theta)$.

BOX 4.2: The breast edge equations: semi-circle model

Using the coordinate system of Figure 4.3 we consider the shape of the breast edge to be semi-circular. With no loss of generality save for assumptions of rotational symmetry about the azimuth, we consider the 1D case where $X = 0$ and Z is perpendicular to the chest-wall so that the breast edge can be described by: $Y(Z_0) = a \pm \sqrt{(a^2 - Z_0^2)}$, where $a = \frac{H}{2}$ and Z_0 is the Z-coordinate relative to the edge of the inner breast edge, i.e. $Z_0 = Z - Z_{edge}$. Figure 4.4 shows the two cases for when we are inside the breast. The case **A1** shows the ray travelling through both breast and breast edge, for angles of $0 < \theta < \theta_H$ where $\theta_H = \tan^{-1} \frac{H}{|Z_0|}$ the extra-focal rays must travel through a thickness of breast tissue and a thickness of breast edge tissue so that:

$$h_{fat}(\theta) = \frac{Z_0}{\cos \theta} + \frac{Z_{intersect}}{\cos \theta}$$

and $Z_{intersect}$ is the intersection of the ray and the breast edge which occurs at:

$$Z_{intersect} = \frac{m(a - c) \pm (m^2 a^2 - c^2 + 2ac)^{0.5}}{(1 + m^2)}$$

where $m = \tan \theta$ and $c = Z_0 \tan \theta$. For the points which satisfy case **A2**, some of the extra-focal rays will come through tissue which is within the uniform breast thickness and some through the breast edge area. These rays are from θ_H to $\frac{\pi}{2}$ and the thickness of the breast is simply: $h_{fat}(\theta) = \frac{H}{\sin \theta}$ Outside the $h_{int} = 0$ line, there are angles that have a free line-of-sight to the pixel (x, z), see case **B1** in Figure 4.4. In fact, these angles are from 0 to θ_{limit} where θ_{limit} is the angle of the tangent to the breast curve which passes through the pixel. The tangent to the bottom half of the breast which passes through the point $(Z_0, 0)$ that is required passes through the point:

$$Z_{tangent} = \frac{2a^2 Z_0}{Z_0^2 + a^2}$$

and thus:

$$\theta_{limit} = \tan^{-1} \frac{Z_{tangent}}{(a^2 - Z_{tangent}^2)^{0.5}}$$

So, that for $0 < \theta < \theta_{limit} : h_{fat}(\theta) = 0$. Case **B2** in Figure 4.4 reveals that for some of the angles of interest the x-ray path is purely through the breast edge. We now need the two intersection points of the ray with the breast edge semi-circle, i.e. $(Z_{intersect\ 1}, Y_{intersect\ 1})$ and $(Z_{intersect\ 2}, Y_{intersect\ 2})$. The two Z coordinates are given by:

$$Z_{intersect} = \frac{m(a - c) \pm (m^2 a^2 - c^2 + 2ac)^{0.5}}{(1 + m^2)}$$

with $m = \tan \theta$, $a = \frac{H}{2}$ and $c = -\tan \theta Z_0$. And thus:

$$h_{fat}(\theta) = ((Z_{intersect\ 1} - Z_{intersect\ 2})^2 + (Y_{intersect\ 1} - Y_{intersect\ 2})^2)^{\frac{1}{2}}$$

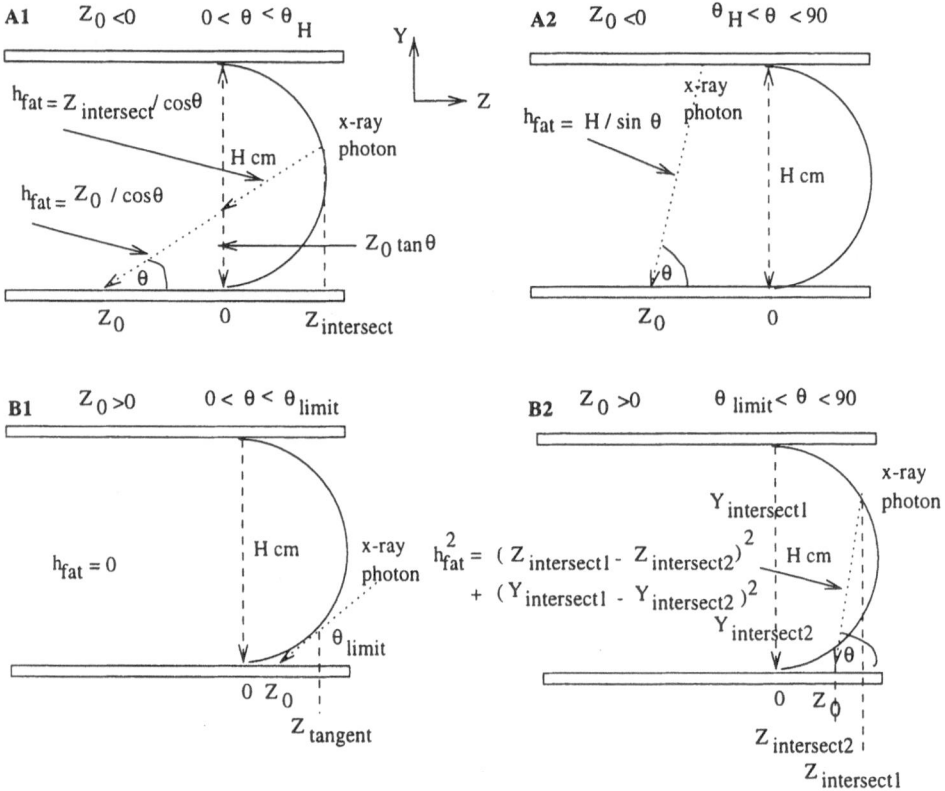

Figure 4.4. This shows the length of breast tissue that extra-focal x-rays have to pass through to reach a point well inside the breast (top pictures) and a point within the breast edge (bottom pictures). See Box 4.2 for a definition of θ_H and θ_{limit}. In the top picture there are two cases: on the left the x-ray needs to travel through the breast and the breast edge, and on the right the x-ray needs to travel through just the breast. In the bottom picture, there are also two cases: on the left we show how some extra-focal is able to reach the film-screen directly with no attenuation and on the right we show the x-rays passing through some proportion of the breast edge. The thicknesses of tissue are marked onto the diagrams. Only the extra-focal coming through thin amounts of breast tissue will reach the film-screen combination and this will therefore be at low angles where the breast is mostly fatty thus we model the breast as fat for the purposes of extra-focal radiation.

BOX 4.3: Advanced extra-focal radiation equation

Using Equation 4.1 and then substituting in the breast edge equations from Box 4.2 allows us to write a more specific equation for the extra-focal component at each pixel:

$$E_e^{imp}(x,z) = 2\pi E_{extra}^{imp} \int_0^{\frac{\pi}{2}} e^{-\mu_{fat}h_{fat}(x,z,\theta)}T(\theta)d\theta$$

$$= 2\pi E_{extra}^{imp} \left(\int_0^{\theta_{limit}} T(\theta)d\theta + \int_{\theta_{limit}}^{\frac{\pi}{2}} e^{-\mu_{fat}h_{fat}(x,z,\theta)}T(\theta)d\theta \right)$$

$$(4.2)$$

where θ_{limit} is the angle of the tangent to the breast edge curve and for cases **A1** and **A2**, $\theta_{limit} = 0$.

BOX 4.4: Determining the extra-focal constant E_{extra}^{imp}

Let the curve with $h_{int} = 0$ and $h_{fat} = H$ be $C_{h_{int}=0}$. Since we know where that curve is from the breast edge we have an estimate of the extra-focal component there:

$$\forall (x,z) \in C_{h_{int}=0} \bullet E_e^{imp}(x,z) = E_{pse}^{imp}(x,z) - E_s^{imp}(x,z) - E_p^{imp}(x,z)$$

The scatter estimate comes from Chapter 3, E_{pse}^{imp} comes from the image and E_p^{imp} comes from knowing that $h_{int} = 0$ and $h_{fat} = H$. We use the average of E_e^{imp} along the $C_{h_{int}=0}$ curve and Equation 4.2 with $\theta_{limit} = 0$ to determine the constant:

$$E_{extra}^{imp} = \frac{\overline{E_e^{imp}(C_{h_{int}=0})}}{2\pi \int_0^{\frac{\pi}{2}} e^{-\mu_{fat}h_{fat}(x,z,\theta)}T(\theta)d\theta} \qquad (4.3)$$

BOX 4.5: Computing extra-focal

(1) Determine the projected breast edge and thus the $h_{int} = 0$ curve using the technique described in Chapter 5, this gives the breast edge radius a.

(2) Determine the extra-focal constant E_{extra}^{imp} using the inner projected breast edge curve and Equation 4.3.

(3) Compute the extra-focal at each pixel using the constant, the breast edge and Equation 4.2 and the equations in Box 4.2.

(4) Check the computation by integrating the extra-focal constant over π and dividing by the incident radiation to give the percentage of the amount of extra-focal radiation to focal radiation.

4.6. Summary and Results: Computing extra-focal

Box 4.5 summarises the steps involved in computing the extra-focal component and how to estimate the percentage of the total radiation that is extra-focal. Figure 4.5 shows two examples of the extra-focal component computed using our model. They show that, as expected, the extra-focal radiation is high at the breast edge but falls rapidly inside the breast falling to zero if the breast is large enough. Figures 4.6 and 4.7 show profiles that may be compared with those reported by Lam and Chan.

Incorporating all the assumptions above, the percentages that we have computed indicate that extra-focal radiation is of the order of 6-10% of the total radiation. This is on the low side of the estimate made in [13, 27] which state that extra-focal can make up to 15% of the total radiation, but since it is unclear what systems they were discussing and how they measured extra-focal we conclude that 6-10% is reasonable. We now go on to show how we compute breast thickness and, as a consequence, the projected breast edge.

EXAMPLES OF EXTRA-FOCAL RADIATION

Original image   Energy imparted   Extra-focal component

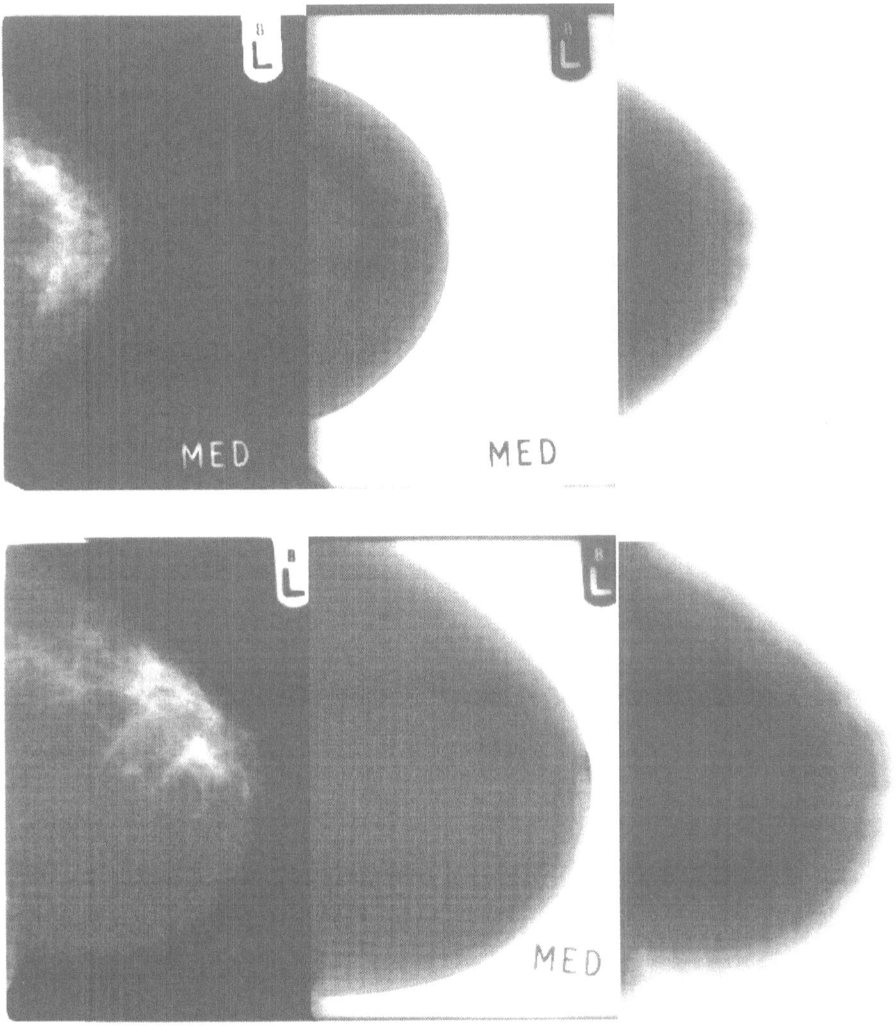

Figure 4.5.   These images show examples of extra-focal radiation computed using our model. The images on the left are the original mammograms, in the middle are the energies imparted to the intensifying screen and on the right are the extra-focal components. The brightness is proportional to energy. Note that the bottom example shows that extra-focal has no effect near the chest wall for such a large breast. The results of our model compare favourably with published results. In particular, the penetration of the extra-focal into the breast appears accurate as does the total extra-focal radiation compared to focal-radiation.

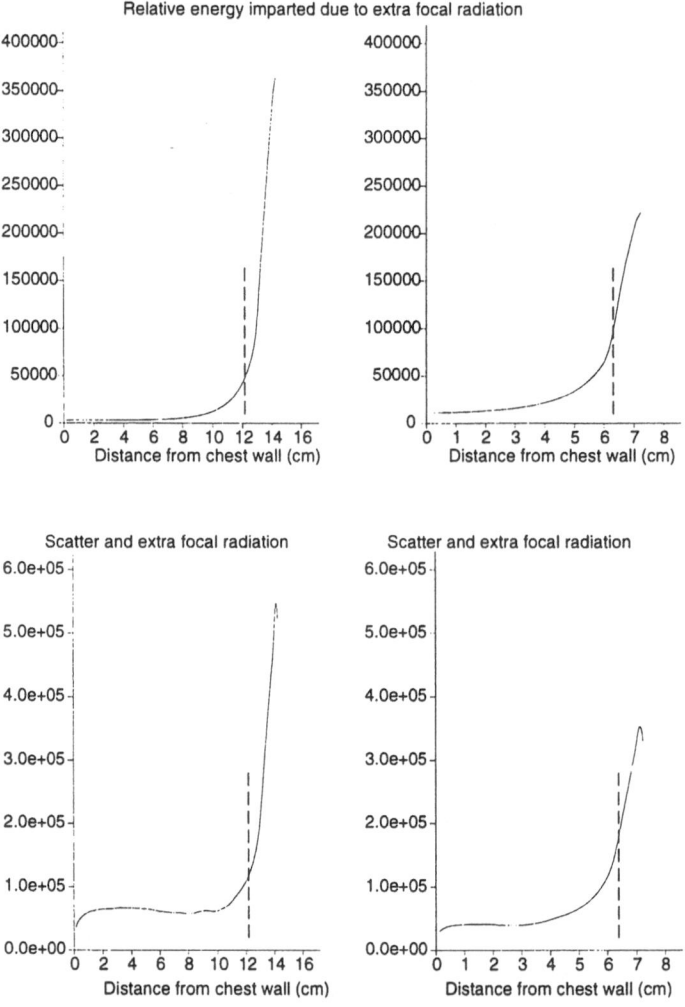

Figure 4.6.   The top profiles show the variation of extra-focal radiation from the chest wall out towards the nipple and the bottom ones the variation of scatter plus extra-focal. The left profiles are from a breast with consistent breast thickness up to 12cm from the chest-wall, and on the right up to 6.5cm. The difference in the magnitude between left and right reflect that the left profiles are from a much thicker and larger breast. Note the rapid fall-off of the extra-focal as the breast tissue begins to attenuate it and the similar penetration to that reported by Lam and Chan [156] and shown in Figure 4.2. The profiles on the right, from the smaller breast are particularly comparable showing similar penetration and rise of extra-focal towards the breast edge. Note the decrease near the chest wall of the scatter and extra-focal as scatter drops off due to it only coming from one side.

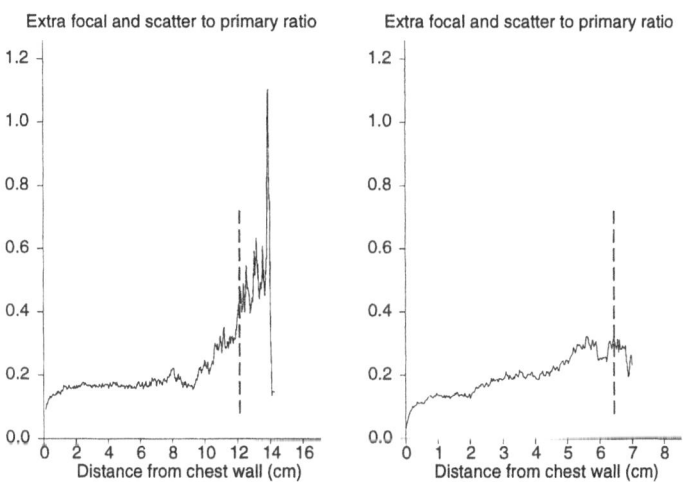

Figure 4.7. This shows the combined scatter and extra-focal to primary ratio for two breasts. The left breast has constant thickness to 12cm, and on the right up to 6.5cm. The thickness of the left breast is 7cm and the right breast is 4.7cm. The graphs are comparable to Figure 4.2 except these ones are for real mammograms when a grid has been used.

CHAPTER 5

ESTIMATING THE THICKNESS OF A COMPRESSED BREAST

5.1. Introduction

Many recent mammography systems have built-in analogue or digital thickness meters but their accuracy and precision are currently wanting [29]. In clinical practice, most existing systems do not have such indicators. Burch and Law [29] have reported putting lead markers on the top compression plate and then using the magnification of the separation between these markers to estimate breast thickness, a technique replicated by Smith et al. [225]. However, although their results appear promising, with an average accuracy of the order of 2mm or so, and with a maximum error of 4.9mm, analysis of the projective equations reveals that the method is far from stable: a change in the projected measure of just 1mm produces a change in breast thickness estimate of at least 2.4mm. Furthermore, in many cases, the lead markers were reported to be not visible on the film due to scatter and sometimes were projected onto other lead markers or the breast. Moreover, this technique does not allow for retrospective estimation of breast thicknesses which is crucial for estimating the accumulated radiation dose.

In this chapter we propose a robust and accurate method for estimating the compressed breast thickness from a mammogram using image processing and modelling techniques [120]. The estimation is based upon the existence of the "breast edge", a fatty area around each breast where the breast thickness steadily reduces to zero. Determining that area using image processing provides us with enough data to estimate the breast thickness when calibration data such as the tube voltage and exposure time are known. The proposed technique does not involve adding markers and can be applied to mammograms taken previously.

The chapter starts by explaining exactly what we mean by the breast edge, and how we can use it to estimate breast thickness. We then rephrase these explanations in terms of h_{int}. The crucial step in estimating the breast thickness is to determine a smooth curve in the breast image where the breast tissue is all fat. To do this requires a measure of roughness and we explain the motivation for our choice of a fractal measure. Our algorithm is outlined with implementation details before we show a number of typical results which demonstrate that our method is at least as accurate as Burch

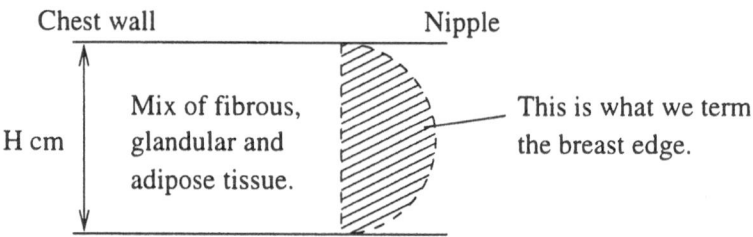

Figure 5.1.   We model the breast as having constant thickness up to the start of the so-called breast edge. At this point the breast thickness rapidly decreases to zero. We model the breast edge as being homogeneous and to consist mostly of fat.

and Law's. The projected breast edge determined by our technique is crucial to the estimation of extra-focal radiation described in Chapter 4.

5.2. What is the breast edge?

During mammography, the breast is compressed between two supposedly parallel flat plates. The compression causes the breast to spread out, so that over most of the plate the breast is of equal thickness. However, towards the edge of the breast the breast bulges like a balloon and there is a not a straight vertical edge; Figure 5.1 shows this schematically. This bulge is what we term the breast edge.

The breast tissue is enveloped in two layers of fibrous tissue, the deep layer overlying the muscle, and the very thin superficial layer beneath the skin. The superficial layer is separated from the skin by 0.5 to 2.5cm of subcutaneous fat or areolar tissue. Joining the layers to the skin are fine fibrous ligaments (Cooper's ligaments). From this, it is reasonable to assume that what we have called the breast edge consists entirely of fat, though we recognise that in localized regions, particularly near the nipple and near the ligaments, this will not be strictly true.

Figure 5.2 shows a schematic of the breast for a cranio-caudal view mammogram. The arc denoted by the letter E lies right on the edge of the breast as seen from the x-ray source, that is, an x-ray from the source tangentially touches the breast before reaching E. There is very little attenuation of the x-ray beam anywhere along E. Along the arc denoted by the letter D, there is a greater thickness of tissue than at E, but still relatively little attenuation, since this is the breast edge and most of the breast tissue is fat. Along the arc C, there is H cm of fat so that the x-ray attenuation

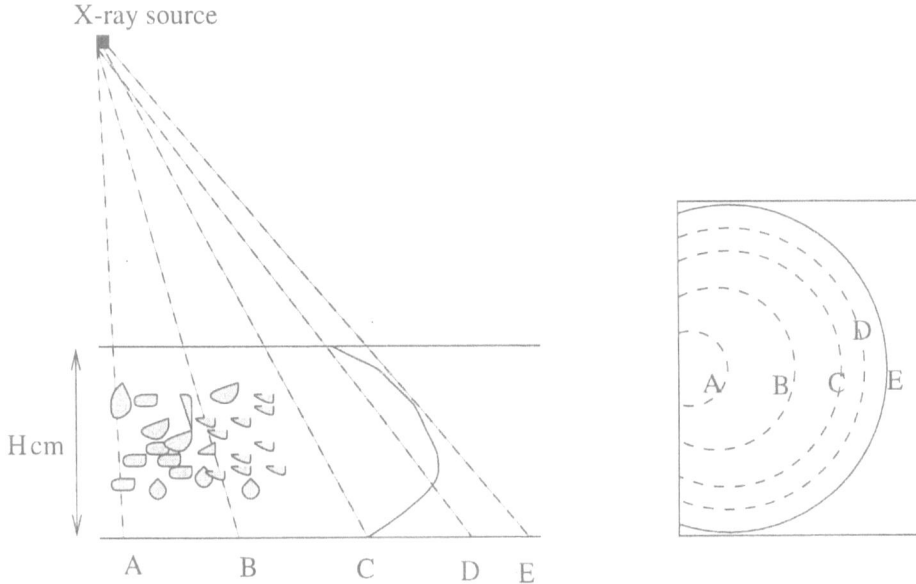

Figure 5.2.   This is a schematic of a cranio-caudal mammogram. Note that the picture is not to scale. The left picture shows the breast, while the right picture is the mammogram. The shaded areas are meant to represent volumes of interesting tissue. The picture shows the reduction in x-ray attenuation and thickness of breast tissue as the nipple is approached. See the text for a full explanation.

is quite large but it is still uniform along the arc. This all changes along arcs A and B, where there is a heterogeneous mixture of tissues. The x-ray attenuation along these arcs can vary from being due to H cm of fat to almost H cm of interesting tissue.

Our method of determining breast thickness H is based-upon delimiting the projected breast edge from the interior of the breast. That is, we seek to determine the arcs C and E in Figure 5.2. Recall that in Chapter 3 we gave a method to segment the breast from the background and hence determine the smooth arc E on the basis of the film densities. If we then mark all the pixels which are slightly brighter than those on E we get another smooth curve, since we are still in the homogeneous breast edge. This may be arc D. Eventually, we reach arc C, which is still smooth, since it is just within the homogeneous breast edge region. If we continue to mark pixels which are slightly less dark, we start to mark pixels within the interior of the breast. These could be anywhere and numerous since the interior is a heterogeneous mix of tissues. Thus we see that the arc that delimits the interior of the breast (arc C) is the extremum of the smooth iso-intensity curves. From our model, it is also clear that the breast tissue between arc C and the x-ray source comprises H cm of fat. Thus, if we can find C, and if we have a good model of the mammographic imaging process, we can use the pixel values along C to estimate the amount of fat which must have been between the pixels along C and the x-ray source and thus we have the breast thickness H.

5.3. Using the h_{int} representation to locate the breast edge

There are two potential approaches to finding the curve which delimits the breast interior and then estimating the breast thickness. One is to find the smooth curve by using the original pixels values which are produced by the digitiser. The imaging process is then simulated using different breast thicknesses until the predicted pixel value matches that which we find on the smooth curve. The second approach, and the one we take, is to take a rough initial estimate of the breast thickness and then to generate the h_{int} representation that we introduced in Chapter 2. Analysis of the h_{int} representation enables us to determine how the estimate of the breast thickness should be changed. When the h_{int} values are generated using an accurate breast thickness, we find that within the projected breast edge there is so little attenuation that there cannot even be H cm of fat within that region. For these regions we set $h_{int} = 0$ and then determine what thickness of fat alone would give us the observed attenuation. Figure 5.3 shows some examples of the breast edges found by marking those pixels that have $h_{int} = 0$.

Since the compression plate typically slants by up to 0.5cm from the chest-wall out to the nipple we need to compensate the image for it in someway before we perform the h_{int} computation. The approach we take is to effectively add a wedge of fat to the breast by adjusting the mammographic image using monoenergetic modelling assumptions.

Our method of determining H is to start with an underestimate of the breast thickness and then to compute the h_{int} representation. We mark those pixels that have $h_{fat} = H, h_{int} = 0$ and compute a measure of how rough the curve that those pixels represent is (we explain how we do this in the next section). Initially, the h_{int} values will be too high and there will be no pixels with $h_{int} = 0$. As H increases, we start to detect more and more pixels with $h_{int} = 0$ and these pixels will represent a smooth curve. This continues until the internal breast region is reached at which point the roughness measure ought to rise dramatically to indicate a rougher curve. Performing the computation this way rather than just using the

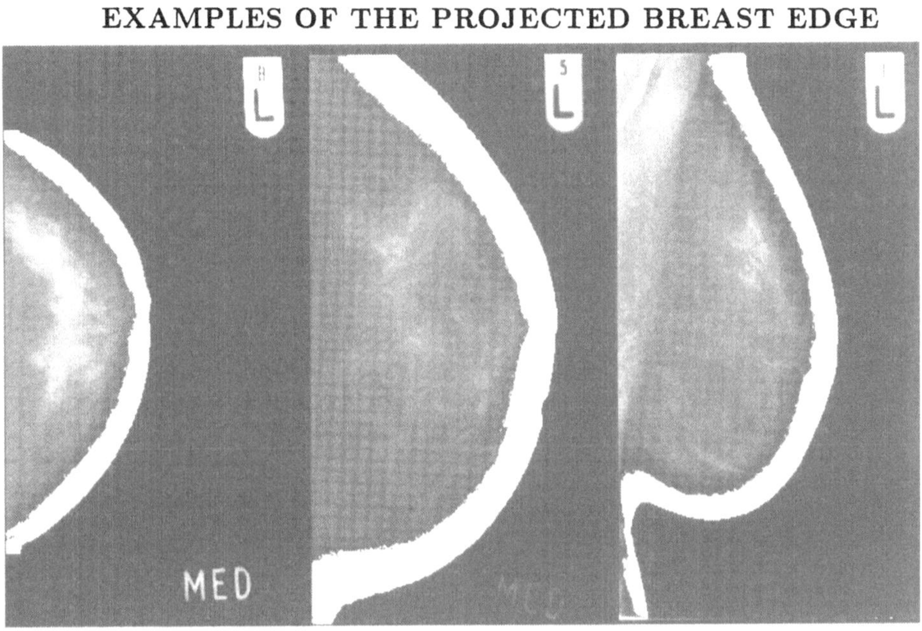

EXAMPLES OF THE PROJECTED BREAST EDGE

Figure 5.3. The bright white areas represent the so-called breast edge. This is where the breast starts to decrease from its constant thickness H and the attenuation is no longer enough even to be of H cm of fat. The inner edge of the projected breast edge region is mathematically quite smooth.

pixel values in the original image and looking for iso-intensity curves allows us to be more accurate since we can use H to predict scattered and extra-focal radiation. It also enables us to check that the algorithm is working properly using any of a number of useful metrics which can be computed using the h_{int} values. One example is that if we start with many points that have $h_{int} > H$ then the value of H is far too low and we should increase it dramatically rather than increase it in small steps. Another example is that if we find more that 20% of the breast as being within the projected breast edge, then we have increased H too far. Figure 5.4 shows pictorially how the computation progresses and Figure 5.5 shows real examples of the breast edge as H varies.

When skin thickening occurs in a breast, the edge of the breast becomes denser and this results in a higher x-ray attenuation around the edge. Potentially, this could be sensed as being a smooth $h_{int} = 0$ line for an erroneous breast thickness. However, since it would be a localized region of the breast edge it should not affect our finding of the interior breast region.

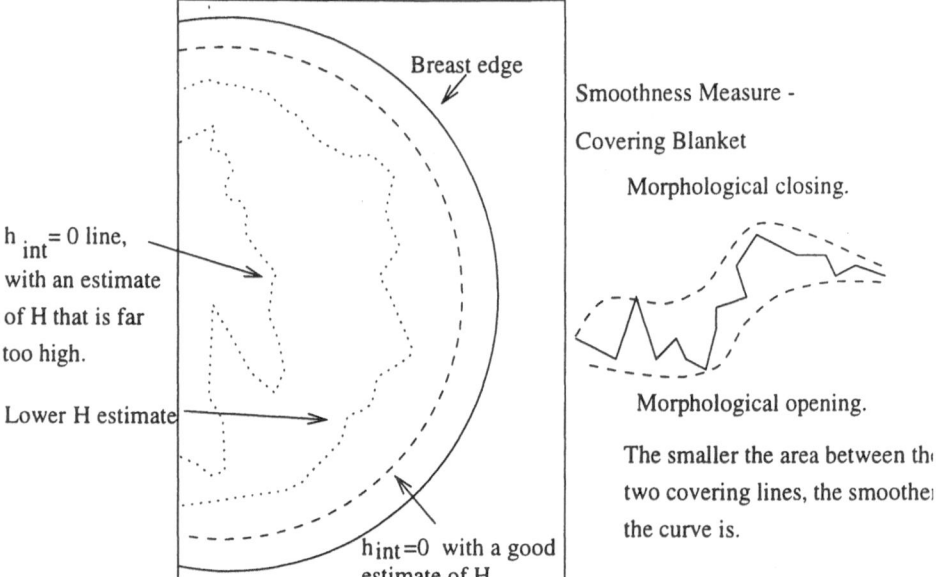

Figure 5.4.   One way of estimating the breast thickness is to determine what value of H gives a satisfactory $h_{int} = 0$ curve. This curve is meant to be around the edge of the breast where the breast thickness drops sharply away, and the breast consists mostly of fat. Consequently, we expect the $h_{int} = 0$ curve to be present, complete and smooth. At low values of H the values of h_{int} are too high, and there in no $h_{int} = 0$ curve. As H increases the curves appear and are smooth but then they become rough. We measure the roughness using the covering blanket concept which is shown on the right of this picture and described fully in the text.

5.4. An appropriate roughness measure

All that remains is to devise a roughness measure for the $h_{int} = 0$ curve that enables us to determine when that curve has reached the interior of the breast. As we start with an underestimate of H the roughness measure should initially be low and should then rise as the $h_{int} = 0$ curve becomes rougher. Figure 5.6 illustrates this.

There are several possibilities for such a roughness measure. One approach is to use a mathematical measure such as the average curvature, or variance in curvature, or an estimate of the Lipschitz dimension. Although these are nice in theory, they are complicated by the discrete nature of digital images.

A second approach is to use an estimate of a fractal characteristic of the curve. Xie and Brady [262] point out that a fractal curve has two parameters: fractal dimension and D-dimension, and show that for estimating

CHANGE IN THE BREAST EDGE WITH H

| 3.4cm | 5.4cm | 6.0cm | 6.4cm |

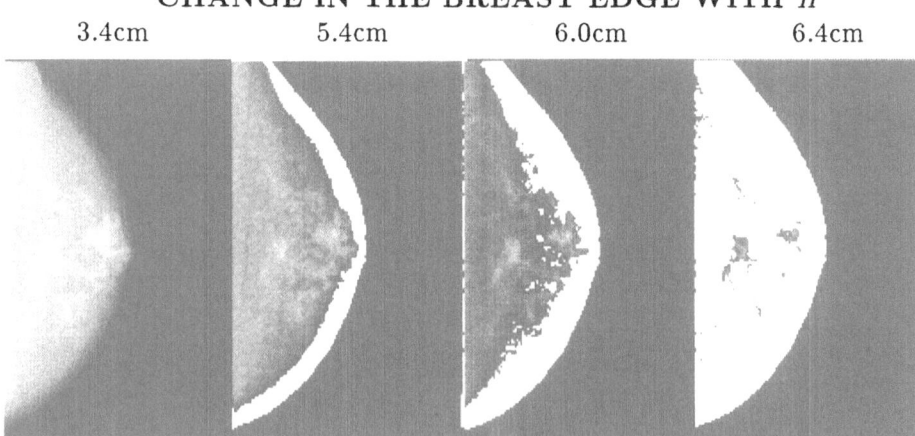

Figure 5.5. This shows images with luminance proportional to h_{int} except for the bright white breast edge which is where $h_{int} = 0$. The breast thicknesses tried are marked above each image. The first value, 3.4cm, is far too low - there is no breast edge; the second value, 5.4cm is just about right - there is a substantial breast edge and a smooth internal edge; the last two estimates are far too high - the projected breast edge has become ragged.

image textures the latter is more reliable, stable and gives better discrimination. Image texture is closely related to the concepts of roughness and smoothness so that this observation is directly relevant to our work. Xie and Brady also give an elegant technique to estimate the D-dimension: "the covering blanket" which is based upon morphological operations [101, 200]. To compute the measure, two further curves are created from the $h_{int} = 0$ curve: one from opening the $h_{int} = 0$ curve and one from closing it (see Figure 5.4). An opening operation creates a smaller curve which is smoother than the original, whilst a closing operation creates a larger curve which is smoother than the original. The area contained between the two curves is a measure of roughness: the larger the area the rougher the curve. We use as our morphological operator a 5 pixel by 5 pixel disk and we always perform the thickness estimation on 300 micron resolution images.

Although the area between the curves is related to roughness, it is also directly related to the total length of the curve, so we need to normalise the measure and make it dimensionless by dividing by the length of the curve. Note that the area is not related to any concept of radius of the curve so that that does not need to be accounted for. Taking all these considerations into account, we define:

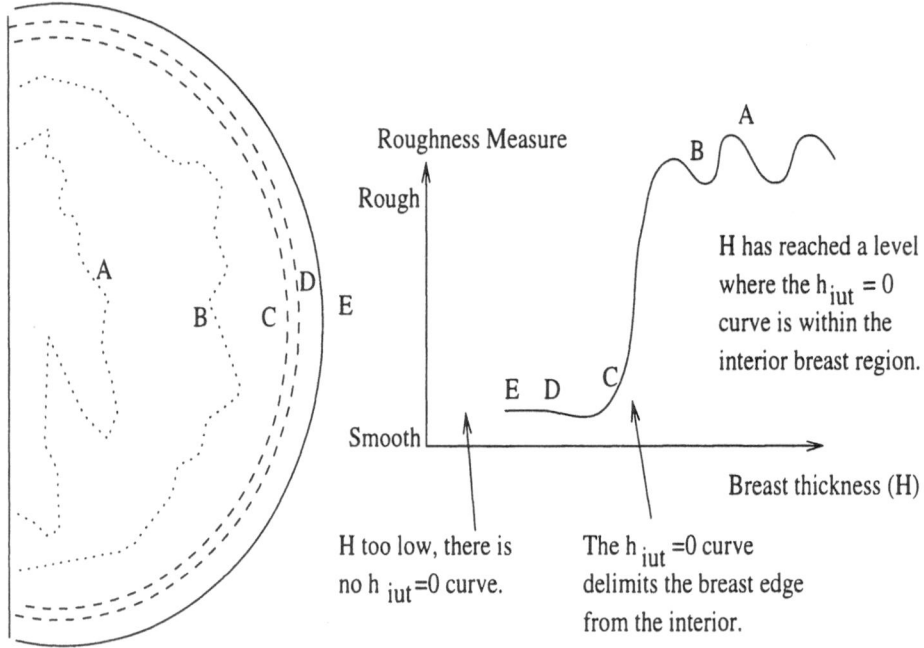

Figure 5.6.   We desire a roughness measure that reflects the roughness of a curve. As breast thickness increases we expect to see a large jump in the measure just after the breast thickness that we require. In this picture, the curves marked A-E would ideally have the roughness measures as shown on the right.

$$\text{Roughness} = \frac{\text{Number of pixels enclosed by closing and opening of } h_{int} = 0}{\text{Number of pixels on } h_{int} = 0 \text{ curve}}$$

$$(5.1)$$

When this measure increases above a threshold we stop increasing H. We use a value of 1.3 and have found this to be sufficient for every image that we have examined.

In our estimate of breast thickness, we detect the smooth curve which delimits the interior breast region. The presence of Cooper's ligaments in the image, which is quite unusual, would affect only a section of the curve and only slightly the overall roughness measure. The increased density of tissue around the nipple just means that the curve is not a semi-circle but a more irregular shape that is still smooth. Indeed, we intend to use the fact that the curve is less regular to detect the position of the nipple.

5.5. An initial estimate of breast thickness

There are several ways of forming an initial estimate of breast thickness from the calibration data and image. One exploits the fact that near the chest wall there is low scatter and the breast tends to be fatty so one can assume $h_{int} = 0, h_{fat} = H$. From the energy imparted we can estimate H. Another way is to assume that near the breast edge we have pure fat and some nominal, high scatter-to-primary ratio. To date, we have proceeded by estimating an initial value for the breast thickness using a film density that we know to be outside the breast and the calibration data; this always gives an underestimate of the actual breast thickness.

Bounds on the breast thickness can also be estimated. These can be used to check that the method is not trying infeasible breast thicknesses. The lower bound on H is related to the minimum attenuation apparent within the breast image. To achieve such low attenuation requires a certain minimum thickness of breast tissue. The minimum possible H occurs if the breast tissue has very low fat content so that $h_{int}=H$ (i.e. highly attenuating). An upper bound on H can be determined in exactly the same way except that we use the maximum attenuation and consider the breast to be nearly all fat.

5.6. Summary and Results: Estimating H

Box 5.1 summarises the algorithm to estimate the breast thickness H. We have observed and measured the projected breast edge on hundreds of different images from different sites from around the world. Figures 5.3 and 5.7 show typical breast edge extents. For both cranio-caudal and medio-lateral oblique mammograms the breast edge is consistently about 10% of the total area of the projected breast. This is one of a number of useful metrics which can be used to determine if the algorithms are working properly.

To test our estimate of breast thickness we performed a series of tests at the Breast Care Unit within the Churchill Hospital in Oxford. The mammography machine that was used was an IGE Senographe which has a foot-controlled compression device. A volunteer measured the breast thicknesses during mammography by hand near the chest-wall. She felt that her measurements were accurate for cranio-caudal images (within ±0.30cm) but far less accurate for medio-lateral oblique images (within ±0.50cm) since the position of the woman's arm on the machine severely hampers the measurement. Figure 5.8 shows two examples of the roughness measure and its variation with breast thickness H.

Breast thickness measurements were taken for cranio-caudal mammograms at assessment clinics at the Churchill Hospital in Oxford on three different occasions over a period of 6 months. A total of 32 cranio-caudal

---

BOX 5.1: Estimating compressed breast thickness

(1) Segment the breast part of the image as explained in Chapter 3, Page 70

(2) Find an underestimate of H

(3) Generate the approximate h_{int} values using simple approximations to scatter and extra-focal at the breast edge

(4) Find all the $h_{fat} = H, h_{int} = 0$ pixels and make them into a curve

(5) Compute the roughness of the curve using the covering blanket

(6) If the roughness is above a threshold:
$\qquad$ then decrease H and stop
$\qquad$ else increase H and go to (3)

The increase or decrease in H in step (6) is 0.1cm. We need to decrease H before we stop in order to get back to a smooth $h_{int} = 0$ curve.

---

mammograms with measurements were collected and digitised, the 32 were 16 pairs of left and right breasts. The women were aged from 51 to 65. The measured thicknesses ranged from 3.4 to 7.0cm with an average of 5.55cm. The average absolute difference between the left and right measured breast thicknesses was 0.39cm. Comparisons between measured and estimated thicknesses revealed an average absolute error of 0.22cm including a single exceptional error of 0.71cm. Burch and Law's average accuracy of 0.2cm appears to be the average relative accuracy rather than the average absolute error and so our technique compares favourably. There is no apparent relation between breast composition or breast thickness and the difference in estimated and measured breast thicknesses with the errors varying mostly between 0 and 5% with a maximum error of 10%.

Medio-lateral oblique mammograms were collected at a screening clinic. A total of 22 medio-lateral oblique mammograms were collected. The women were aged 51 to 71. The measured thicknesses ranged from 3.0 to 7.0cm with an average size of 5.09cm. The average absolute difference between the left and right breasts was 0.25cm. The average absolute error for medio-lateral images using our technique was much higher than for cranio-caudals at 0.44cm, but this almost certainly reflects the dubious nature of the thickness measurements for the medio-lateral oblique images rather than our technique. This is supported by the fact that the breast edges were again around 10% of the total breast area and that 90% of the estimates using

FURTHER EXAMPLES OF THE BREAST EDGE

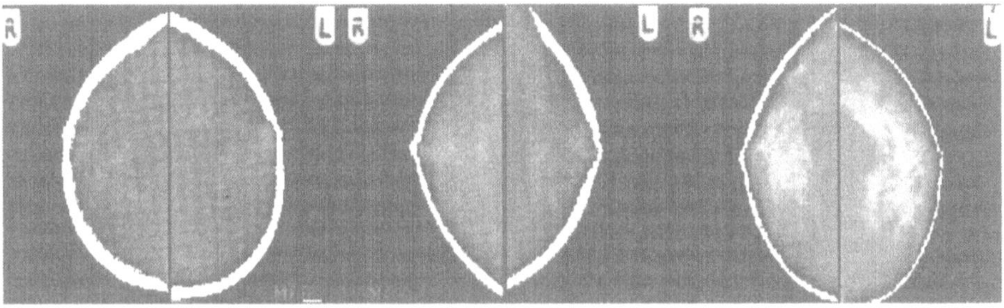

Figure 5.7. This picture shows further examples of breast edges, i.e. areas where $h_{int} < 0$, these are shown in bright white. These examples are from a different data-base to the images shown in figures (5.3) and (6.2) In these cases the breast edges are slightly curtailed since the digitiser used had a maximum density of 3.2, compared to 4.0 for the newer databases.

our technique were under-estimates suggesting a systematic problem such as consistent over-measurement.

We also estimated the breast thicknesses from mammograms for which we had little calibration data. In these cases we would typically have the tube voltage and mAs value but not our usual film-screen calibration (a 14 step wedge). Instead, we used the standard calibration data collected by the Breast Care Unit itself, film-screen gradient and speed, to predict how our step wedge would appear. Over a set of such uncalibrated cranio-caudal mammograms we found an average close to the national average. In the few cases where we have calibrated mammograms and uncalibrated ones from previous screenings the breast thicknesses were within 0.5cm.

The chapters so far have explained the h_{int} representation and how we estimate it using calibration data and models of scattered and extra-focal radiation. In this chapter we considered estimation of breast thickness, a crucial part of the calibration data. The next chapter analyses the effects of errors in the calibration data, such as H, on the h_{int} values.

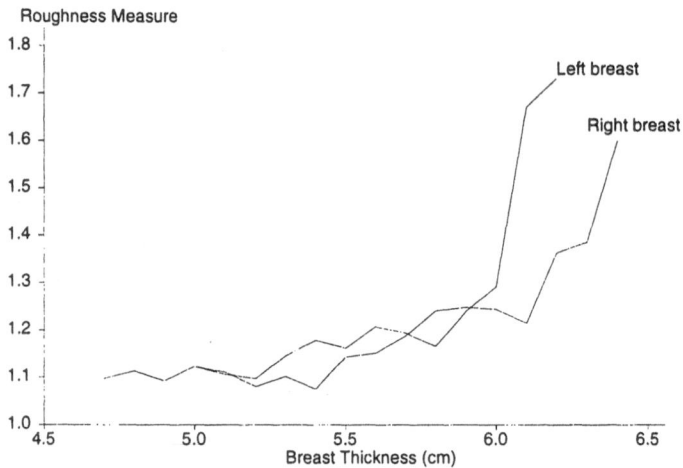

Figure 5.8.   The horizontal axis shows the breast thickness in cm. The vertical axis shows the roughness measure as described in the text. The higher the value, the rougher the curve is. We set a threshold to stop increasing the breast thickness at a roughness value of 1.3. This graph shows the variation of the roughness parameter for left and right breasts of the same woman in the cranio-caudal view. In these cases the measured thicknesses were 6.0cm and the estimated thicknesses 5.9 and 6.1cm.

CHAPTER 6

MODEL VERIFICATION AND SENSITIVITY

6.1. Introduction

In the preceding chapters we have shown how to generate the h_{int} representation for a mammogram using mathematical models of the imaging process. In this chapter we seek to further verify our modelling using practical results and to perform a more theoretical study looking at the sensitivity of the h_{int} values as the calibration data is varied. Consequently, the first part of the chapter should be accessible to a wide readership, whilst the latter part is more mathematical and can be skipped by readers who are less interested in the mathematical detail.

6.2. Practical verification of modelling

Once a mammographic image has been transformed into an h_{int} image there are (at least) seven tests **V1-V7** which we can perform to verify the modelling:

V1: The computed breast thickness should be accurate.
V2: There should be a "breast edge" on each mammogram.
Both these tests were passed in Chapter 5, where our method for estimating the breast thickness H was explained. We also found that not only did the breast edge exist but that it was a consistent proportion of the total imaged breast size.

V3: h_{int} at each pixel must be less than the breast thickness H.
This has been found to hold in hundreds of examples, i.e. we do not get $h_{int} > H$ when the correct calibration data and breast thickness are used. We note, however, that the presence of calcification could potentially lead to localized estimates of h_{int} that exceed H, since we exclude the possibility of microcalcifications in the estimation of h_{int}. Indeed, it might be that values of h_{int} that are high relative to the surrounding values could be used to detect calcifications! We explore this in detail in Chapter 11.

V4: The h_{int} values within the dense pectoral muscle should increase towards H.

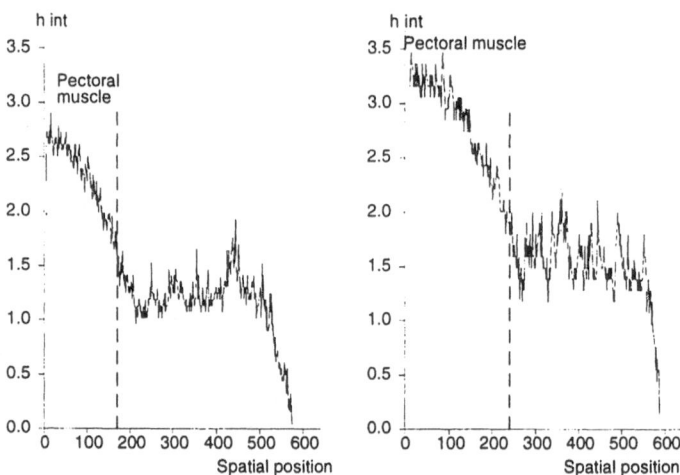

Figure 6.1. These two graphs show profiles of the h_{int} values across two medio-lateral oblique images. The graph on the left is from a breast with thickness 3.5cm and on the right the thickness is 4.9cm, the pectoral muscles are as marked.

This test requires high h_{int} values in the pectoral muscle when a medio-lateral oblique mammogram is being analysed. Figure 6.1 shows profiles across the h_{int} images of just two of the many medio-lateral oblique images that have been processed. The profiles clearly show the large increase in h_{int} as the pectoral muscle is crossed. They also show that the values approach H.

V5: The percentage of interesting tissue should rise or fall
        according to breast composition.
Figure 6.2 shows some examples of mammograms and the percentages of interesting tissue computed:

$$\text{Percentage of interesting tissue} = 100 \times \frac{V_{int}}{V_{total}} = 100 \times \frac{V_{int}}{V_{int} + V_{fat}},$$

where V denotes volume. In the examples that we have seen the percentage of interesting tissue has proven to be quite consistent between left and right breasts. As the figure caption explains, the percentages do also rise and fall as expected, though sometimes the *visual* appearance of a mammogram can be deceptive. For example, a breast might be under-exposed and therefore very bright when in fact the breast itself is fatty. A much

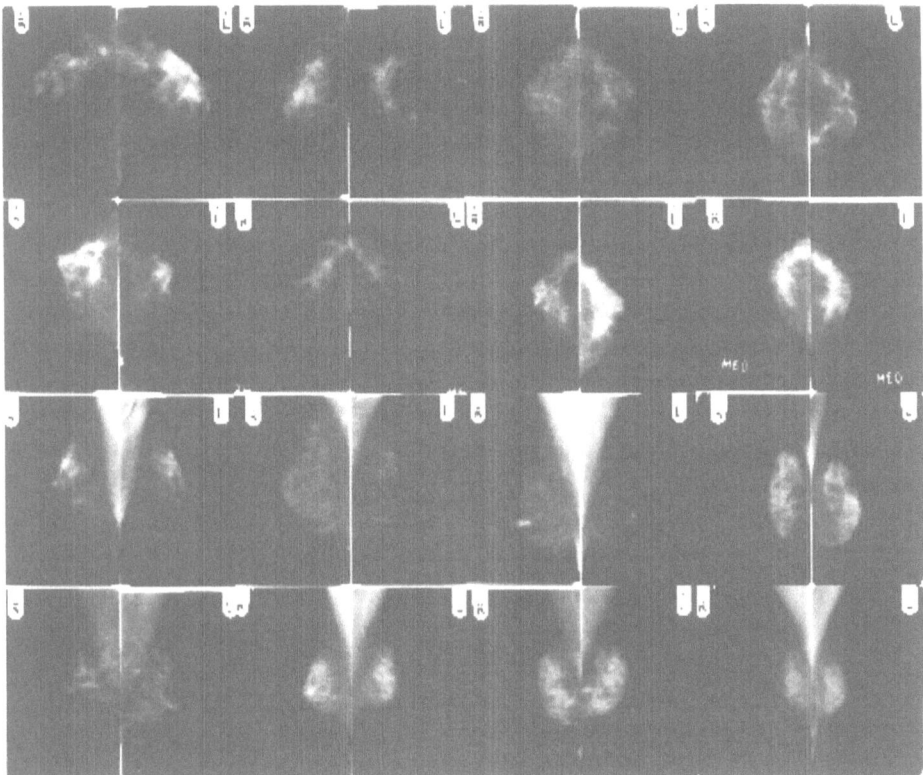

Figure 6.2.   These are 16 pairs of mammograms that represent a selection from our databases. The percentage of interesting tissue for the left and right breasts is very similar despite varying breast thicknesses so we only give one percentage here. The top 8 pairs and bottom 8 pairs are ordered from top-to-bottom and from left-to-right in ascending order of percentage of interesting tissue: The top row has the following percentages. 7, 9, 11, 13; the second row: 13, 15, 22, 27; the third row: 22, 23, 25, 34 and the fourth row: 41, 42, 43, 55. Considering the cranio-caudal images first, the percentages generally match well with visual appearance but there are exceptions. For example, the percentages suggest that the pair at the start of the second row are less dense than the pair to the right, and yet visually the first pair are far brighter. However, the first pair were compressed 0.5cm less than the other pair but the exposure times were nearly identical. Similar arguments can be made about the medio-lateral oblique mammograms where the percentages again correlate with visual perception except for a couple of exceptions.

better comparison would be visual degree of involution and computed percentage of interesting tissue. If such comparisons are favourable, then the percentage of interesting tissue could be used to sort easy-to-diagnose from hard-to-diagnose mammograms.

The percentages of interesting tissue that we have been finding for cranio-caudal mammograms are low compared to the standard breast used for radiation dose calculations (which is usually deemed to consist of 50% interesting tissue and 50% fat by mass). This is partly due to dose work assuming a flat breast edge, whereas here a volume of fat has been added

to represent the curved breast edge. However, as Figure 6.2 shows, if the
pectoral muscle is included the percentage of interesting tissue rises substantially, and can be around 50%. One of the problems in comparing the
percentage of interesting tissue is that it is particularly sensitive to errors
in measuring H; a small increase in H causes a large increase in the overall
breast volume estimate, whilst reducing the volume of interesting tissue.
Two further problems in matching percentages between the breasts exist.
One is that as the breast is compressed blood appears to be compressed
out of it, reducing the interesting tissue content. The other problem is that
some digitisers only record film densities up to a film density of 3.0, so that
the breast edges on some images might be curtailed leading to underesti-
mates of total breast volume - if the edge is included in the estimation.
Note that this does not trouble the algorithm to find the breast edge as
described in Chapter 5 since the film densities of interest there are usually
below 3.0.

V6: The h_{int} values estimated from two images of the same breast
at different compressions should correspond on a pixel basis and
be the same on a global basis.

This test deals with mammograms of the same breast performed at different compressions, the work which provided these mammograms can be
found in Chapter 9. The computed values of interesting tissue for those
mammograms compared remarkably well for mammograms taken of the
same breast at different breast compressions. In fact, we use h_{int} to view
tissue dispersion, see Figure 9.6. Also, the total percentages of interesting
tissue were found to be within 1% for the mammograms taken at different
compressions.

V7: The h_{int} values estimated for the same breast at different
times should be similar.

To prove this test, we would ideally take two mammograms over time, compute the h_{int} representations and then subtract one from the other to reveal
no change in h_{int} and thus its invariance. Unfortunately, breasts change over
time but estimation of H, as explained in Chapter 5, relies heavily on h_{int}
and there we've seen that over time our H estimates vary only by 0.5cm,
suggesting an invariant representation. We return to this issue in Chapter
13.

We conclude the first part of the testing by noting that several of the
tests require opposite effects. For example, **V4** requires high h_{int} values
which can be achieved by decreasing H, whereas **V2** requires low h_{int} values which can be achieved by increasing H. To satisfy all the tests simul-
taneously appears difficult, but in the hundreds of images that have been

processed all the tests have been passed every time. Clearly, the h_{int} representation is strongly supported by these tests and it provides a platform for reliable enhancement and analysis of mammograms which is Part II of this book. Of course, the compressed breast thickness H is a key parameter in estimating h_{int}, and so we now turn to an analysis of the sensitivity of h_{int} to errors in H and other parameters. However, the analysis is quite mathematical and some readers may choose to skip it. We can summarise the results of the next section as follows: first, most errors give rise to uniform shifts up or down in the h_{int} values. If we have accurate calibration, then we can use the absolute h_{int} values as quantitative features. Otherwise, it is better to use features that involve local differences or gradients to remove any calibration-induced uniform shifts in the h_{int} values. The h_{int} measurement has now been performed on many mammograms from diverse populations. In all cases the model has held up and returned entirely feasible values of h_{int} and H. The robustness of the image analysis techniques to be discussed in Part II of the book is eloquent proof of the usefulness of h_{int}.

> This next section can be omitted by readers who are less interested in a mathematical proof of the robustness of the h_{int} generation.

6.3. Theoretical sensitivity analysis

Calculation of h_{int} values from breast images requires a great deal of calibration data and estimation. Here we reconsider this process and consider the effects of errors in the data on the h_{int} values. In this way, we hope to identify the crucial variables and the effects of errors and hence control (or at least account for) them.

Many of the variables involved in the theoretical calculations are relatively stable. However, some have different values at different photon energies and it is extremely difficult to estimate how they might change; although each system could be calibrated. For these reasons, we make no attempt at analysing changes in h_{int} when the screen absorption $S(\mathcal{E})$, grid transmittance $G(\mathcal{E})$ and incident energy spectrum $N_0^{rel}(\mathcal{E})$ vary, although the latter varies when we change the tube voltage. Changes in these variables tend to cancel out due to their presence in several equations. Other variables can be measured accurately (e.g. the compression plate thickness, h_{plate}), and others are universally accepted constants (e.g. linear attenuation coefficient of lucite, $\mu_{luc}(\mathcal{E})$). So, the analysis reduces to consideration of: breast thickness (H), time-of-exposure (t_s), photon flux (ϕ), tube voltage (V_t), linear attenuation coefficients of fat and interesting tissue (μ_{fat}, μ_{int}), the speed of the film-screen system and the gradient of the film-screen characteristic curve and scatter estimate. Note that the film-screen characteristics become important in the estimate of the imparted energies, and also that H plays a role in the estimation of the scatter component E_s. To simplify matters, we note that extra-focal radiation has most effect near the breast edge, not over the bulk of the image and so can be assumed minimal for much of what follows although in effect its similarity to scatter means that the analysis for scatter applies equally to extra-focal.

Recall from the previous chapters that $h_{int}(x, y)$ is computed by adjusting the value at each pixel until the theoretical primary energy matches the measured primary energy. The polyenergetic nature of the incident x-ray beam, and the resulting integral equation for the theoretical energy makes analytical analysis impossible, but simplifying to a hypothetical monoenergetic beam removes many of the variables. In the analysis that follows, we use a mixture of analysis of the hypothetical monoenergetic case, supported by numerical analysis in the polyenergetic case.

Analytical analysis using monoenergetic arguments

In the monoenergetic simulation, the theoretical primary energy (Equation 2.4) becomes:

$$E_p^{imp}(x, y) = \phi(x, y) A_p t_s \mathcal{E} \ S \ G \ e^{-\mu_{luc} h_{plate}} \ e^{-h_{int}(x,y)(\mu_{int} - \mu_{fat}) - H \mu_{fat}}$$

Rearranging to give an explicit equation for h_{int}:

$$h_{int}(x, y) = \frac{H \mu_{fat}}{\mu_{fat} - \mu_{int}} + \frac{\ln E_p^{imp}(x, y) - \ln(\phi(x, y) A_p t_s \mathcal{E} SG e^{-\mu_{luc} h_{plate}})}{\mu_{fat} - \mu_{int}}$$

$$(6.1)$$

The average incident photon energy for a typical x-ray tube is 16.036keV at 25kVp, 16.610keV at 28kVp and 16.954keV at 30kVp. The average exiting photon energy from the breast is higher than the average incident energy since photons at lower energies are more greatly attenuated. Table 6.1 shows the value of the denominator in Equation 6.1 over a range of energies. A useful, but not critical, observation is that the denominator has a value of around -0.5 for the energy values with which we are mostly interested:

$$\mu_{fat} - \mu_{int} \approx -0.5 \qquad (6.2)$$

Breast thickness, H

An error in the estimate of breast thickness results in an error in the estimation of the scatter component and an error in the analysis of the primary energy. We estimate the thickness as set out in the previous chapter, where we saw that our method is generally accurate to within ±0.2cm,

$\mathcal{E}$	μ_{int}	μ_{fat}	$\mu_{int} - \mu_{fat}$	$\mathcal{E}$	μ_{int}	μ_{fat}	$\mu_{int} - \mu_{fat}$
15	1.635	0.832	0.803	23	0.594	0.362	0.232
16	1.381	0.718	0.664	24	0.546	0.340	0.205
17	1.184	0.628	0.556	25	0.505	0.322	0.183
18	1.028	0.558	0.470	26	0.471	0.307	0.164
19	0.903	0.502	0.401	27	0.441	0.293	0.148
20	0.802	0.456	0.346	28	0.416	0.282	0.134
21	0.719	0.419	0.301	29	0.393	0.272	0.122
22	0.651	0.388	0.263	30	0.374	0.263	0.111

TABLE 6.1. The left most columns show photon energy; the second shows the linear attenuation coefficient (cm^{-1}) for "interesting" tissue; the third column shows the linear attenuation coefficient for fat; the fourth column shows the difference between the coefficients. This difference is an important variable in many equations. The energy range of most interest is between 16 and 20keV as the vast majority of x-ray photons lie within this range.

which compares favourably with other techniques (that have additional drawbacks [29]).

Let H' be the estimated breast thickness with h'_{int} the resulting h_{int} values. Then taking the monoenergetic simplification and subtracting Equation 6.1 for H and H':

$$h'_{int}(x,y) = h_{int}(x,y) + \frac{(H'-H)\mu_{fat}}{\mu_{fat} - \mu_{int}} + \frac{\ln E_p^{imp'}(x,y) - \ln E_p^{imp}(x,y)}{\mu_{fat} - \mu_{int}}$$

$$= h_{int}(x,y) + \frac{(H'-H)\mu_{fat}}{\mu_{fat} - \mu_{int}} + \frac{\ln\left(\frac{E_{ps}^{imp}(x,y) - E_s^{imp'}(x,y)}{E_{ps}^{imp}(x,y) - E_s^{imp}(x,y)}\right)}{\mu_{fat} - \mu_{int}} \quad (6.3)$$

We shall show that the change in scatter component has little effect compared to the error in H and that the total error only causes a uniform decrease/increase of h_{int} values, i.e. $h'_{int}(x,y) = h_{int}(x,y) + $ error. This kind of effect is acceptable in practice since almost every use that we will make of h_{int} requires taking its spatial gradient or subtraction of a background component and this removes any uniform decrease/increase in value:

$$h'_{int} - h_{int}^{background'} = (h_{int} + \text{error}) - (h_{int}^{background} + \text{error})$$

$$= h_{int} - h_{int}^{background}$$

Concentrating on the last part of Equation 6.3, we can simplify it:

$$\frac{E_{ps}^{imp}(x,y) - E_s^{imp'}(x,y)}{E_{ps}^{imp}(x,y) - E_s^{imp}(x,y)} = \frac{E_p^{imp}(x,y) + E_s^{imp}(x,y) - E_s^{imp'}(x,y)}{E_p^{imp}(x,y)}$$

$$= 1 + \frac{E_s^{imp}(x,y)}{E_p^{imp}(x,y)} - \frac{E_s^{imp'}(x,y)}{E_p^{imp}(x,y)} \qquad (6.4)$$

From the work of Carlsson et al.[32] (Table 3.1) we know that for any block of breast tissue of a certain composition there is an approximately linear relationship between the scatter-to-primary ratio and breast thickness. From their values we deduce that the rate of change of the scatter-to-primary ratio with breast thickness is about 0.02 per cm, so Equation 6.4 can be written:

$$\frac{E_{ps}^{imp}(x,y) - E_s^{imp'}(x,y)}{E_{ps}^{imp}(x,y) - E_s^{imp}(x,y)} = 1 + 0.02(H - H')$$

Equation 6.3 thus becomes:

$$h'_{int}(x,y) = h_{int}(x,y) + \frac{(H' - H)\mu_{fat}}{\mu_{fat} - \mu_{int}} + \frac{\ln(1 + 0.02(H - H'))}{\mu_{fat} - \mu_{int}}$$

In the energy range of most interest μ_{fat} is greater than 0.5 (see Table 6.1). Moreover, in practice $|H - H'| < 0.5$cm, so that $\ln(1 + 0.02(H - H'))$ is negligible and we can remove the third term from the equation leaving:

$$h'_{int}(x,y) = h_{int}(x,y) + \frac{(H' - H)\mu_{fat}}{\mu_{fat} - \mu_{int}}$$

Rewriting this equation using error terms we get:

$$h_{int}^{error}(x,y) = H^{error} \times \frac{\mu_{fat}}{\mu_{fat} - \mu_{int}}$$

The amplifying term, $|\frac{\mu_{fat}}{\mu_{fat} - \mu_{int}}|$ is always greater than 1.0 for the energy range of interest (see Table 6.1) and is of the order of 1.2. This means that H^{error} has a relatively important effect on the calculation of h_{int}. However, the equation also suggests that h_{int} is linearly related with H^{error}. This can be shown in the polyenergetic case by considering specific values or by studying histograms of the h_{int} image. Table 6.2 shows the change for various different h_{int} values in different circumstances in the polyenergetic case. Given H and a poor estimate H' the error in h_{int} is independent of h_{int}, i.e. an error in H gives a uniform decrease/increase of h_{int}.

H	H'	h_{int}	h'_{int}	H	H'	h_{int}	h'_{int}
4.0	3.0	1.0	2.15	6.0	5.0	1.0	2.18
		2.0	3.17			2.0	3.20
		3.0	4.15			3.0	4.22
	3.5	1.0	1.53			4.0	5.24
		2.0	2.54		5.5	1.0	1.54
		3.0	3.55			2.0	2.55
	4.5	1.0	0.31			3.0	3.56
		2.0	1.29			4.0	4.57
		3.0	2.28		6.5	1.0	0.28
	5.0	1.0	Neg			2.0	1.27
		2.0	0.67			3.0	2.25
		3.0	1.65			4.0	3.23
					7.0	1.0	Neg
						2.0	0.63
						3.0	1.60
						4.0	2.57

TABLE 6.2. This shows the h'_{int} values calculated when a poor breast thickness estimate H' has been entered. The first column shows the actual breast thickness and the second shows the estimated breast thickness. The third column shows the actual h_{int} thickness and the fourth shows the thickness estimated from the estimated breast thickness. The error in h_{int} is near constant for each circumstance as predicted by the monoenergetic analysis.

Time of exposure (t_s) and photon flux (ϕ)

Consider an error in the measurement of the time of exposure (e.g. through an error in the mAs value) so that t_s is the actual value and t'_s the measured value. The value of h_{int} using t'_s is, in the monoenergetic case:

$$h'_{int}(x, y) = \frac{H\mu_{fat}}{\mu_{fat} - \mu_{int}} + \frac{\ln E_p(x, y) - \ln(\phi(x, y) A_p t'_s \mathcal{E} SGe^{-\mu_{luc}h_{plate}})}{\mu_{fat} - \mu_{int}}$$

$\frac{t_s}{t_s'}$	h_{int}^{error}	$\frac{t_s}{t_s'}$	h_{int}^{error}
0.500000	1.386294	1.100000	-0.190620
0.600000	1.021651	1.200000	-0.364643
0.700000	0.713350	1.300000	-0.524728
0.800000	0.446287	1.400000	-0.672944
0.900000	0.210721	1.500000	-0.810930
1.000000	0.000000		

TABLE 6.3. The left columns show the error in the time-of-exposure t_s value whilst Δh_{int} gives the corresponding change in the h_{int} value.

Subtracting this from Equation 6.1 and substituting in the value from Equation 6.2 we get:

$$h_{int}'(x,y) - h_{int}(x,y) = \frac{\ln\left(\frac{t_s}{t_s'}\right)}{\mu_{fat} - \mu_{int}}$$

$$h_{int}^{error} \approx -2.0\ln\left(\frac{t_s}{t_s'}\right)$$

Two points should be noted here. The first point is that the error is again a uniform decrease/increase. The second is that with a 10% error (i.e. $\frac{t_s}{t_s'} = 0.9$ or $\frac{t_s}{t_s'} = 1.1$) the change in h_{int} is ± 0.2cm, which is quite small in dense breasts, but might be significant in fatty breasts, or fatty areas of any breast. Table 6.3 shows the error versus $\frac{t_s}{t_s'}$. This result also holds for errors in measurement of photon flux (ϕ), i.e. replace $\frac{t_s}{t_s'}$ by $\frac{\phi}{\phi'}$.

Tube voltage (V_t)

The tube voltage can be changed by the radiographer and might even be adjusted automatically on some machines. Changing the tube voltage is sometimes done on the grounds that the breast "feels dense", or "feels fatty", or on the basis of previous mammograms. Decreasing the tube voltage increases image contrast since the attenuation coefficients of the relevant tissues are better differentiated at lower energies, but the radiation dose increases. The tube voltage is noted down on the woman's records for every mammographic examination.

Table 6.4 shows the variation in the h_{int} value as the tube voltage is changed for various film densities and a breast 6.5cm thick. The changes

D	h_{int}		
	25kVp	28kVp	30kVp
1.0	2.792	4.803	6.470
1.3	2.348	4.234	5.763
1.6	1.965	3.751	5.165
1.9	1.550	3.235	4.534
2.2	1.186	2.788	3.996
2.5	0.765	2.278	3.387

TABLE 6.4. In this example the breast has a thickness under compression of 6.5cm. The value on the left shows the film density and the top row shows the respective tube voltages. The values in the table show the value of h_{int} which would be allocated to each film density.

appear to be related directly to the change in kVp:

$$h'_{int}(x, y) = h_{int}(x, y)(1 + \alpha \times (V_t - V'_t)),$$

where α is some constant. Although it is possible, it is not likely that the kVp will be noted down wrongly by the radiographer. Therefore, we are more concerned with fluctuations in the actual kVp rather than with a wrong nominal tube voltage being entered. Prior et al. [205] report that in their experiments the tube voltage was typically 1kVp lower than the nominal recorded and that is consistent with measurements performed at our site.

Film-screen calibration data (β, γ)

The film-screen system consists of the x-ray film, intensifying screen and film processing. The system response is traditionally measured by creating a characteristic curve, or H-D curve. We create such a curve using a step wedge and we measure the gradient of the linear part, γ. We also compute the energy imparted to the screen to give a film density of 1.0 as our measure of system speed. In order to analyse errors in the data, we assume a linear characteristic curve:

$$D(x, y) = \gamma \log_{10} \beta E_{ps}^{imp}(x, y)$$

Tests in our laboratory have revealed a variation in γ of between 2.6 and 3.1. The film-screen curve is known to vary, especially with the temperature that the film processing is performed at. One of the major advantages of directly digital mammography is likely to be the uniformity of the processing.

The primary energy imparted can be written in terms of the total energy imparted and the scatter-to-primary ratio:

$$E_p^{imp}(x,y) = \frac{E_{ps}^{imp}(x,y)}{1 + \frac{E_s^{imp}}{E_p^{imp}}(x,y)}$$

Substituting in the linear film density equation:

$$E_p^{imp}(x,y) = \frac{\frac{1}{\beta}10^{D(x,y)/\gamma}}{1 + \frac{E_s^{imp}}{E_p^{imp}}(x,y)} \tag{6.5}$$

We assume that the scatter-to-primary estimate stays the same when an erroneous value γ' is used, so that the primary becomes:

$$E_p^{imp'}(x,y) = \frac{\frac{1}{\beta}10^{D(x,y)/\gamma'}}{1 + \frac{E_s^{imp}}{E_p^{imp}}(x,y)} \tag{6.6}$$

Divide Equation 6.6 by Equation 6.5:

$$\frac{E_p^{imp'}(x,y)}{E_p^{imp}(x,y)} = 10^{D(x,y)(\frac{1}{\gamma'}-\frac{1}{\gamma})}$$

Using Equation 6.1, we thus see that the error in h_{int} is related to the film density:

$$h_{int}^{error}(x,y) = \frac{\ln\left(\frac{E_p^{imp'}(x,y)}{E_p^{imp}(x,y)}\right)}{\mu_{fat} - \mu_{int}}$$
$$= -2.0\ln 10^{D(x,y)(\frac{1}{\gamma'}-\frac{1}{\gamma})}$$
$$= -2.0(\ln 10)D(x,y)(\frac{1}{\gamma'}-\frac{1}{\gamma})$$

Table 6.5 shows typical errors. The errors are not uniform since the error depends on D. It is clear that γ is an important parameter.

The error in β is much easier to predict, using the same arguments as for γ and letting $\beta = \eta\beta'$ be the error relationship we see:

$$h_{int}^{error}(x,y) = h_{int}'(x,y) - h_{int}(x,y) = -2.0\ln\frac{\beta}{\beta'} = -2.0\ln\eta$$

γ'	$D(x,y)$	h_{int}^{error}	γ'	$D(x,y)$	h_{int}^{error}
2.8	1.0	-0.110	3.2	1.0	0.096
	1.5	-0.164		1.5	0.144
	2.0	-0.219		2.0	0.192
	2.5	-0.274		2.5	0.240
	3.0	-0.328		3.0	0.287

TABLE 6.5. This shows the error in h_{int} when the real value of γ is 3.0. As can be seen the error increases with film density. This happens since the higher the film density, the higher the energy imparted and so the higher the error

η	h_{int}^{error}	η	h_{int}^{error}	η	h_{int}^{error}
0.7	0.714	0.9	0.211	1.2	-0.364
0.8	0.447	1.1	-0.190	1.3	-0.525

TABLE 6.6. This shows the error in h_{int} when there is an error in β, which is related to film-screen speed. The error relation is $\beta = \eta\beta'$ where β' is the erroneous value. A value for η of 1.3 indicates a film that requires 30% less exposure to reach a certain film density, so that it's a faster film.

Table 6.6 shows the error in h_{int} related to η. This time the error is a uniform decrease/increase of the h_{int} values.

Attenuation coefficients

The h_{int} calculation is based upon the premise that breast tissues can be classified into 3 classes since the linear attenuation coefficients group well. Table 2.2 shows the linear attenuation coefficients reported by Johns and Yaffe [137]. The calculation has at present used the mean values of the linear attenuation coefficients. In this section we vary the coefficients to the reported extremes and see the effects on the h_{int} calculation. Note that we assume that the coefficients are the same throughout any one breast.

Table 6.7 shows some variations in linear attenuation coefficients and the

$\overline{h\mu_P}$	Variation	$\mu_{int}(18)$	$\mu_{int}(20)$	$\mu_{fat}(18)$	$\mu_{fat}(20)$	h_{int}
2.5	min,min	1.014	0.791	0.538	0.441	0.527
	mean,mean	1.050	0.820	0.558	0.456	0.347
	max,max	1.137	0.884	0.585	0.476	0.113
3.0	min,min	1.014	0.791	0.538	0.441	1.694
	mean,mean	1.050	0.820	0.558	0.456	1.471
	max,max	1.137	0.884	0.585	0.476	1.116
3.5	min,min	1.014	0.791	0.538	0.441	2.937
	mean,mean	1.050	0.820	0.558	0.456	2.666
	max,max	1.137	0.884	0.585	0.476	2.182
4.0	min,min	1.014	0.791	0.538	0.441	Over 4
	mean,mean	1.050	0.820	0.558	0.456	3.942
	max,max	1.137	0.884	0.585	0.476	3.321

TABLE 6.7. The first column gives a practical attenuation coefficient, the breast thickness is 4.0cm. The second column gives the variation in the attenuation coefficients for that row, e.g. min,min means that we are using the minimum values for both the interesting tissue and fat attenuation coefficients. The next four columns give the actual values used at two energies (18 and 20keV). The final column gives the h_{int} value that would be computed. As might be expected, variations in the linear attenuation coefficients of the tissues give rise to large fluctuations in the h_{int} values.

effect on h_{int}. As expected from Equation 6.1, relatively small variations in the coefficients gives relatively large deviations in the h_{int} values and these deviations are not simply a uniform decrease/increase. However, if we could assume that the differences between the two sets of attenuation coefficients is constant between breasts then we are able to show a uniform error in h_{int} in the monoenergetic case. That is, we assume that:

$$\mu_{fat} - \mu_{int} = \mu'_{fat} - \mu'_{int}$$

This assumption might be reasonable when one considers that the linear attenuation coefficient is related to the density of the material, the atomic number of the material, and the photon energy.

Recall the monoenergetic equation for h_{int} (Equation 6.1), and put in the erroneous values of the linear attenuation coefficients:

$$h'_{int}(x, y) = \frac{H\mu'_{fat}}{\mu'_{fat} - \mu'_{int}} + \frac{\ln E_p^{imp}(x, y) - \ln(\phi(x, y)A_p t_s \mathcal{E} S G e^{-\mu_{luc} h_{plate}})}{\mu'_{fat} - \mu'_{int}}$$

$\overline{h\mu_P}$	Variation	$\mu_{int}(18)$	$\mu_{int}(20)$	$\mu_{fat}(18)$	$\mu_{fat}(20)$	h_{int}
2.5	max,max	1.137	0.884	0.585	0.476	0.113
	constant1	1.000	0.747	0.448	0.339	1.215
	constant2	1.050	0.800	0.498	0.248	1.380
3.0	max,max	1.137	0.884	0.585	0.476	1.116
	constant1	1.000	0.747	0.448	0.339	2.288
	constant2	1.050	0.800	0.498	0.248	2.286
3.5	max,max	1.137	0.884	0.585	0.476	2.182
	constant1	1.000	0.747	0.448	0.339	3.434
	constant2	1.050	0.800	0.498	0.248	3.192
4.0	max,max	1.137	0.884	0.585	0.476	3.321
	constant1	1.000	0.747	0.448	0.339	Over 4
	constant2	1.050	0.800	0.498	0.248	Over 4

TABLE 6.8. The first column gives a practical attenuation coefficient, the breast thickness is 4.0cm. The second column gives the variation in the attenuation coefficients for that row. constant1, constant2 represent constant shifts in the attenuation coefficients from the max,max row. The next four columns give the actual values used at two energies (18 and 20keV). The final column gives the h_{int} value that would be computed. $\mu_{int} - \mu_{fat}$ is preserved in these cases and the h_{int} values shift by a more constant factor than when the difference between the attenuations coefficients is not held constant.

Subtracting this from the equation with the true values and using the above assumption yields:

$$h'_{int}(x, y) = h_{int}(x, y) + \frac{(\mu_{fat} - \mu'_{fat})H}{\mu_{int} - \mu_{fat}}$$

The addition term is constant for any one image. Table 6.8 shows a polyenergetic simulation where the attenuation coefficients have this "constancy" property.

It is clear that the h_{int} values depend strongly upon the linear attenuation coefficients and that there might well be errors in h_{int} introduced that are not simply a uniform decrease/increase across the entire image. In any case, using the mean linear attenuation coefficients will minimise the errors and the results from the verification tests earlier suggest that in practice using the mean values works well.

Scatter and extra-focal estimate

An erroneous estimate of extra-focal radiation has the same effect as an erroneous estimate of scatter, so here we consider only errors in the scatter estimate. We've already covered the error in the scatter estimate due to an error in H in the breast thickness section, in this section we look at effects of errors in the scatter estimate due to errors in the model. Let the correct scatter estimate be E_s^{imp} and let $E_s^{imp'}$ be the erroneous one, then the erroneous h_{int} term is given by:

$$h'_{int}(x,y) =$$

$$\frac{H\mu_{fat}}{\mu_{fat} - \mu_{int}} + \frac{\ln(E_{ps}^{imp}(x,y) - E_s^{imp'}(x,y)) - \ln(\phi(x,y)A_p t_s \mathcal{E} S G e^{-\mu_{luc}h_{plate}})}{\mu_{fat} - \mu_{int}}$$

Combining this with the correct h_{int} expression and rearranging gives us:

$$h'_{int} = h_{int} + 2.0\ln\left(\frac{E_{ps}^{imp}(x,y) - E_s^{imp}(x,y)}{E_{ps}^{imp}(x,y) - E_s^{imp'}(x,y)}\right)$$

E_{ps}^{imp} alters across the image so that the effect of an error in the scatter estimate is hard to predict, but we can be sure that the error is not a simple uniform decrease/increase. To get some idea of the error we'll take some example values. Assume that the scatter-to-primary ratio is 0.15, which is a good average figure:

$$\frac{E_s^{imp}}{E_p^{imp}} = 0.15$$

Then:

$$E_{ps}^{imp} = E_s^{imp} + E_p^{imp} = 7.67 E_s^{imp}$$

Let's take a constant multiplicative error in E_s across all values:

$$E'_s = \eta E_s^{imp}$$

Then:

$$h'_{int} \approx h_{int} + 2.0\ln\left(\frac{6.67}{7.67 - \eta}\right)$$

Table 6.9 shows this equation evaluated for values of η. The errors are relatively small.

η	h_{int}^{error}	η	h_{int}^{error}
0.7	-0.088	1.1	0.030
0.8	-0.059	1.2	0.061
0.9	-0.030	1.3	0.092
1.0	0.000		

TABLE 6.9. This table shows the variation in h_{int} with a multiplicative error (η) in the scatter estimate for a typical situation within the breast.

6.4. Summary: Sensitivity

Bringing all the monoenergetic simplifications together allows us to consider the total error in the h_{int} computation:

$$
\begin{aligned}
h'_{int}(x,y) \approx\ & h_{int}(x,y) \\
+\ & 1.2(H - H') \\
+\ & 2.0\ln\left(\frac{t'_s}{t_s}\right) \\
+\ & \alpha \times h_{int}(x,y) \times (V_t - V'_t) \\
+\ & 4.6D(x,y)(\frac{1}{\gamma} - \frac{1}{\gamma'}) \\
+\ & 2.0\ln\frac{\beta'}{\beta} \\
+\ & 2.0\ln\left(\frac{6.67}{7.67 - \frac{E'_{scatter}}{E_{scatter}}}\right)
\end{aligned}
$$

We've seen that the first two terms have the most effect for a certain percentage error. For, say, a 10% error, they typically cause a shift in h_{int} of twice that of the other errors. It is difficult to predict the total error, especially since the errors are independent. Obviously, given certain circumstances the error in h_{int} will be overwhelming but, crucially, if that happens it will be detectable.

However, it also appears that most errors give shifts in the h_{int} values that are uniform across the image. When h_{int} is computed, H is adjusted until the breast edge has appropriate values and is suitably smooth. This adjustment of H leads to feasible h_{int} values - effectively compensating for any errors. But this does mean that only the differences in the h_{int} values should be used quantitatively, the absolute values cannot be trusted **unless** careful calibration has taken place. Our work suggests that careful calibration is possible, and results from qualitatively comparing percentages of interesting to visual appearance are very promising. Furthermore, the adjustment of H to compensate for all calibration errors leaves the potential for implausible values of H, either too high or far too low. The h_{int} measurement has now been performed on many mammograms of breasts from diverse populations. In all cases, the model has held up and returned entirely feasible values of h_{int} and H.

To conclude: if we have accurate calibration then we can use the absolute h_{int} values as quantitative features. Otherwise, use features that involve local differences or gradients to remove any calibration-induced uniform decreases/increases in the h_{int} values.

PART II

Exploiting The h_{int} Model

CHAPTER 7

IMAGE ENHANCEMENT

7.1. Introduction

As the mammographic model was being developed, a number of image de-grading factors became evident. These included: scattered radiation, beam hardening, glare and possible over or under exposure. These motivate the model-based image enhancement and restoration algorithms proposed in this chapter. The h_{int} representation lies at the heart of our approach and enables us to simulate any projective x-ray examination. If $D(x, y)$ is the original (2 dimensional) film density image, and $h_{int}(x, y)$ is the (2.5 dimensional) interesting tissue surface, then enhancement processes can be represented in terms of the two steps:

$$D_{given}(x, y) \longrightarrow h_{int}(x, y) \longrightarrow D_{enhanced}(x, y)$$

The first step normalises the data, by removing image generation specific information such as the time-of-exposure and allows quantitative measures of breast tissue to be attained from which we can simulate any projective mammographic examination. The second step replaces the imaging parameter values by those desired; simulation without the degrading factors produces enhanced images.

Because the algorithms are based on the physics of the imaging process they are less likely to introduce artifacts than conventional algorithms and are far more predictable. Furthermore, since users understand how the algorithms work they are better placed to diagnose from the enhanced image.

A repertoire of enhancement modules has been implemented as a radiography aid **Xmammo**. Figure 7.1 shows the **Xmammo** user-interface to the algorithms: every algorithm is presented using terms that are familiar in radiology. Of course, we cannot accurately simulate x-ray examinations for which the required data is simply not present in the original mammogram; but we can simulate the x-ray examination accurate to the original data. Also, it should be noted that we do not seek to perform exact simulations: our goal is to enhance the image, so, for example, we do not introduce a noise contribution.

We begin the chapter with a discussion of the optimal display of mammographic images on a computer terminal. The optimal display should

XMAMMO

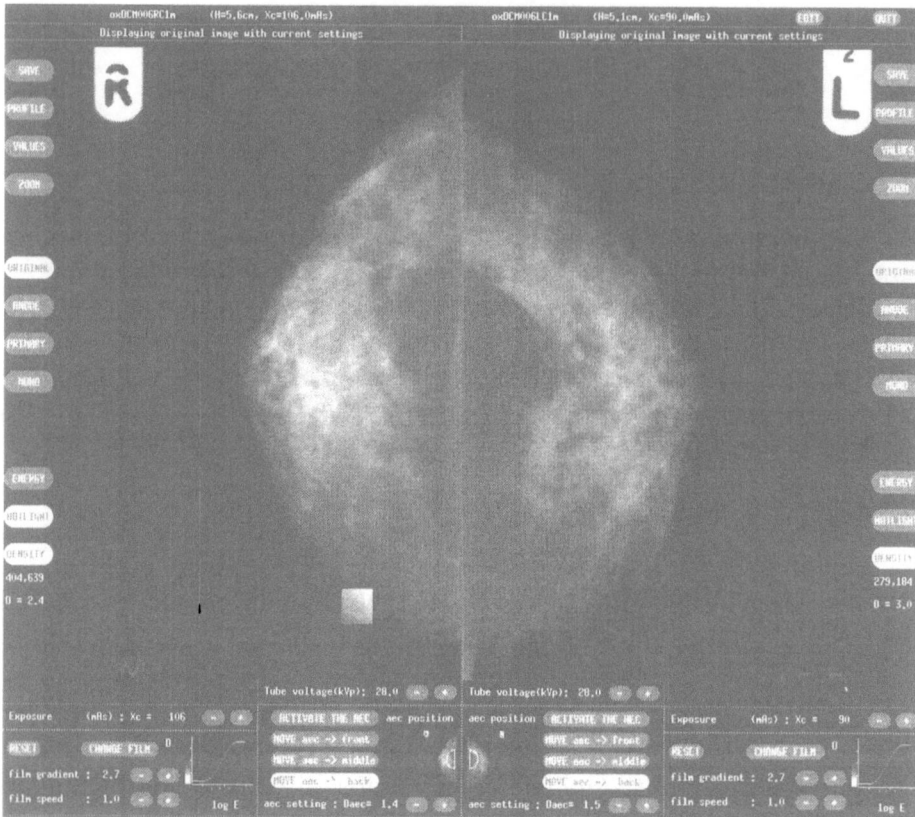

Figure 7.1. This is an example of the **Xmammo** user-interface to our model-based image processing algorithms. The user-interface uses terms from the users own domain terminology so that the user is familiar with, and knows what to expect, from each button.

approach the appearance of a mammographic film on a light-box therefore we focus on the luminance that the computer terminal displays. The next section deals with adjusting the time-of-exposure to counter over- or under- exposure. We then give examples of correction for the unsharpness introduced due to glare and digitisation. We end by showing the effects of changing tube voltage and simulating a scatter-free monoenergetic examination.

7.2. Simulating light-box appearance

Most mammographic images are stored in the computer with the value at each pixel related linearly to film density. Simply displaying such images on a computer screen presents an image quite unlike how the original mammogram appears on a light-box. When a film is viewed using a light-box, the eye receives the light transmitted through the film and this is exponentially related to film density. The light transmitted through the film is also directly proportional to the intensity of the illuminating light (i.e. the light-box). In practice the illuminating light varies over the light-box, but for our simulations we assume constant illumination.

To simulate the appearance of a mammogram on a light-box we need to display the digital images so that the luminance at each pixel on the screen is set to be directly proportional to the light transmitted through the film in the corresponding area. This means that if an area on the film displayed on a light box is twice as bright as another area (i.e. has twice the light being transmitted through the film), then that area in the digitally displayed image is also twice as bright (i.e. has twice the luminance). In order to achieve this we need to consider how a display device maps from pixel value to luminance. Box 7.1 contains the mathematics relating to simulating a light-box.

Currently, most display of digital images takes place on cathode ray tubes (CRTs). A device driver converts the pixel value to a voltage for input to the tube in a linear fashion, but there is a non-linear relationship between input voltage and luminance specified by a variable commonly called gamma (Γ). Typically, there is an approximately square relationship which makes the bright parts of the image have more contrast at the cost of making the dark parts of the image look almost black. Since mammograms are typically quite dark it is crucial that this mapping be considered when displaying them on a computer screen. The mapping varies between screens but it is relatively simple to calibrate each monitor. Box 7.2 shows the relevant equations and Figure 7.2 shows examples of image display with and without "gamma correction". Further processing is required to overcome "veiling glare" (or internal scattering) and modulation transfer which cause a blurring effect on images displayed on CRTs [17, 18, 135].

There is one last issue to be discussed, namely discretization, which becomes especially important when displaying 8-bit transmitted light images. If we map a film density image to a transmitted light image then the film density range from 2 to 3 is compressed into just 20 pixel values. If processing is now done on the image to make that range visible (such as we propose in the next section) then false contouring will become a problem unless the original pixel values are used. This is yet another way in which

---

BOX 7.1: Simulating a light-box

The light transmitted $T_l(x,y)$ through a radiographic film is related to the illuminating light I_l and film density $D(x,y)$ in the area corresponding to (x,y) is

$$T_l(x,y) = I_l 10^{-D(x,y)}, \qquad (7.1)$$

We consider I_l to be spatially constant. We seek to display the mammogram such that the luminance L at each pixel is directly proportional to the light transmitted through the film:

$$L(x,y) = \alpha T_l(x,y) \qquad (7.2)$$

BOX 7.2: Luminance and pixel value

The device driver converts the pixel value in an image to a voltage:

$$V(x,y) = \eta P(x,y) \qquad (7.3)$$

The relationship between input voltage and luminance is, assuming a black level of 0:

$$L(x,y) = V(x,y)^\Gamma = (\eta P(x,y))^\Gamma \qquad (7.4)$$

The value of Γ is usually between 1.8 and 2.4. The Γ of a monitor can either be measured using a photometer or can be estimated by comparing a binary image to a greyscale image [203]. Rearranging Equation 7.4 and substituting in Equations 7.1 and 7.2 gives the transform required to get luminance directly proportional to transmitted light:

$$P(x,y) = (\frac{\alpha^{\frac{1}{\Gamma}}}{\eta} I_l^{\frac{1}{\Gamma}}) 10^{-D(x,y)/\Gamma} \qquad (7.5)$$

The first part of this equation is simply a constant, call it $\phi = (\frac{\alpha^{\frac{1}{\Gamma}}}{\eta} I_l^{\frac{1}{\Gamma}})$. We choose ϕ based upon the standard light-box as follows. Film densities of between 0.25 and 2.25 are said to be the useful film density range on a mammogram. That is, the light transmitted through a film with densities between 0.25 and 2.25 is usually discernible on a light-box. The dynamic range for that situation is 100. Unfortunately, although theoretically the dynamic range of the television screen is infinite, in practice it is around 40. This comes from $\frac{L_{max}}{L_{min}}$ when the luminances are perceivable. Thus, in order to retain the relationship between transmitted light and luminance we have to compromise in our display of the transmitted light images. This is made easier by the realisation that most film densities are over 0.6, but we have to be careful since low film densities are usually significant (e.g. calcification). Mapping film densities of $D_{min} = 0.6$ to a pixel value of 255 gives us the constant (assuming here that $\Gamma = 2.0$):

$$\phi = 255 10^{D_{min}\frac{1}{\Gamma}} = 507.76$$

This mapping puts a film density of 2.25 to a pixel value of 19 which is perceivable on a screen with "normal brightness".

DISPLAYING A MAMMOGRAPHIC IMAGE

| Original film density image | Transmitted light image no gamma correction | Transmitted light image with gamma correction |

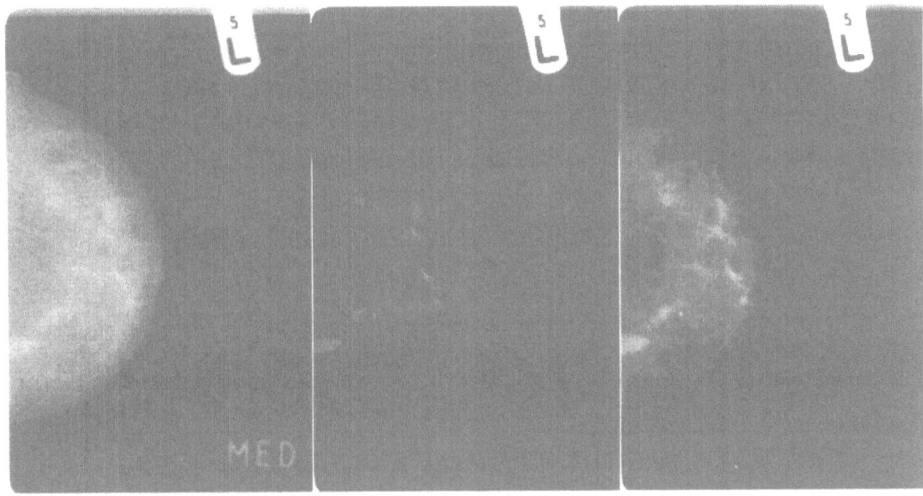

Figure 7.2.   The image on the left is the output from a digitiser displayed directly onto the screen. This image has pixel values linearly related to film density and so is unlike a mammogram on a light-box. The middle image shows a film density image transformed to show the light transmitted through the film. In this case, the image has not been compensated for the approximately square relationship between pixel value and luminance which introduces contrast into bright areas of the image whilst making the dark areas practically black. The image on the right has been compensated for the CRT transform so that the luminance is directly proportional to the light transmitted through the film at each point.

non-model based enhancement algorithms can be led astray.

Radiologists sometimes use a "hot-light" to view the breast edge and other dark areas on a mammogram. A hot-light is easily simulated by simply considering it to be an increase in the illuminating light over a small area. Figure 7.3 shows an example of the hot-light simulation and Box 7.3 shows the mathematics.

BOX 7.3: Simulating a hot-light

A hot-light can be easily simulated by increasing I_l in Equation 7.5. Let I_l' be the new illuminating light, and let P' be the new pixel value, then:

$$P'(x,y) = \left(\frac{I_l'}{I_l}\right)^{\frac{1}{\Gamma}} P(x,y) \qquad (7.6)$$

Typically the hot-light is 20 times brighter than the main part of the light box, in which case with $\Gamma = 2.0$, the equation becomes:

$$P'(x,y) = 4.47 \times P(x,y)$$

Of course this transform does not have to be applied just to a small area, it could be used to simulate a change in brightness of the whole light-box.

SIMULATING A HOT-LIGHT

Figure 7.3.   This shows the result of simulating a hot-light some 20 times as bright as a normal light-box. The hot-light is used to examine dark areas of the breast for signs such as skin-thickening.

7.3. Simulating different exposures

As explained during the development of the analogue model, the automatic exposure control (AEC) is meant to control the amount of radiation
reaching the film under a dense area of the breast, and to terminate the
exposure when a certain average film density has been reached in the area.
The AEC on the GE Senographe, for example, is a half-cylinder with a
radius of 3.5cm and our radiologists' have it set to give an average film
density of between 1.4 and 1.6. The automatic exposure control can give
poor results due to limitations in x-ray detection, beam hardening, reciprocal law failure and poor positioning [81] (see Chapter 2). To overcome
beam hardening, breast thickness tracking has to be built into the AEC
in order that it can adjust. Introduction of the AEC into mammography
reduced the number of retakes from 15% down to 1%. In this section we
explain two ways of increasing/decreasing the exposure and show how to
simulate the corresponding changes in the mammographic images.

To correct a mammographic image for under- or over-exposure, it can
be changed to simulate manipulation of the mAs exposure value. Let X_c
mAs be the exposure at which the original mammogram was performed,
and let X_c' mAs be the new exposure value. The energy imparted to the
intensifying screen is directly proportional to the time of exposure so that
we can write:

$$E^{imp}(x,y) = X_c E^{imp\ nd}(x,y) \qquad (7.7)$$

where we use E^{nd} to represent that part of the signal not related to time of
exposure (the nd stands for not-dependent). The energy imparted at (x,y)
with the new exposure can be written similarly:

$$E^{imp'}(x,y) = X_c' E^{imp\ nd}(x,y) = \frac{X_c'}{X_c} E^{imp}(x,y)$$

Figure 7.4 shows an original mammographic image performed with an
exposure of 68mAs and the result of simulating an increase in exposure
to 80mAs and a decrease to 56mAs. The transformed image was created
by calculating the new energy imparted values $E^{imp'}$ and re-applying the
relationship depicted in the film-screen characteristic curve to find the film
density.

Instead of manually adjusting the exposure, the action of an automatic
exposure control can be modeled. We model the action of the AEC as
aiming to produce an average film density in a certain area as shown mathematically in Box 7.4. This simple model of the AEC is not affected by
beam hardening because it works on the values within the film itself; it is
thus an idealised AEC. A model for the AEC that takes account of beam
hardening can be derived using h_{int}.

CHANGING THE TIME-OF-EXPOSURE

80mAs	68mAs	56mAs
Increase	Original	Decrease

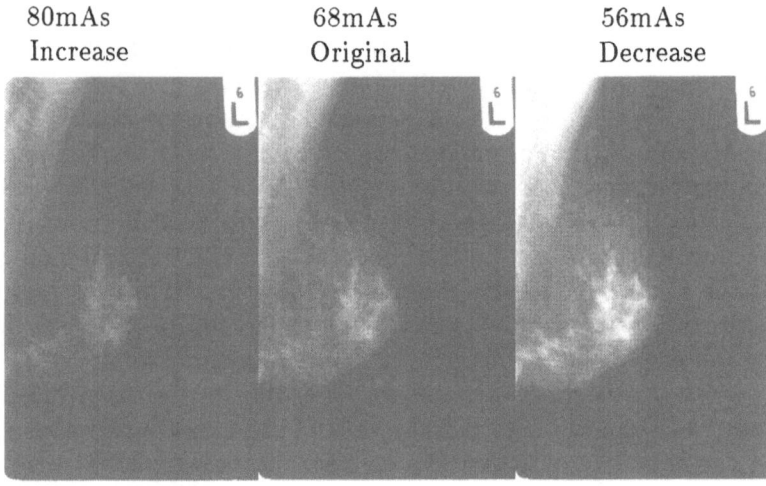

Figure 7.4. The middle image is the original mammogram with an exposure of 68mAs. The image on the left is a simulation of an exposure of 80mAs and the image on the right is a simulation of an exposure of 56mAs.

As well as adjusting the setting of the automatic exposure control, it is also possible to adjust its position. The automatic exposure control unit can typically be fixed into any one of three positions underneath the breast, Figure 7.5 shows the positions. To model a change in AEC position is a simple process of changing the position of the area over which the average energy is calculated. Figure 7.6 shows the effect on an actual mammogram of varying the exposure by changing the AEC position.

The simulation of increasing/decreasing exposure described in this section not only idealises the functioning of the automatic exposure control unit, but also the mammographic process: in practice, an increase in exposure would reduce the quantum noise, and a decrease in exposure would increase the quantum noise. Using straight-forward/elementary mathematics we can analyse the image changes with exposure, see Box 7.5.

BOX 7.4: Theoretical automatic exposure control

Let $\overline{E}_{AEC}^{imp}$ be the average energy imparted to the screen in a radiographer selected area $\mathcal{A}$, corresponding to the automatic exposure control position, with n the total number of pixels in $\mathcal{A}$, and E^{imp} the energy imparted corresponding to the pixel (x, y):

$$\overline{E}_{AEC}^{imp} = \frac{1}{n} \sum_{(x,y) \in \mathcal{A}} E^{imp}(x, y) \qquad (7.8)$$

Let $\overline{E}_{AEC}^{imp'}$ be the average energy imparted required, and let $E^{imp'}(x, y)$ be the energy imparted at each pixel which obtains this average. The automatic exposure control setting might equally be set by specifying an average film density, this value giving $\overline{E}_{AEC}^{imp'}$ when converted to energy imparted. In the new image, $\overline{E}_{AEC}^{imp'}$ is the average of the new energies imparted in the area $\mathcal{A}$:

$$\overline{E}_{AEC}^{imp'} = \frac{1}{n} \sum_{(x,y) \in \mathcal{A}} E^{imp'}(x, y) \qquad (7.9)$$

Divide this equation by Equation 7.8:

$$\sum_{(x,y) \in \mathcal{A}} E^{imp'}(x, y) = \frac{\overline{E}_{AEC}^{imp'}}{\overline{E}_{AEC}^{imp}} \sum_{(x,y) \in \mathcal{A}} E^{imp}(x, y) \qquad (7.10)$$

From Equation 7.3 it is known that increases/decreases in overall exposure have a multiplicative, rather than additive effect on each individual energy imparted. Thus the following relationship must hold for some λ:

$$E^{imp'}(x, y) = \lambda E^{imp}(x, y) \qquad (7.11)$$

If $\lambda > 1.0$ then the exposure is increased, if $\lambda < 1.0$ then the exposure is decreased. Combining Equation 7.10 with 7.11 we find λ:

$$\lambda = \frac{\overline{E}_{AEC}^{imp'}}{\overline{E}_{AEC}^{imp}} \qquad (7.12)$$

POSITIONS OF THE AEC

Back   Middle   Front

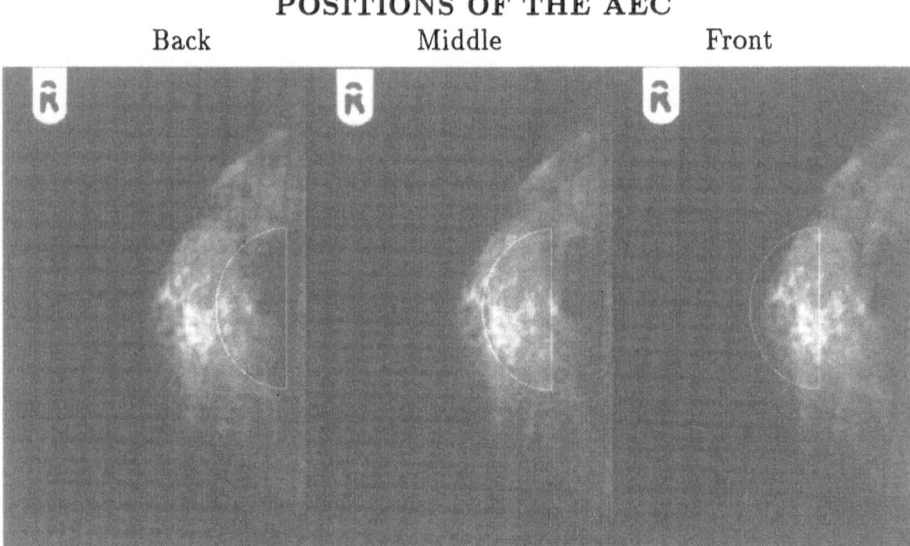

Figure 7.5.   This shows the three possible positions of the automatic exposure control beneath the breast. In this example the middle position is clearly best since it is there that most of the densest tissue lies. The most forward position would give a very low exposure since part of the AEC unit is visible to the x-ray tube.

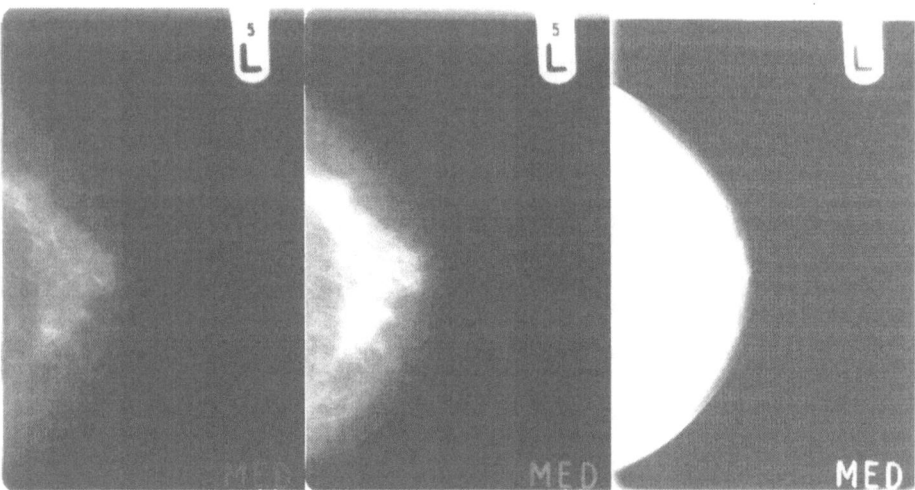

Figure 7.6.   The AEC position is changed and the x-ray process simulated; the exposure varied from (back to front): 144mAs, 82mAs and 15mAs. With the AEC in the forward position it becomes exposed to direct radiation.

BOX 7.5: Analysing the image changes with exposure

The effect of increasing/decreasing the exposure can be partly analysed by examining the effect on the individual transmitted light values. Combining Equation 7.1 and the linear film-screen curve equation gives:

$$T_l'(x, y) = \frac{I_l}{(\beta E^{imp'}(x, y))^\gamma},\qquad(7.13)$$

where T_l' represents the transmitted light through the film after the increase/decrease in the exposure and β and γ are the linear film-screen variables. Let λ be the multiplicative factor by which the imparted energies were changed:

$$E^{imp'}(x, y) = \lambda E^{imp}(x, y)$$

Substitute this into Equation 7.13:

$$\begin{aligned}
T_l'(x, y) &= \frac{I_l}{(\beta \lambda E^{imp}(x, y))^\gamma} \\
&= \frac{I_l}{(\beta E^{imp}(x, y))^\gamma \lambda^\gamma} \\
&= \frac{T_l(x, y)}{\lambda^\gamma}
\end{aligned}$$

If $\lambda > 1.0$ then the exposure is being increased and the intensity of the light transmitted through the film falls; if $\lambda < 1.0$ then the exposure is being decreased and the intensity of the light transmitted through the film rises. If $\gamma \approx 3$, doubling the exposure ($\lambda = 2$) reduces the transmitted light values by a factor of 8. The effect of different exposures can also be viewed in terms of the range of transmitted light. Let $T_{l\ range}$ be the initial transmitted light range:

$$\begin{aligned}
T_{l\ range} &= T_{l\max} - T_{l\min} \\
&= \frac{I_l}{(\beta E^{imp}_{min})^\gamma} - \frac{I_l}{(\beta E^{imp}_{max})^\gamma}
\end{aligned}$$

Substituting in the new imparted energies gives the new transmitted light range:

$$\begin{aligned}
T_{l\ range}' &= T_{l\max}' - T_{l\min}' \\
&= \frac{I_l}{(\beta E^{imp}_{min})^\gamma \lambda^\gamma} - \frac{I_l}{(\beta E^{imp}_{max})^\gamma \lambda^\gamma} \\
&= \frac{1}{\lambda^\gamma} T_{l\ range}
\end{aligned}$$

Taking the example above, doubling the exposure ($\lambda = 2$) reduces the range of transmitted light by a factor of 8.

7.4. Correcting for unsharpness

The two primary sources of unsharpness are intensifying screen glare and digitising the x-ray film. In Chapter 2, we presented our model of glare, while Davies [54] presents the modulation transfer functions for a scanning microdensitometer, CCD camera and a laser scanner similar to the one which we use. We use the modulation transfer function presented by Davies in order to remove the blur due to the digitiser. Figure 7.7 shows the results of the corrections for the glare and digitiser.

EXAMPLE OF GLARE REMOVAL

Original image   Glare removed

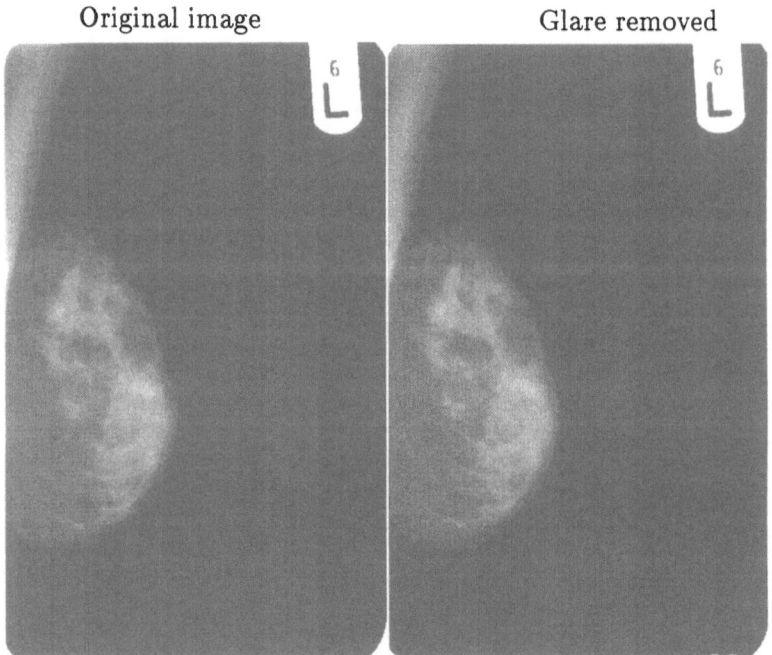

Figure 7.7.   The image on the left is the original mammogram. The image on the right has had the blur due to intensifying screen glare and the digitiser removed.

7.5. Simulating a scatter-free examination

Using the scatter and extra-focal models, the primary component of the energy imparted can be determined and it is the primary that contains most information. In order to generate an image which the radiologist can understand more easily it is necessary to convert the primary component back to the form in which the radiologist usually sees it. Unfortunately, simply looking up the film density corresponding to the primary component from the film characteristic curve is not suitable, since the primary component by itself is not large enough to expose the film to give a viewable image (the film would be effectively under-exposed). The approach we propose is to apply the automatic exposure control model to amplify the signal. The amplified energy imparted is converted to a film density using the same film characteristic curve as the original. The scatter removal algorithm developed here is essentially a local high-pass operation, and this indicates that we can be certain that calcifications, if present, will be enhanced, despite not being included in the breast model. Figure 7.8 shows an example of a scatter-removed image with calcifications. Figure 7.9 shows an example of the removal of the effects of scatter on a whole mammogram.

EXAMPLE OF SCATTER REMOVAL

Original image   Scatter removed

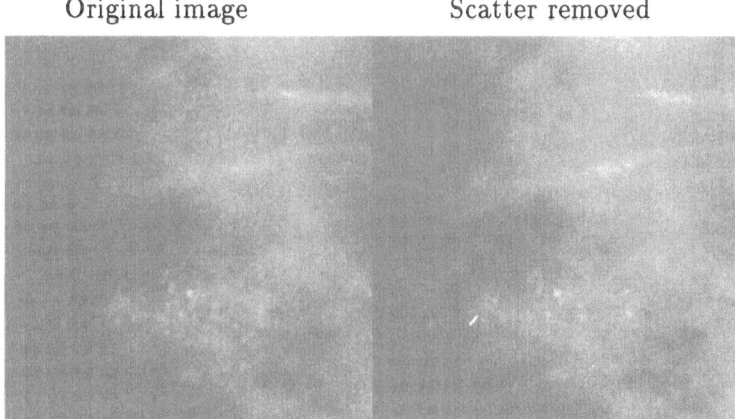

Figure 7.8. The image on the left is the original mammogram. The image on the right has had the effects of scattered radiation removed. After the scatter component was removed the model of the automatic exposure control was used to properly expose the film.

EXAMPLE OF SCATTER REMOVAL

Original image   Scatter removed

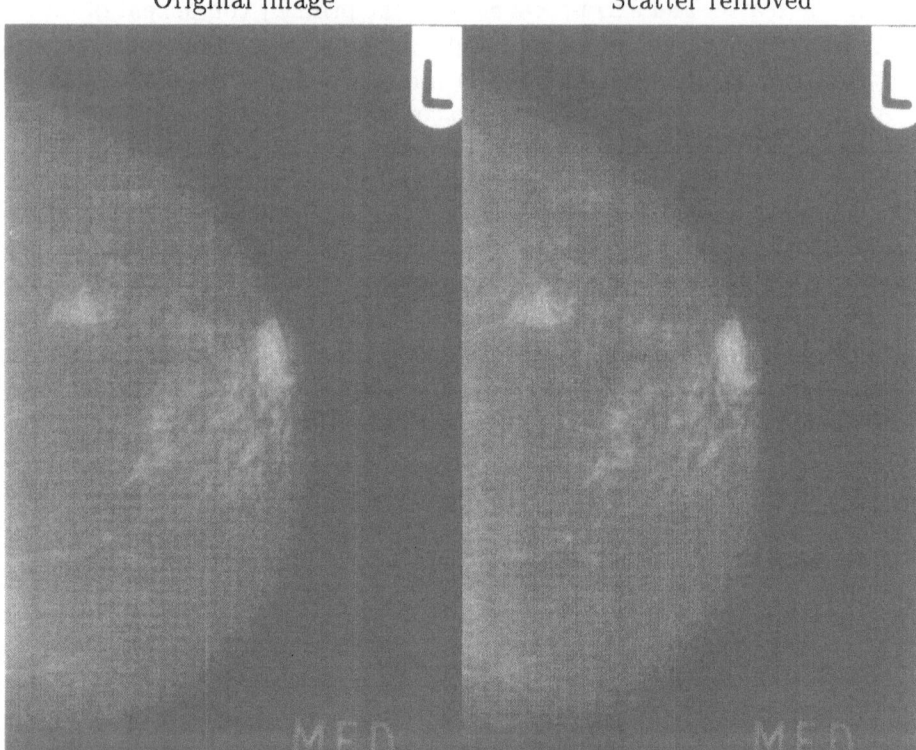

Figure 7.9.   The image on the left is the original mammogram. The image on the right has had the effects of scattered radiation removed. After the scatter component was removed the model of the automatic exposure control was used to properly expose the film.

7.6. Simulating a different x-ray source

There are two reasons why changing the energy distribution of the x-ray photons might produce enhanced images. The first is that although beam filtering takes place, the beam used in mammography is still basically polyenergetic and contrast is therefore lowered in areas of high attenuation. As noted in Chapter 2 this is termed beam hardening, and arises because as the beam passes through the breast, lower energy photons are absorbed or scattered, while the higher energy photons continue and are harder to attenuate. The second reason is that the x-ray tube components and voltage are chosen to produce a beam to give high contrast between different tissues whilst keeping the dosage low [134, 150, 185, 220, 230, 261]. The lower the energy of the beam, the greater the difference between the linear attenuation coefficients and the greater the contrast. However, the lower the energy, the greater the linear attenuation coefficient and thus the greater the radiation absorbed in the breast. We can ignore radiation dose since we are simulating an examination, and thus can use the photon energy distribution which is best for image quality .

The standard x-ray tube voltage for mammography, in the UK, is 28kVp. The radiographers are able to change this as appropriate if inspection of previous mammograms of the same breast reveals it to be excessively dense or fatty. We simulate the effects of changing the tube voltage. The difficult part of this operation is to calculate the scatter component at the new voltage. Though this is entirely feasible, currently rather than do this using the model of scatter, we estimate the new scatter component from the old scatter component, because this makes for a faster computer program. Box 7.6 shows the mathematics and Figure 7.10 shows an example of changing the tube voltage from 28kVp to 25kVp.

BOX 7.6: Changing the tube voltage

Ignoring extra-focal, the total energy imparted can be written:

$$E^{imp}_{ps\,V_{tube}} = E^{imp}_{p\,V_{tube}} + E^{imp}_{s\,V_{tube}} = E^{imp}_{p\,V_{tube}}(1 + \frac{E^{imp}_{s\,V_{tube}}}{E^{imp}_{p\,V_{tube}}})$$

Carlsson et al. [32] show that scatter-to-primary ratios do not change much between 25 and 30 kVp, and thus it is reasonable to assume that for two voltages V_{tube} and V'_{tube} within this range:

$$\frac{E^{imp}_{s\,V_{tube}}}{E^{imp}_{p\,V_{tube}}} = \frac{E^{imp}_{s\,V'_{tube}}}{E^{imp}_{p\,V'_{tube}}} \qquad (7.14)$$

Given this, we can write the total energies imparted at two different voltages in terms of each other:

$$E^{imp}_{ps\,V'_{tube}} = \frac{E^{imp}_{p\,V'_{tube}}}{E^{imp}_{p\,V_{tube}}}E^{imp}_{ps\,V_{tube}} \qquad (7.15)$$

We could approximate the ratio between the primaries at the different tube voltages and assume that the total number of incident photons is the same between the voltages to estimate the new imparted energy. However, if some time delay is allowable then we can use the known values of h_{int} to work out the ratio. To create a mammographic image, a film-screen characteristic curve is used to calculate the film density attained.

CHANGING THE TUBE VOLTAGE
28kVp   25kVp

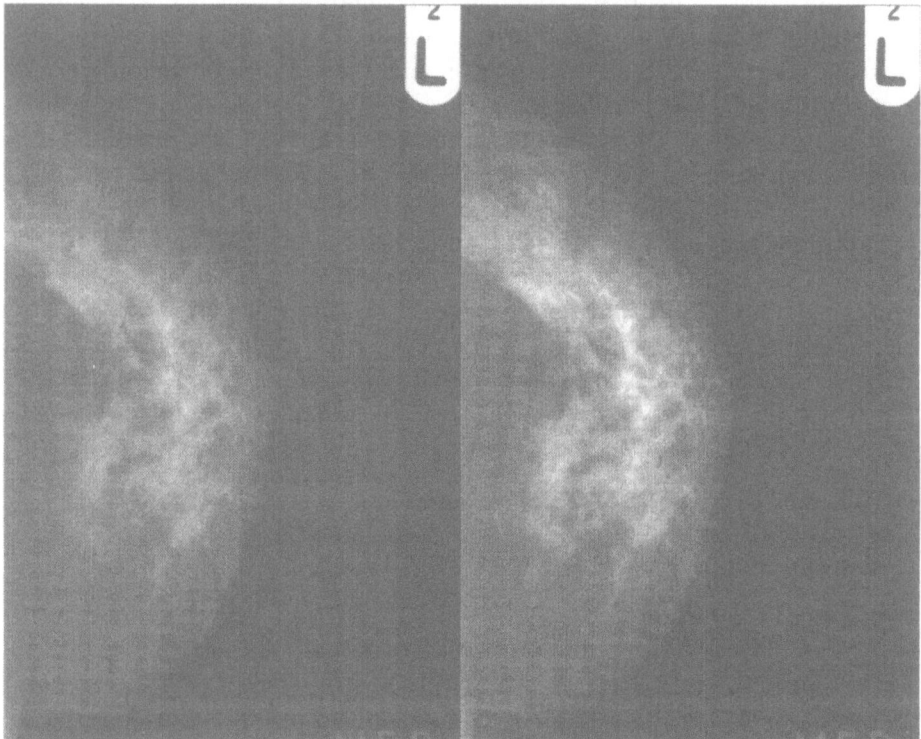

Figure 7.10.   The image on the left is the original mammogram taken at 28kVp. The image on the right is the mammogram simulated to appear as if the tube voltage was 25kVp. In practice, lower tube voltages incur greater radiation dose to the breast but give higher contrast.

Next we simulate a scatter-free monoenergetic examination . This time we use the h_{int} values explicitly. The chosen photon-energy for this examination is crucial to the contrast displayed in the final image because the difference in the linear attenuation coefficients is heavily dependent on the photon energy as can be seen by looking at the equations in Box 7.7. In practice, a low photon energy causes excessive radiation dose to the breast but contrast is greatest at the low photon energies. However, the problem with high contrast is that it does not allow a large range of values to be shown. The problem can be overcome to some extent by altering the value of exposure, to show a particular range of interest.

It is possible to automate the choice of photon energy and exposure by

---

BOX 7.7: Simulating a scatter-free monoenergetic examination

Let $\mathcal{E}$ be the photon energy chosen for the monoenergetic simulation, then the primary component of the signal at pixel (x, y) is given as follows:

$$E_p^{imp}(x, y) = N_0 \mathcal{E} e^{-\mu h(x, y; \mathcal{E})},$$

where N_0 is the number of photons, and $\mu h(x, y; \mathcal{E})$ is the estimate of the attenuation found from knowledge of h_{int} for the pixel and the linear attenuation coefficients at the appropriate energy. This equation can be expanded to illustrate the effect of the chosen energy on the simulation :

$$
\begin{aligned}
E_p^{imp}(x, y) &= N_0 \mathcal{E} e^{-\mu h(x, y; \mathcal{E})} \\
&= N_0 \mathcal{E} e^{-(\mu_{int}(\mathcal{E}) h_{int}(x, y) + \mu_{fat}(\mathcal{E}) h_{fat}(x, y))} \\
&= N_0 \mathcal{E} e^{-(\mu_{int}(\mathcal{E}) h_{int}(x, y) + \mu_{fat}(\mathcal{E})(H - h_{int}(x, y)))} \quad (H \text{ cm thick}) \\
&= N_0 \mathcal{E} e^{-H \mu_{fat}(\mathcal{E})} e^{-(\mu_{int}(\mathcal{E}) - \mu_{fat}(\mathcal{E})) h_{int}(x, y)} \quad (\text{rearrange})
\end{aligned}
$$

$$(7.16)$$

Across any image, the only factor in this equation that changes is $h_{int}(x, y)$ thus the value of $\mu_{int}(\mathcal{E}) - \mu_{fat}(\mathcal{E})$ is vital. Taking the film to be linear and assuming a perfect intensifying screen enables us to see the effects of different source photon energy:

$$D(x, y) = \gamma \log_{10} \beta E_p^{imp}(x, y)$$

In the simulation we keep the same film gradient (γ) as the original film. Note that β (which is related to system speed) and the number of incident photons (N_o) are multiplicative constants across the image, so that the value of β is of no great concern since the number of photons is to be manipulated by the automatic exposure control model. In terms of the final image, the amount of light transmitted through the theoretical film, T_l can be written as follows:

$$T_l(x, y) = \frac{I_l}{(\beta E_p^{imp}(x, y))^\gamma},$$

where I_l is the illuminating light intensity. Substituting Equation 7.16 in shows the importance of γ:

$$T_l(x, y) = \frac{I_l}{(\beta N_0 \mathcal{E})^\gamma} e^{H \mu_{fat}(\mathcal{E}) \gamma} e^{(\mu_{int}(\mathcal{E}) - \mu_{fat}(\mathcal{E})) h_{int}(x, y) \gamma} \quad (7.17)$$

---

performing an operation similar to an automatic exposure control. If the gradient of the characteristic curve (γ) is known, there are four unknowns in the monoenergetic equations. If values can be chosen then these unknowns can be computed as shown in Box 7.8.

BOX 7.8: Choosing photon energy and exposure time

Firstly, combine Equations 7.16 and 2.5:

$$
\begin{aligned}
D(x,y) &= \gamma \log_{10}(\beta N_o \mathcal{E} e^{-H\mu_{fat}(\mathcal{E})} e^{-(\mu_{int}(\mathcal{E})-\mu_{fat}(\mathcal{E}))h_{int}(x,y)}) \\
&= c - (\log_{10} e)(\mu_{int}(\mathcal{E}) - \mu_{fat}(\mathcal{E}))h_{int}(x,y)\gamma
\end{aligned}
$$

where

$$
c = \gamma \log_{10} \beta N_0 \mathcal{E} e^{-H\mu_{fat}(\mathcal{E})}
$$

The four unknowns are $h_{int}(x,y)$, $D(x,y)$, c and $\mathcal{E}$. If two values of h_{int} are to be set to two specific film densities, then the two unknowns k and $\mathcal{E}$ can be calculated. For example, one possible mapping of the maximum h_{int} is to a film density of 0.6 (the minimum film density displayable). Another possible mapping is the average h_{int} across the image to a film density of 1.5 (the usual AEC setting).

Notice that Box 7.7 uses the fact that the breast is H cm thick. As explained earlier, the breast thickness at the edge decreases rapidly and gives a low attenuation measure which is unaccountable for even by H cm of pure fat. We consider these areas to consist of pure fat and the attenuation found in this area is mapped to a thickness of fat only. The monoenergetic photon beam in the simulation is attenuated theoretically by this thickness of fat before reaching the film-screen combination at the breast edge.

Figure 7.11 shows an example of a monoenergetic examination at 18keV and Figure 7.12 shows the result of theoretically performing a monoenergetic examination on an image at three different photon energies: 15keV, 18keV, 24keV. At the low photon energies there is far too much contrast and the image is saturated, as the energy rises the contrast is reduced and the entire image can be viewed without saturation. Figure 7.13 shows a segment taken from a mammographic image before and after monoenergetic simulation. This contains microcalcifications which have been verified by a radiologist, and they have been greatly enhanced.

7.7. Summary: Image enhancement

In this chapter we have detailed several model-based image enhancement routines and explained the benefits that such an approach brings. We could perform exhaustive testing of these routines with regards to their benefit to the practising clinician but such testing is expensive and time-consuming. One of the key benefits of our approach is that before progressing to such expense we can be certain of the basic idea.

MONOENERGETIC SIMULATION
Polyenergetic (28kVp)   Monoenergetic (18keV)

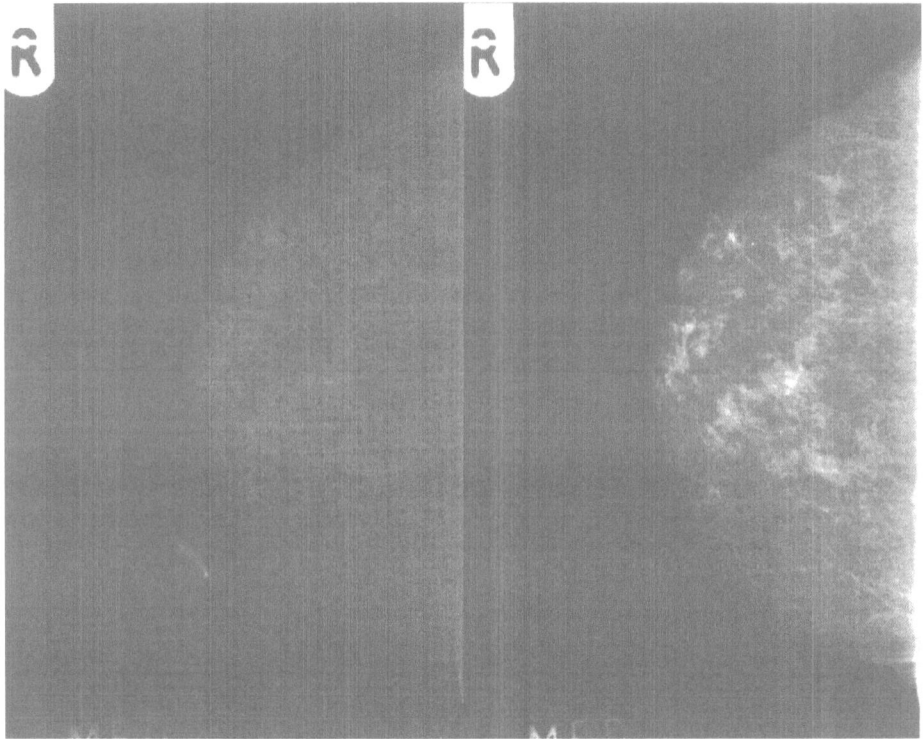

Figure 7.11. On the left is an original mammographic image. The breast was 5.55cm thick, the time of exposure was 0.705 seconds and the tube voltage 28kVp. On the right is a monoenergetic simulation at 18keV. There is some obvious shot noise in the image which can be removed during processing using the technique outlined in Chapter 11.

MONOENERGETIC SIMULATIONS
15keV   18keV   24keV

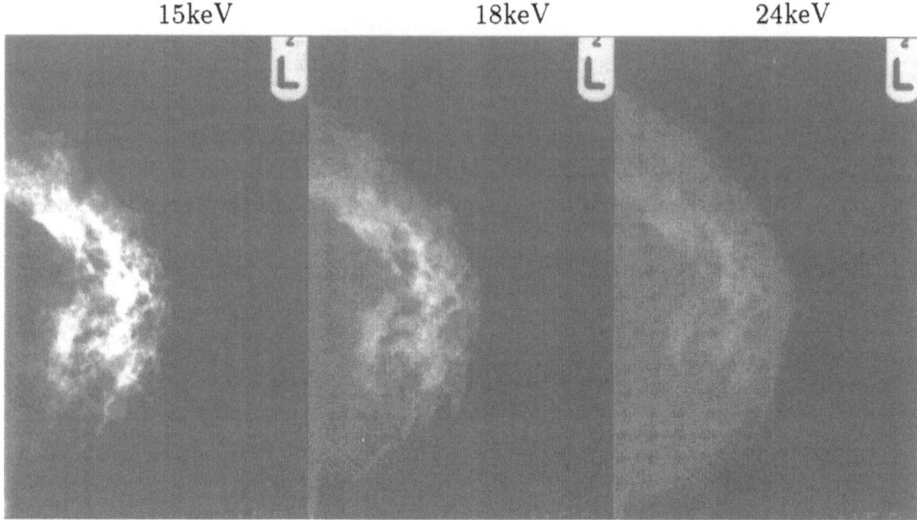

Figure 7.12.   This shows the result of different photon energies in the monoenergetic simulation, with the automatic exposure control set to give an average density of 1.5. The left image is for a photon energy of 15keV, the middle is 18keV and the right is 24keV. As the photon energy increases the contrast is reduced, and the dynamic range decreases allowing the image to be viewed without saturation.

Polyenergetic (28kVp)   Monoenergetic (18keV)

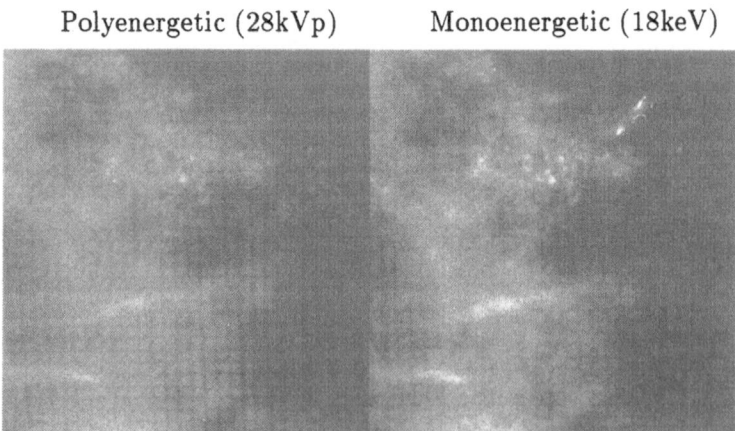

Figure 7.13.   The image on the left is the original mammogram. The image on the right is the result of a monoenergetic simulation at 18keV. The original is the same as shown in Figure 7.8 with and without scatter-correction.

CHAPTER 8

DISEASE SIMULATION

8.1. Introduction

We've shown how we can generate the h_{int} representation for any mammographic image and we've seen how each facet of the imaging process can be manipulated to enhance and restore the image. In this chapter, we present results that show how the h_{int} surface can be transformed prior to re-display in order to simulate change in anatomical structure or breast tissue. In particular, we simulate: the appearance of masses of various types in various contexts; microcalcifications; macrocalcifications; curvilinear structures. These simulations can be represented by:

$$D_{original}(x,y) \rightarrow h_{int}(x,y) \rightarrow h'_{int}(x,y) \rightarrow D_{simulated}(x,y).$$

The first and last steps are the same as in the previous chapter. First, we normalise the image by cutting out all the original imaging parameters and in the last step we choose a set of new parameters to display the transformed image. In this chapter we concentrate on the middle step which effectively transforms the breast tissue.

We contend that by realistically simulating anatomical structures we gain insight into:

- The 3D shape of anatomical structures found within the breast;
- The effects on anatomical structures of physical compression from different directions;
- The way that abnormal (both malignant and benign) structures interact with the local tissues;
- The tissue composition of anatomical structures.

This information will be useful for image processors in that it will help in devising reliable and robust features for image analysis, but it will also provide information to radiologists about the 3D shapes and compositions of abnormalities. Additionally, since tumours are rarely seen in a breast screening clinic the ability to summon up simulations on demand could be a powerful teaching tool as well as proving useful in testing image analysis algorithms.

8.2. Cysts

In this section we show how to use the h_{int} surface to simulate how a cyst might appear in a mammogram. The mammogram we use is from a real asymptomatic woman. Our aim is to show what the image would look like if a cyst were to develop in the breast. To make the point as simply as possible, in an initial experiment, we model the cyst simply as a sphere. Let $h_{int}^{cyst}(x, y)$ be the corresponding interesting tissue values, where the value at (x, y) represents the thickness of interesting tissue above that spatial position within the cyst. This thickness is found by multiplying the thickness of the sphere $h_{thick}^{sphere}(x, y)$ by a "mass composition value":

$$h_{int}^{cyst}(x, y) = h_{thick}^{sphere}(x, y) \times \text{mass composition}$$

The mass composition value represents the proportion of interesting tissue to fatty tissue within the cyst; this is assumed uniform throughout the cyst. In our preliminary experiments, it appears that this value should be lower for cysts than malignant masses. This conforms to the description of benign masses tending to be of "lower density" than malignant masses.

The simulation starts with the breast image being converted to its interesting tissue surface representation which we call h_{int}^{breast} here. Let S be the set of pixels that the sphere covers when projected onto the image, then the new surface is given as follows:

$$h_{int}^{breast\prime}(x, y) = \begin{cases} h_{int}^{breast}(x, y), & (x, y) \notin S \\ h_{int}^{breast}(x, y) + h_{int}^{cyst}(x, y), & (x, y) \in S \end{cases}$$

Note that in doing this, we are implicitly assuming not only that the cyst develops separately from the breast tissue, but that it doesn't displace interesting tissue either, only fat. Although this might be appropriate for benign lesions, it is unlikely to be correct for malignant lesions, where in radiology parlance, "masses pull in the surrounding tissues" which can lead to "architectural distortions".

Having added in the appropriate h_{int}^{cyst} values, the mammographic imaging process is then simulated to show how the new $h_{int}^{breast\prime}$ surface would appear. Figure 8.1 shows the result from two such simulations using mass compositions of just 0.5. Figure 8.2 shows the result from imposing a mass into the left breast with the shape of the cyst from the right breast and a mass composition of 0.4.

8.3. Malignant masses

Malignant lesions tend to have more irregular outlines than cysts. Currently, to simulate a malignant mass we simply extract an outline malignant mass shape from one image, and "place it" into the h_{int} surface of

SIMULATION OF A CYST
Genuine cyst   Simulated cysts

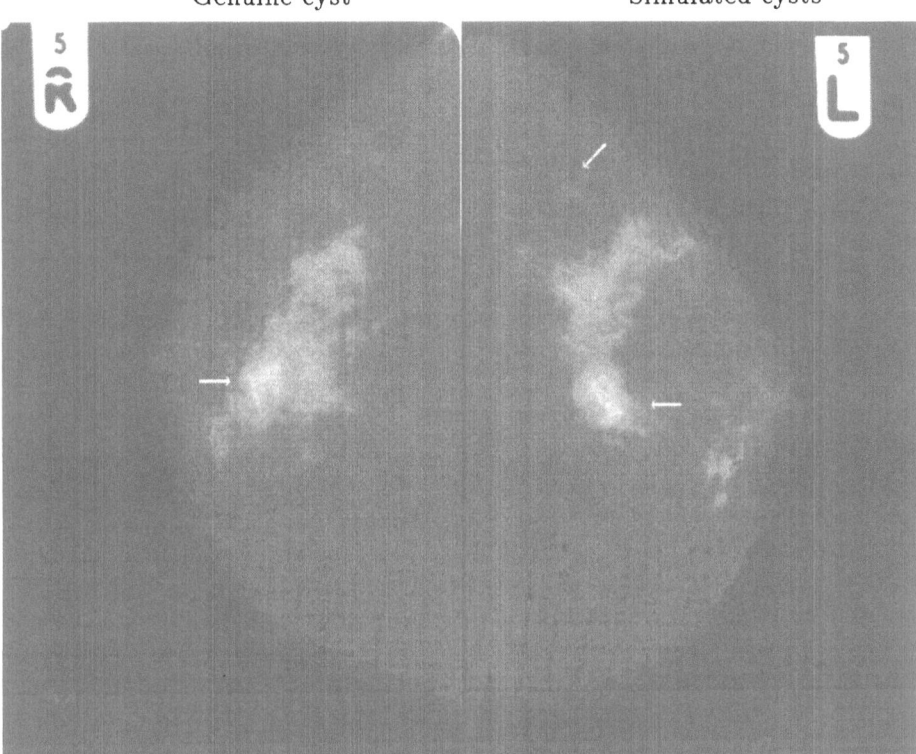

Figure 8.1.   In the right breast there is a round cyst immersed in fibroglandular tissue just behind the nipple. In the left breast there have been two spheres implanted with mass compositions of 0.5. Towards the top of the breast there is a 1cm diameter sphere, and near the middle of the breast theres a 2cm diameter sphere.

another breast image. The underlying three-dimensional shape of the mass is again assumed to be spherical. This shape is implemented using binary morphological erosion to define layers within the mass, and then the spherical model is used to find the thickness of the mass for each layer. This thickness is multiplied by a mass composition value to attain the thickness of interesting tissue due to the mass. Malignant masses probably consist almost entirely of interesting tissue and we've seen that mass composition values of over 0.9 provide realistic results. Figure 8.3 shows an example of a simulation of a malignant mass. Current work considers simulating spicules and automatically computing the mass composition value.

SIMULATION OF A CYST

Genuine cyst   Simulated cyst

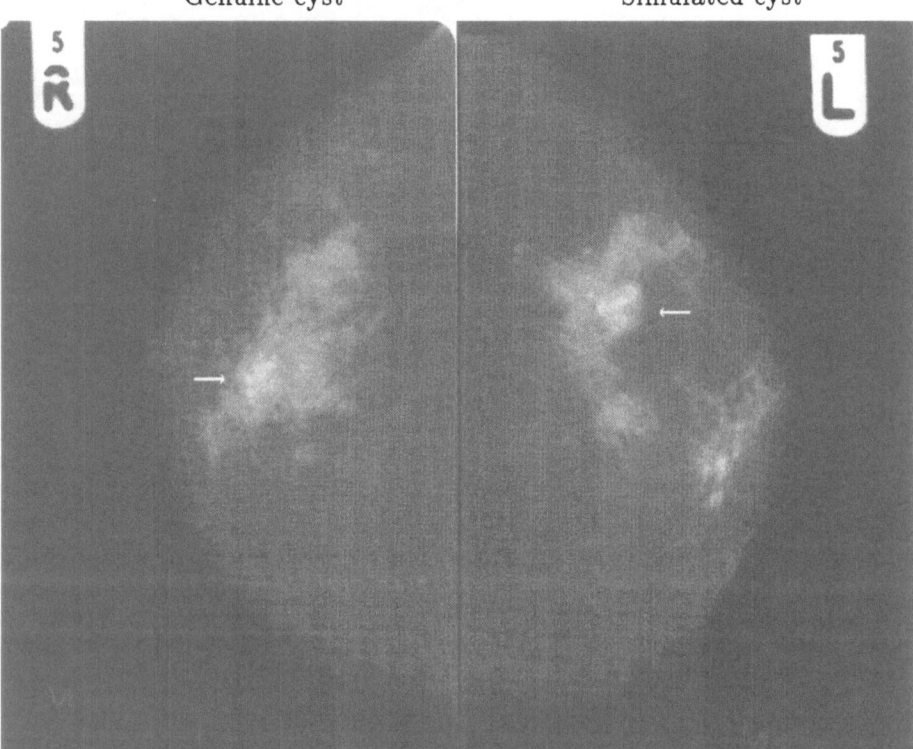

Figure 8.2.   In the right breast there is a round cyst immersed in fibroglandular tissue just behind the nipple. The shape of this cyst was manually extracted and then a 3D model of the cyst was formed by rotating the shape to form a volume of revolution. At each pixel within the cyst we now have a total thickness, we multiply that thickness by a mass composition value (in this case we used 0.4) to get the thickness of interesting tissue within the cyst at that pixel. These thicknesses were then added to the h_{int} surface of the left breast and the x-ray process simulated to produce the simulated cyst just above the centre of the left breast.

SIMULATION OF A MALIGNANT MASS

Simulated mass   Genuine mass

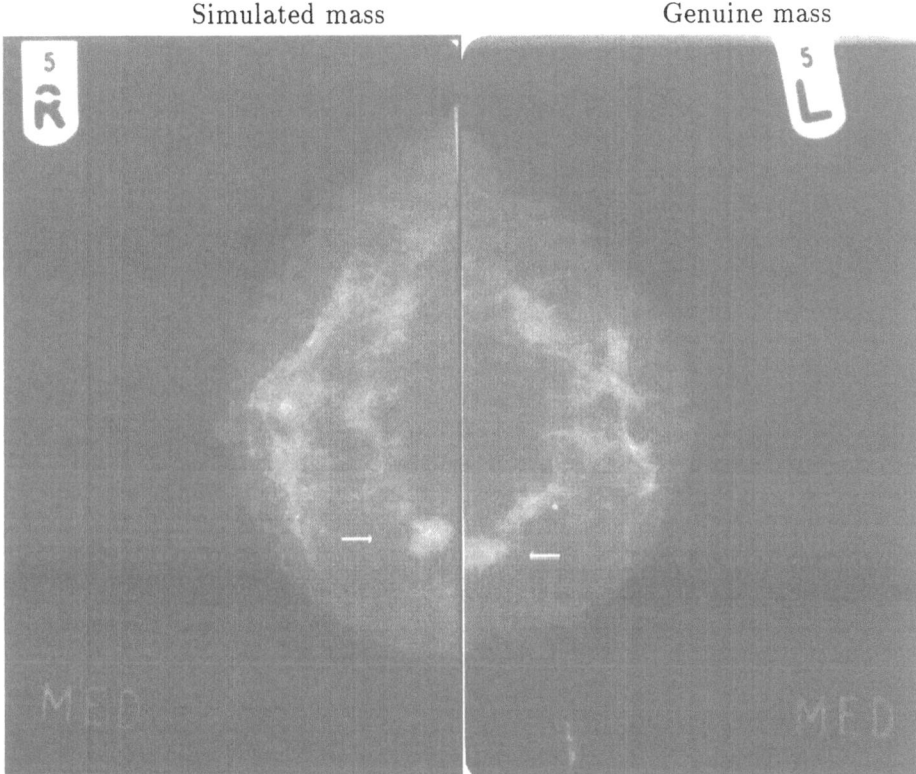

Figure 8.3.   In the right breast there is a malignant mass near the chest wall. The shape of the mass was manually extracted and a 3D model was formed by eroding the mass into layers and then estimating the height of the mass in each layer from a spherical model. This height was then multiplied by a mass composition value. We've found that high values have to be used for malignant masses (in this case 1.0), whereas benign masses require lower values to be realistic. The 3D model was then added to the h_{int} surface for the right breast and the x-ray process simulated.

8.4. Curvilinear structures

Further simulations involve much smaller anatomical structures, namely curvilinear structures (CLS). Simulating various size structures and matching with actual images allows models of the CLS to be proposed and their appearance in images and responses to feature detectors calculated. These models can be used to support the work discussed in Chapter 12. CLS modelled with elliptical cross-sections are shown in Figure 8.4.

SIMULATION OF CURVI-LINEAR STRUCTURES

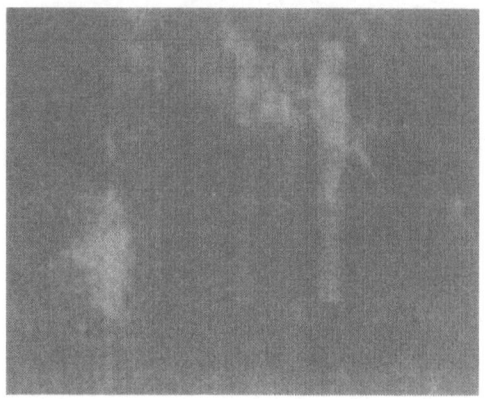

Figure 8.4.   In this example four linear structures have been "implanted" into the breast and a polyenergetic x-ray simulation performed. The linear structure on the left apparently passes through the area of increased density (brightness) much as a vessel might if it were really above or below the tissue volume that is projected onto that area. The four implanted structures all have elliptic cross-sections of varying radii. Varying the cross-sectional model allows us to investigate the effects of breast compression on curvilinear structures by comparing the simulations with real images.

8.5. Calcifications

Figure 8.5 shows examples of simulating calcifications. Calcifications push the x-ray model to its limits due to their high x-ray attenuation and small size. For example, calcifications implanted into breasts without modelling glare appear far too sharp and bright to be realistic. Figure 8.6 shows simulations of coarse calcifications.

SIMULATION OF MICROCALCIFICATIONS
Original   "Real" model   Spherical model

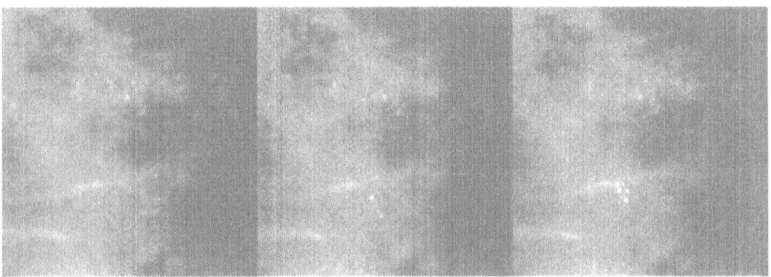

Figure 8.5. The image on the left is a sample at 100 microns of an original mammographic image containing microcalcifications. Using the rise in attenuation at the site of the microcalcifications it is possible using the h_{int} representation to estimate the thickness of the microcalcification. In this example the largest calcification is estimated to be 250 microns in thickness at its peak. Using the thickness, simulated calcifications were added to the lower part of the image and then the x-ray process was simulated. The middle image shows the result of the x-ray simulation. The image on the right shows the result of adding to the original h_{int} image several 200 micron spherical calcifications along with a few 100 micron ones which are hardly visible.

SIMULATION OF MACROCALCIFICATIONS

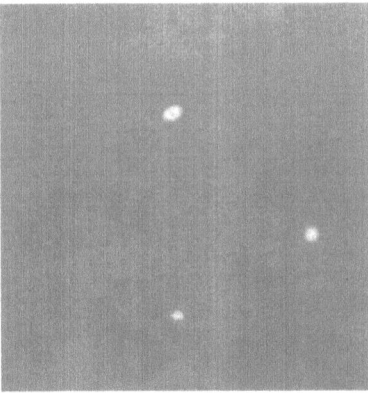

Figure 8.6. This 100 micron image has a genuine coarse calcification towards the top. The other two bright shapes are simulated using a sphere and ellipse as basic models. The thickness of calcification is taken to be 1.5mm maximum for each of the two simulated ones.

BOX 8.1: Disease simulation

(1) Compute the h_{int}^{breast} values for the mammogram

(2) Choose a disease shape, 3D model and mass composition value and then compute h_{int}^{object}

(3) Add h_{int}^{object} to h_{int}^{breast} to give the new "altered" h_{int} values

(4) Simulate an x-ray examination

8.6. Summary: Disease simulation

We have shown how disease simulation can take place using the h_{int} representation and this is summarised in Box 8.1. More realistic simulation will involve understanding the complex shapes that some objects present which in itself is an immensely interesting research area and one which will benefit enormously from disease models. The other key area for realistic simulation is breast compression and that is the topic of the next chapter.

CHAPTER 9

BREAST COMPRESSION

9.1. Introduction

This chapter analyses the effects of breast compression in mammography. There are three key reasons for our interest:

(i) We believe that it might be possible to determine hardness of tissue and tissue connectivity on the basis of knowing how the tissue moves and deforms with compression. We describe in this chapter a technique which we have dubbed "differential compression mammography" that aims to show movement and deformation.

(ii) Automated image analysis must be robust to changes in the imaging conditions and to changes in the breast which are not clinically significant. Earlier chapters have dealt with modelling the mammographic imaging process in order to ensure robustness to changes in the imaging condition. In this chapter, we consider robustness to changes in breast compression and show the improvements to image analysis possible using h_{int}.

(iii) Matching between cranio-caudal and medio-lateral oblique mammograms is difficult, not because of the change in viewing angle; but because of the change in direction of the breast compression. We report our initial work[1] on matching between cranio-caudal and medio-lateral oblique image pairs which has already proved to be useful to radiologists, for whom establishing such correspondences turns out to be remarkably hard.

The chapter begins by reviewing the literature on breast compression. We then introduce, and explain with examples, the new technique "differential compression mammography". Then, it is shown how to use h_{int} to aid the examination of mammograms at different compressions. Furthermore, it's shown how using h_{int} should enable image analysis routines to be more robust to compression. Finally, we present a model of compression and show how to use it to determine correspondences.

---

[1]We acknowledge gratefully the key role played by our colleague Yasuyo Kita.

9.2. Literature survey

Although this chapter is primarily about using the changes in the mammograms which occur with different amounts of breast compression, it is
also relevant to questions regarding the amount of compression needed for
mammography. As we said earlier, the benefits of breast compression in
mammography are well known: reduction of motion artifacts by immobilizing the breast and reducing the time-of-exposure; reduction of geometric
blur; reduction of film density range through more uniform breast thickness;
reduction of scattered radiation; improved separation of tissue structures
through increased projected area; dose reduction.

A number of authors have commented on the radiographic effects of
breast compression which they have observed: Roebuck [209] noted how
with magnification mammography the tissues can be displaced differently
and composite shadows can disappear. Peters et al. [197] noted that the apparent size of tension cysts depends on the forcefulness of the compression,
and they suggested that this information might be useful to differentiate
cysts from solid masses. Pennes et al. [196] cited a case where a cyst appeared to rupture due to compression.

Remarkably little has been published about the effect of compression
on the breast itself: Jackson et al. [132] undertook a survey of discomfort
felt, correlating the results with the menstrual cycle; Clark et al.[45] and
Russell et al.[46] measured the pressure applied to the breast during compression; Sullivan et al. [232] measured the force applied and correlated this
with perceived discomfort; Fife [73, 107] surveyed the average dimensions
of the compressed breast; Eklund [65] discussed the vague terms used to
describe breast compression (e.g. "appropriate", "adequate"), arguing that
compression is an art rather than a science. Yancey et al. [264] explained
the difficulty of viewing deep lesions with conventional compression mammography and showed how with an adhesive dressing the breast can be pre-
stretched before compression to aid visualisation; Watmough [252] stressed
the need for safety limits on the compressive force and expressed concern
that breast compression can cause cancer cells, if present, to spread so that
metastasis becomes more likely [253].

The most comprehensive study of the effects of compression on the
breast to date appears to be that of Novak [187], who studied compression
from the perspective of localisation. He drew lines and circles onto breasts
and then noted how they translated, deformed and rotated with cranio-
caudal, lateral-medial and medio-lateral oblique compression. Amongst many
interesting observations, he showed that there is rarely rotation of the breast
during cranio-caudal compression and that the glandular tissue has the
same longitudinal extent in all three views. The model of breast compres-

sion we present later in this chapter uses the work of Novak to justify several assumptions, as does the work in Chapter 13 on matching mammograms.

The only model of the breast which we have been able to find in the literature deals with thermal modelling [189, 190]. Models of soft connective tissues [64, 133, 227], skin mechanics [188] and flow induced deformation of soft tissues [10] have been published and these might form the basis of some prediction of how fibrous and adipose tissue might react/deform when the normal breast is compressed; but we are unaware of any work dealing with glandular tissue or neoplasms. However, this biomechanical approach does yield some interesting ideas. As Terrance Ryan (private communication) notes, fibrous and adipose tissues in the breast are designed for specific functions, notably to resist gravity and to protect the organ; cancerous and other abnormal tissues within the breast are unlikely to have such a role, thereby possibly reacting differently to deforming forces.

There is a surprising lack of literature on breast tissues in fields such as breast reconstruction and brassiere design. The only attempt at gaining any quantitative measure of the breast tissue appears to have been in determining the firmness of the breast after reconstruction in order to gain a measure of fibrous capsule formation. These measures have been derived using calipers [30, 96] and applanation tonometry [176, 95].

Perhaps the published results that are closest to the work contained in this chapter concern ultrasound imaging. Parker et al. [192] found that preliminary results indicate order-of-magnitude differences between the stiffness of different tissue specimens. Ueno et al. [245] looked at measuring compressibility and mobility using ultrasound. They differentiate cysts, cancer and fibroadenomas on the grounds that cysts are soft and mobile, fibroadenomas are usually soft and may be deformed by pressure, whereas cancers are not deformed and do not roll when compressed. Developing an elastic model of large scale breast deformation remains an open problem. We return to ultrasound on Page 346 in Chapter 15.

9.3. Differential compression mammography

Introduction

Differential compression mammography [122, 123, 124, 119] is a novel way of obtaining information about the internal properties of the breast, by comparing mammograms taken with the breast compressed at different thicknesses. For example, a mammogram might be taken with the breast compressed to a thickness of 5 centimetres, followed by a second mammogram with the breast slightly less compressed to a thickness of 5.5 centimetres. The movement and deformation which is seen by comparing these two mammograms is linked to the physical properties of the breast: mammographic signs which do not change position between the two mammograms might be fixed in some manner (e.g. by spicules to the chest wall); mammographic signs whose appearance does not change might represent solid tissue structures (e.g. a malignant tumour). We believe that having more reliable information about the deeper tissues and internal breast structures would aid more accurate diagnosis. Differential compression mammography seems unattractive in practice because it requires a double dose of x-rays. However, the technique developed in Chapter 10 might allow us to halve the dose per x-ray so that the overall effect is to retain the current radiation dose.

Data collection

Women attending an assessment clinic (after referal from a screening round) were asked, in full accordance with ethics committee directives, whether they would volunteer to have an extra mammogram performed at slightly less compression. The procedure of the clinic was as normal except that two cranio-caudal view mammograms were taken for each breast. The first mammogram was taken at full (normal) compression, the compression plate raised slightly and another mammogram taken. Taking the extra mammogram required an additional 30 seconds and since the positions of the features within the mammograms were to be considered, it was important that the breast did not move significantly in this time. The back edge of the mammogram (by the chest wall) provides a reference line with which to measure absolute movement.

The decision to take the mammogram at maximum compression first was based purely on practical considerations: the radiographers felt that they could not easily judge when they were close to the maximum compression without actually reaching it, and the woman involved might reasonably be dismayed to learn after the first mammogram, that a second was to be taken with more compression. The difference in compression had to be large enough to produce differences, while at the same time being small enough to produce a usable quality mammogram. It was found that releasing the compression between 0.5cm and 1cm gave useful results.

When doing any differential study, care must be taken to isolate the effects of the factor being studied from other effects. In this case, the effects of extra compression are confounded with the effects of changing geometry and x-ray exposure. The changing geometry between the two mammograms can cause a small increase in the size of signs in the more compressed mammogram (potentially caused by the signs being further away from the x-ray source), and possibly an amplification or reduction of movement (depending on which way the object of interest moves with respect to the x-ray source). The exposure time is set by the machine's automatic exposure control and will inevitably be far greater in the less compressed case. Although this should give the same average film density above the automatic exposure control, other factors such as scattered radiation will vary. The difference in exposure removes the possibility of directly using the brightness of the areas to see tissue spreading out: if the exposure had been the same, one might have expected to see small bright areas representing normal soft tissue disperse into larger but less bright areas. By now the reader will not be surprised when we recall that using the h_{int} representation we are able to transform the images to show this.

The pairs of mammograms produced in the trial were studied both as films and on a video in which the mammograms in each pair were alternated quickly; this later provides a vivid impression of the movement and deformation which is taking place. The advent and use of digital mammography will make such presentation of the mammograms straightforward (the CD-ROM that accompanies [117] shows one such movie). Some of the features are readily apparent in each mammogram separately but others can only be spotted using the motion cues provided by alternating the images in rapid succession (psychophysically, the illusion of motion from two images presented in rapid succession is known as the "phi-phenomenon" and is effective in that it engages the exquisite human motion perception processes).

Examples

We start with an example which illustrates how essential breast compression is. Figure 9.1 shows two cranio-caudal images of the same breast under different compressions. There is a cyst towards the chest wall which is only obvious with maximum compression.

Figure 9.2 shows two cranio-caudal images of the same breast under different compressions. There is a spiculated mass in the breast. With increased compression the mass does not shift position whilst tissue around it moves appreciably and deforms. Figure 9.3 shows another example of differential compression mammography with a spiculated lesion. This example shows how important compression can be in making a lesion visible. In this case, the lesion appears to be hidden by fibroglandular tissue when the breast isn't firmly compressed.

Figure 9.4 shows another pair of cranio-caudal images of a breast under different compressions. These images are interesting not only because of the changes due to compression but also because of the difference in brightness between the two images due to the changing imaging conditions (i.e. time of

DIFFERENTIAL COMPRESSION MAMMOGRAPHY: CYST

8cm   7cm

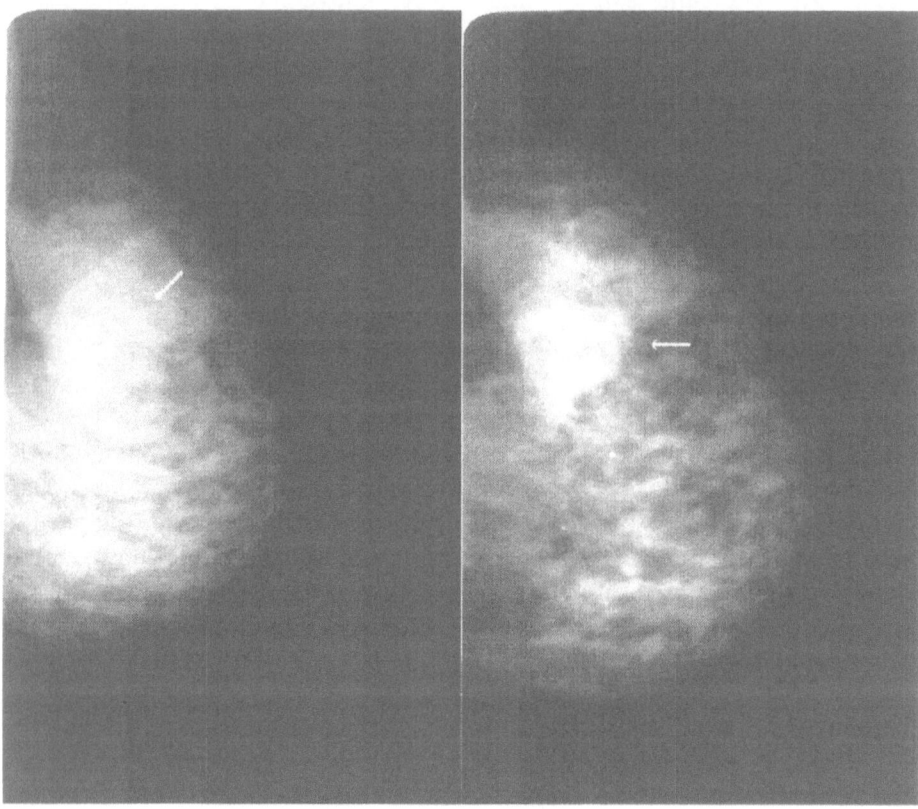

Figure 9.1. These show two mammograms of the same breast under different compressions. On the left the breast is compressed to 8cm, and on the right the breast is compressed to 7cm (these thicknesses were as reported by the radiographers). In this example there is a cyst towards the chest wall which is only obvious in the right image. Some of the features, notably the coarse calcifications, show large movement with compression.

exposure). These two mammograms show that as the breast is compressed blood vessels "disappear". Since blood vessels entering a mass is a sign of increased chance of malignancy, it might be prudent in certain cases to not compress the breast so tightly. This case illustrates one of the problems with mammography: there are many confounding effects. In this case, just because there appears to be no vessels going into the mass doesn't mean that the mass is not malignant, it means that either there are actually no

DIFFERENTIAL COMPRESSION MAMMOGRAPHY:
SPICULATED MASS

6.5cm   6.0cm

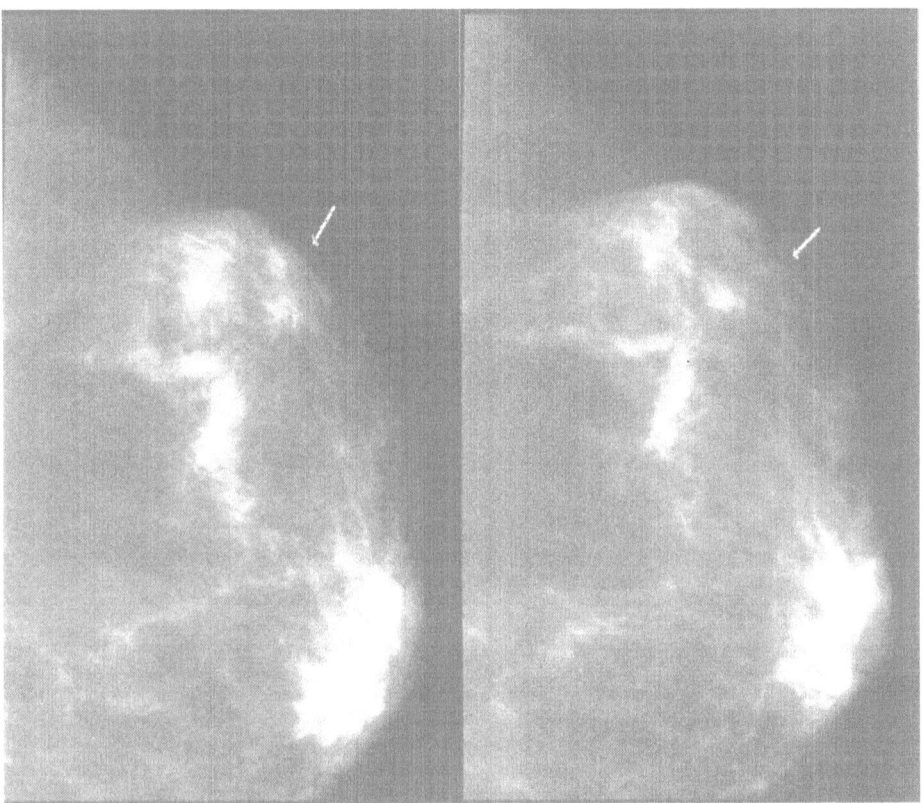

Figure 9.2. These show cranio-caudal view mammograms of the same breast of a 51 year old woman under different compressions. On the left the breast is compressed to 6.5cm, and on the right the breast is compressed to 6cm. In this example there is a spiculated mass which displays relatively little movement compared to the tissue that is positioned next to it. This spiculated mass has spicules which appear to reach the chest wall.

vessels going into the mass or that the breast has been firmly compressed.

Figure 9.5 shows examples of microcalcifications under differential compression. The figure also shows scatter-free monoenergetic simulations at 18keV which show the details more clearly. The cluster obviously changes formation with compression, and the change cannot be due solely to geometry. It is evident from this example that attempts to correlate properties of microcalcification clusters to malignancy (e.g. average distance between

DIFFERENTIAL COMPRESSION MAMMOGRAPHY:
SPICULATED MASS

6.5cm   5.5cm

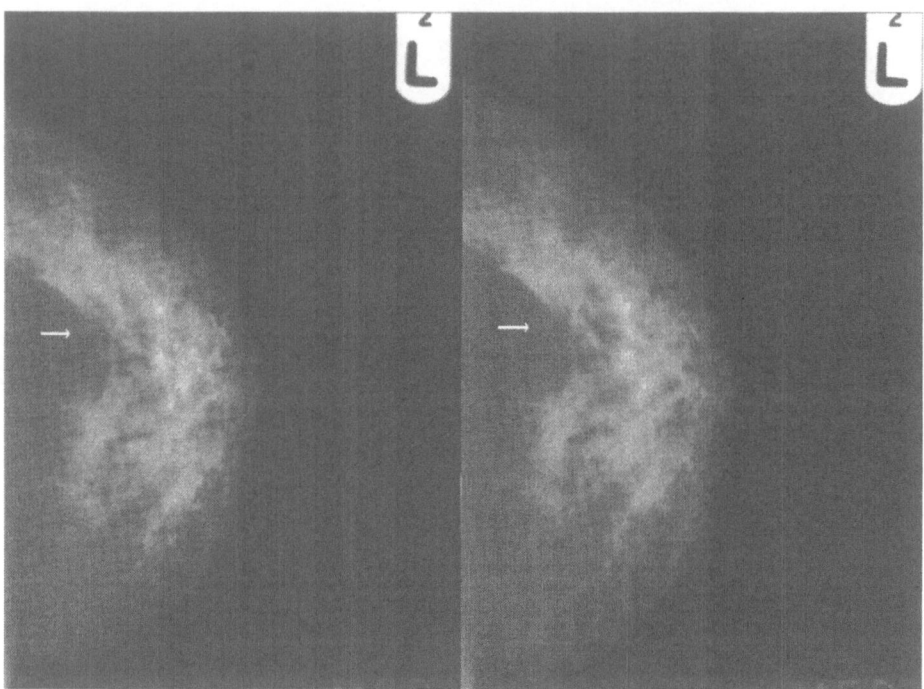

Figure 9.3.   These show cranio-caudal view mammograms of the same breast under different compressions. On the left the breast is compressed to 6.5cm, and on the right the breast is compressed to 5.5cm. There is a spiculated mass close to the centre of the breast image. With the reduction in compression fibroglandular tissue appears to cover the mass somewhat. When viewed as a movie this image presents an impression that the spiculated mass is being held stationary and that the fibroglandular tissue is shifting over it.

particles) should also take account of the effects of compression. This is particularly important if the mammograms being used in the study were performed by more than one radiographer, or were from different centres, since it is highly likely that different compression will be applied.

DIFFERENTIAL COMPRESSION MAMMOGRAPHY: VESSELS

6.5cm   5.5cm

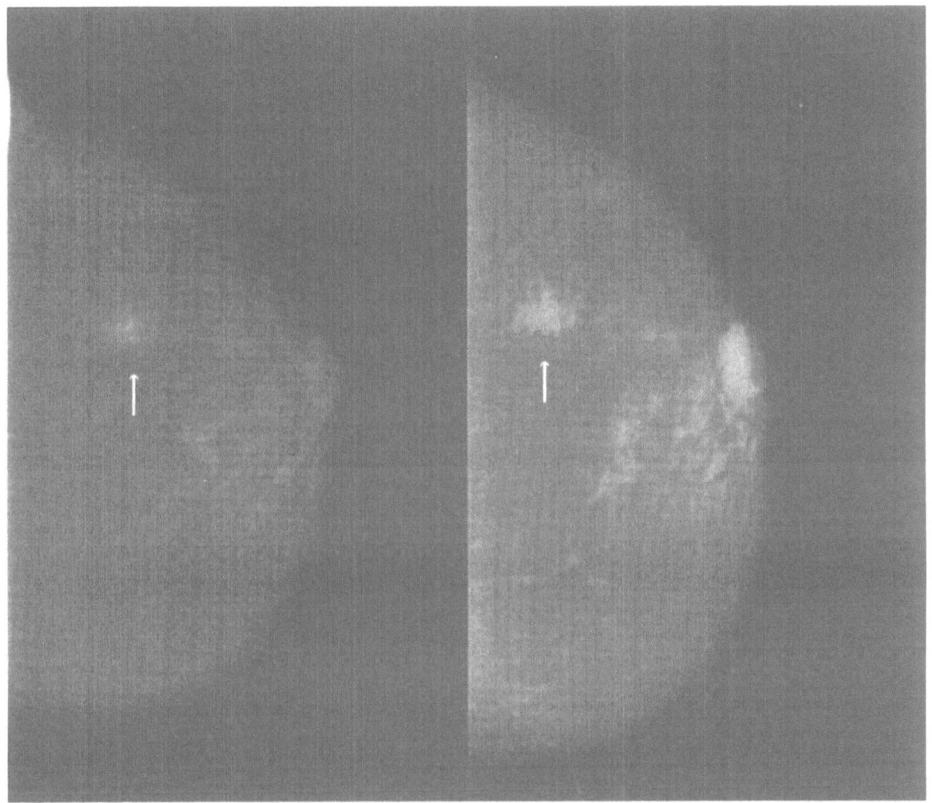

Figure 9.4. These show cranio-caudal view mammograms of the same breast of a 60 year old woman under different compressions. There is a suspect mass in the breast which turned out to be benign. On the left the breast is compressed to 6.5cm, and on the right the breast is compressed to 5.5cm. In this example the blood vessels evident under less compression have practically disappeared in the right mammogram. If increased vascularity is an indicator of cancer it might be better to image the breast under less compression than normal so that vessels going into masses can be visualised on the mammogram.

DIFFERENTIAL COMPRESSION MAMMOGRAPHY:
CALCIFICATIONS

6.1cm   5.4cm

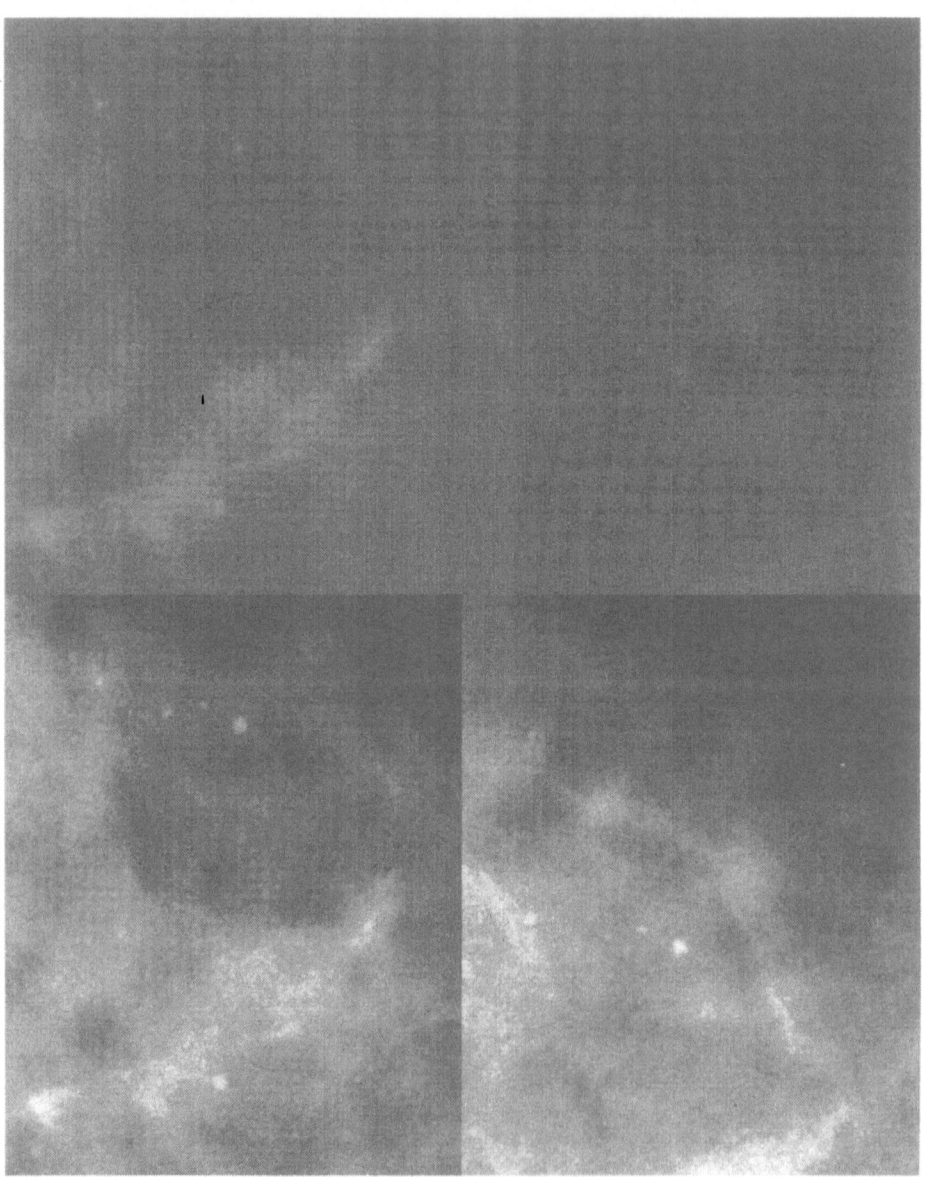

Figure 9.5. The top images show some microcalcifications with maximum compression 5.4cm on the right, and slightly less compression on the left 6.1cm. The lower images are enhanced versions of the top images. See text.

In related work, Brettle et al. [23] have used differential compression mammography to study how fibrous septa move in the breast with compression. They found that they were able to get a good impression of how the septa move and note that there appears to be differences between the movement around ill-defined masses and in normal breasts. For ill-defined masses they noted curved septa becoming straight, indicating tethering.

They note the potential for using differential compression mammography for studying architectural distortion and to look at certain lesions looking benign on ultrasound and ill-defined mammographically. They also observe however, that medullary and mucinous carcinoma rarely tether, so caution should be exercised. The images shown in this chapter have been the images as they appear on a light-box, that is, they are "transmitted light images". As stated in the previous section, the imaging process varies between the mammograms at different compressions so that brightness cannot be used as an indicator of tissue spreading (or not spreading as the case may be). However, if we map the images to h_{int} and then display those images with comparable scaling then we are able to use brightness. Figure 9.6 shows one such pair transformed.

Discussion

Some of the movement observed in differently compressed mammograms is quite dramatic considering the small differences in compression used. These movements are unlikely to be due to any major shift of the breast position between compressions, since that would be noticeable by comparison of the projected breast edge and total projected breast areas. The large movements might explain the difficulty which sometimes occurs when dealing with localisation. The differing motion of features over the mammogram, even when they are projected close to each other, probably comes from them being representative of tissues at different heights within the breast. For example, a superior mass might move far more than an inferior mass.

One aspect which has not been considered in our work to date is symmetry of movement and deformation between left and right breasts. It may well be that, just as mammograms of left and right breasts are checked for symmetry, so the movement and deformation should also be in some way similar. This comparison would be useful even if it only involved observing similar occurrences between left and right breasts.

The study of spiculations as a mammographic sign is particularly interesting because of their apparent "function" in holding a mass onto other breast structures, be it the local tissue or the chest wall. Similarly, two mammograms depicting a mass moving with a great deal of the local tissue

DIFFERENTIAL COMPRESSION MAMMOGRAPHY: h_{int}

5.5cm   5.1cm

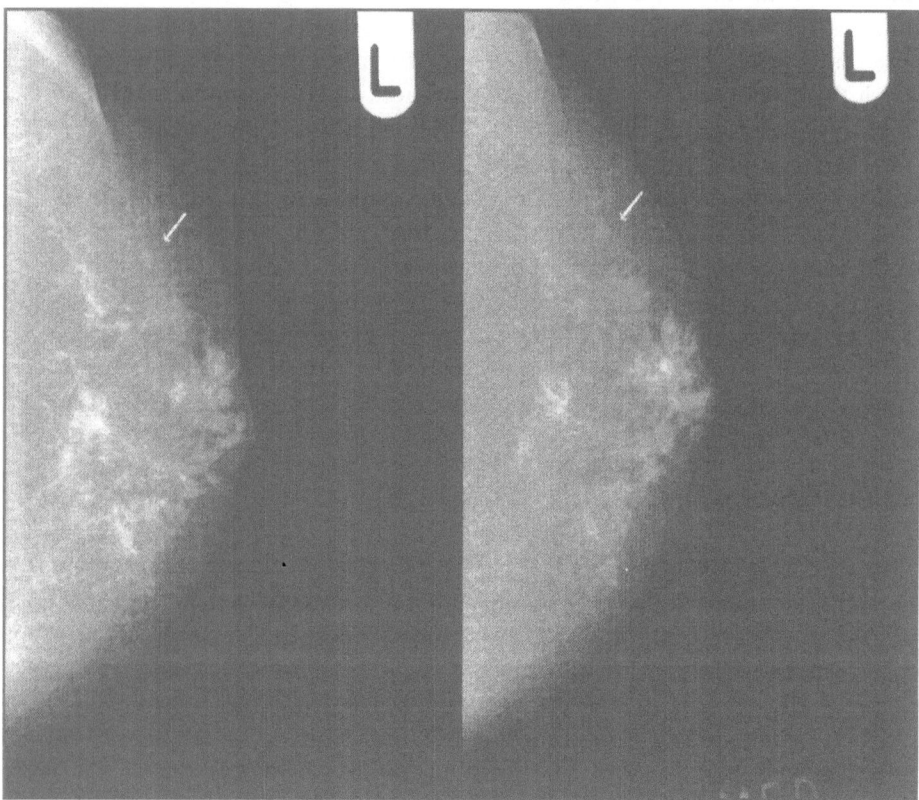

Figure 9.6. On the left the breast is compressed to 5.5cm and the exposure was 91mAs. On the right the breast was compressed to 5.1cm and the exposure was 76mAs. Instead of displaying the original images here we display the h_{int} images scaled and discretized using the same values so that changes in the pixel values have physical significance. In this case we see that, as expected, the image is darker with more compression: there is less h_{int} at each pixel because the breast is spread out. As an example, note the rounded opacity "above and to the left" of the nipple has darkened and larger in projected size. Some of the areas near the nipple get brighter with compression as they overlap each other.

attached to it, or moving relatively independently of the local tissue, might help the radiologist to decide whether a tumour is invasive or *in situ*. This kind of observation could be taken into account in deciding how much of the breast should be removed after diagnosis of cancer.

Magnification mammography goes some way towards taking mammograms at two different compressions, in that radiologists sometimes use it to see whether a particular sign disappears with a different compression. However, this technique doesn't provide a second image for reference, which can be directly compared to the original. It follows that, although gross comparisons can be made, detailed ones cannot. It might be that taking two mammograms with magnification at different compressions provides a much more detailed and explicit picture of the deformation and movement, as well as bringing larger, more specific deforming forces to bear. Whilst this form of differential magnification mammography is interesting, extreme care will have to be taken due to the magnification of size and movement from the changing geometry.

The decision to take mammograms at just two compressions was based solely on ethical grounds due to radiation. Essentially, compression is a continuously variable parameter that we have sampled at two points. We have shown how important the choice of the sample point is, and the additional information made available by a second image. Radiation dose prevents a greater sample set, but such a possibility should be taken into account in any mathematical model of mammography.

9.4. Breast compression and image analysis

We have stressed throughout that transforming a mammogram to the h_{int} representation normalises the mammogram, but further normalisation of the features is necessary for two reasons. The first is that breasts can compress to different thicknesses. The second is that breast composition is highly variable, and an object such as a cyst might be projected onto fat in one image, and onto dense fibroglandular tissue in another. As an example of the susceptibility of features to changes in the background, consider the effect of the breast being less compressed. Figure 9.7 shows a contrast measure on a breast at full and slightly less compression.

Successful normalisation provides consistency in feature values for the same tissue type within the same image and between different images; but also enables differentiation of tissue types. In this section, we look at how we should normalise h_{int} images and feature measurements.

The first point to note is that there has been little research that considers anatomical structure size relative to compressed breast thickness. In the absence of evidence to the contrary, and in the belief that most anatomical structures are from local processes, we assume that disease processes are primarily spatially localised and that feature size is independent of breast thickness H. This means that we should *not* scale the h_{int} images to a standard breast size and then look for a standard size feature; rather we should

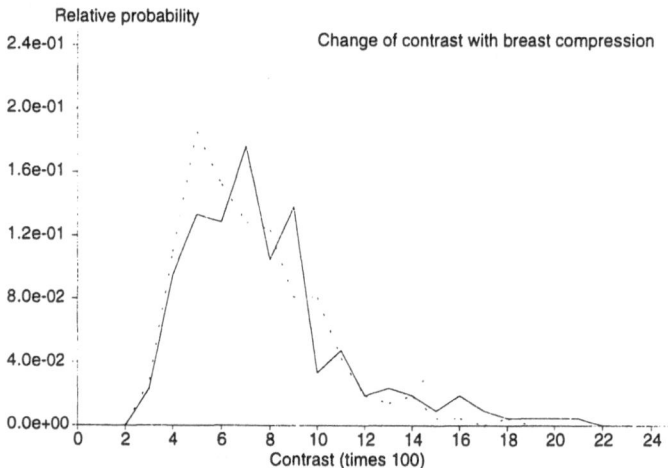

Figure 9.7. This shows the relative distribution of contrast values within a film density image of a volume of fibroglandular tissue. The continuous curve shows the feature distribution on a breast at full compression; the dotted curve shows the feature distribution at less compression.

take the h_{int} images and look for a standard size feature in them.

Another problem with scaling on H is that it can lead to h_{int} values which have little or no relation to the projected spatial size of a feature. For example, a 2cm projected diameter cyst might be mapped to have an apparent depth of 3cm. Indeed, we consider the relationship between projected spatial size and h_{int} value to be of primary importance since it gives an indication of mass density (proportion of interesting tissue to fat) and this might be useful for diagnosis as explained in Chapter 8.

Some simple models of compression are:

M1 Fat compresses and moves, whereas interesting tissue does not compress and remains stationary, where we use "compress" to mean that the tissue deforms;

M2 As **M1** but the interesting tissue moves; but does not compress;

M3 Compression removes a constant value from both h_{int} and h_{fat} across the image. Effectively, this assumes that interesting tissue and fat both compress; but that the interesting tissue does not move.

M4 Both tissue types compress and move.

Model **M1** is the conventional approach to breast compression: "It is only the fat that compresses, the rest stays essentially the same." It can be mod-

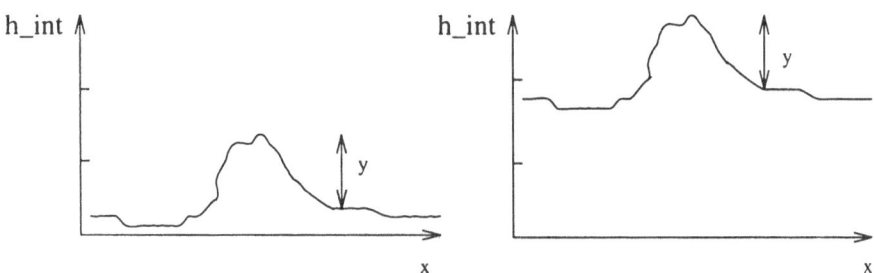

Figure 9.8. Here the same mass is in two different surrounds: one representing a fatty breast (left) and one a dense breast (right). In this scenario many so-called normalised feature measures fail despite the height of the mass above the surroundings (y) being the same.

elled as adding or subtracting a layer of fat from the breast. If this is the case, then any feature measure will return the same value from the h_{int} representation at the different compressions. It is more difficult to predict what happens with model **M2**, since it allows the interesting tissues to overlap after movement. With model **M3**, the effect on the h_{int} representation is equivalent to changes in the surrounding tissue, and that is the issue we now consider.

Breast features might have different tissue surrounds. For example, a mass could be on a fatty surround or a dense surround as demonstrated in Figure 9.8, and in reality in Figure 9.9. Recall the contrast measure defined in Chapter 1:

$$C = \frac{h_{int}^{max} - h_{int}^{min}}{h_{int}^{max} + h_{int}^{min}}$$

Features such as these are exceptionally poor in the situation described since maximum - minimum remains constant, but maximum + minimum is vastly different as the surround changes.

A problem with the h_{int} representation is that the band of tissues that is classed as interesting is too broad. The breast has a great deal of fibrous tissue, which helps to support it and which mostly can be ignored (being irrelevant to diagnosis) although it does give the breast its dense or fatty appearance. We consider large, relatively flat components of h_{int} to be surrounding tissue, and we seek to estimate this component to attain what we term $h_{feature}$:

$$h_{feature}(x, y) = h_{int}(x, y) - h_{surround}(x, y)$$

In Chapter 6, we saw how errors in H lead to uniform decreases/increases in the h_{int} values, so that the definition of $h_{feature}$ actually removes the error since it equally affects both components. Conveniently, this feature

CYST ON VARYING BACKGROUND

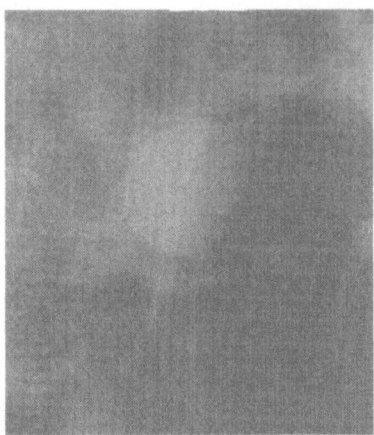

Figure 9.9.   This is a segment from a real mammogram. The cyst appears to be half projected down with dense fibroglandular tissue and half with fatty tissue. In this scenario many feature measures lack consistency.

also fits nicely with model $M3$, so that it should be robust to different compressions. Note, though, that $h_{feature}$ is likely to be near-zero for so-called fatty areas of the breast. As a consequence, feature measurements which are normalised by dividing by a value of $h_{feature}$ might be unstable.

There are several ways to estimate $h_{surround}$. One is to estimate it from the entire breast image, for example, by finding the minimum h_{int} away from the breast edge. Another is to choose window sizes in which to compute the features and to consider h_{min} to be the surrounding level. The correct way to estimate $h_{surround}$ depends upon the definition of surrounding tissue that is being used, and this in turn depends upon the type of feature required. That is, we have to build in some notion of scale.

Due to the range of features and feature sizes in mammograms, it is inappropriate to talk about general feature detection. In this section we deal with features pertinent to detecting masses, in particular cysts, from fatty tissue, seeking feature values that are consistent within an image and between images. The three example images we use are illustrative of our approach.

The three examples we consider involve cysts. Two of them, **C1** and **C2** are of a cyst at different breast compressions. **C1** has the breast compressed to 5.6cm with an exposure of 70mAs, whilst **C2** has the breast compressed to 6.5cm with an exposure of 93mAs. The cyst in these images has surrounding tissue that appears mostly fatty. The third example **C3** has a smaller cyst in an image digitised using a different scanner to the

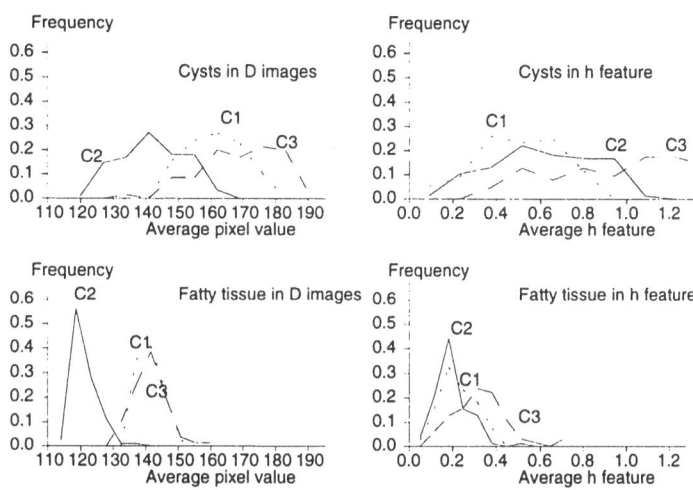

Figure 9.10.   Distributions of mean values in small windows from film density and $h_{feature}$ images of 3 sections from mammograms. Around 100 samples were taken for each example. The values computed on the transformed images show better clustering and differentiation of tissue types.

other two. The breast was 5.8cm thick with an exposure of 89mAs. Again, the surrounding tissue is relatively fatty.

The first observation about cysts is that they often appear denser than fatty tissue. In this case, the attenuation is higher, consequently the image brightness is higher. This suggests using the average value within some window on the image as a feature: higher averages tend to indicate denser tissues. Figure 9.10 shows the distribution of average pixel value in small windows (1.5mm by 1.5mm) in the film density and $h_{feature}$ images for the cyst and fatty tissue in the three examples. Clearly, the average pixel values in the film density images for the fatty tissues are not sufficiently clustered to differentiate purely by thresholding. For the $h_{feature}$ measures, the value of $h_{surround}$ was taken to be the minimum in the large window over which measurements are performed. This is appropriate, because it defines the surrounding tissue. In practice, one might use a large window size that is greater than the maximum expected size of a cyst in order to ensure that some surrounding tissue is covered by the window. The fat values and the cyst values are far better clustered. In particular, the fatty tissue and the cysts in the breast at different compressions are giving almost identical responses, which we would expect given the compression model **M3**.

Fatty tissue has low tissue roughness (there are not many hills in the

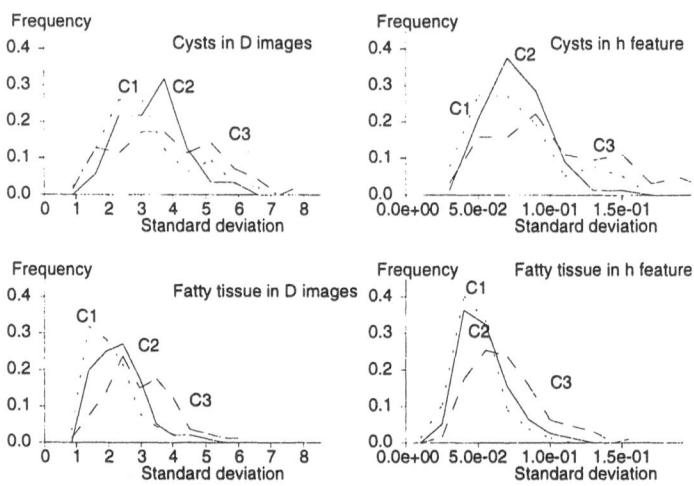

Figure 9.11. Distributions of standard deviation values in small windows from film density and $h_{feature}$ images of 3 breasts. Around 100 samples were taken for each example. Note that the horizontal axis are marked differently, this reflects the fact that the original images are integers whilst the transformed images are floats.

h_{int} representation). There are many possible measures of roughness, many of which are based on the concept of visual contrast, so that the feature gives high response for situations where we have a relatively high peak compared to the background. Although such measures might be appropriate for emulating a radiologist, we are more interested in a measure of the tissue roughness that measures the actual tissue property. For this reason, we again use a simple measure, such as standard deviation. The simplicity of our features derives in part from the task we are considering; but also from not needing to do further normalisation. Figure 9.11 shows the standard deviation distribution from the three film density and $h_{feature}$ images for the cysts and surrounding fatty tissue. The distributions show that the average of the standard deviations is lower for the fatty tissue and that the distributions do overlap for the film density images. However, the distributions in the $h_{feature}$ images are closer than those in the film density images: especially in the case of the breasts at different compressions. It would appear that the $h_{feature}$ values are more robust to breast compression.

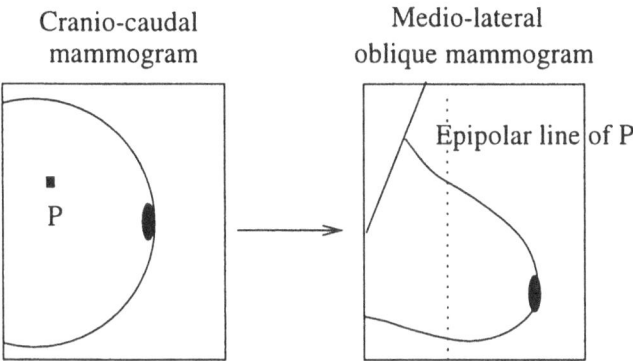

Figure 9.12. If the breast was compressed in the same direction and by the same amount in the two views so that the only change is the angle of view then the correspondence problem becomes one of "wide angle stereo". This is a problem often encountered in computer vision [70] and methods are available that would map a point in one view onto a line (the epipole) in the other view as shown above. The epipole shows likely positions in the other view. Radiologists, with whom we have conducted trials seem to use such a straight line epipolar approximation based around the nipple. In fact, it is far more likely that the epipole is curved and that is what we develop in this section.

9.5. Matching between views

The two views of the breast that are usually taken at a UK breast care unit are cranio-caudal (CC) and medio-lateral oblique (MLO). The geometry of mammography is straight-forward, with the system following the usual projective equations of a pin-hole camera system: the x-ray source can be considered to be a point-source emitting a collimated cone of rays which pass through, or are attenuated by an object and then form an image on the image plane. However, there is a fundamental problem with the geometry since the medio-lateral oblique mammogram can be taken at an angle at the radiographer's discretion typically between 35 and 60 degrees and this angle is not routinely noted down. Usually, short, stocky women are imaged with angles less than 45 degrees, whilst tall, thin women have angles over 45 degrees.

If the only change between the two views was the angle, then the problem of correspondence is the same as in "wide-angle stereo" [70], Figure 9.12; but the problem becomes considerably more complicated due to breast compression. We have developed a method to predict where in a medio-lateral oblique mammogram the potentially corresponding positions of a point marked in the cranio-caudal mammogram are. The crucial step in our approach is a model of breast compression, which, though simple, proves to out-perform radiologists on outline images. Our method also allows estimation of the 3D location of objects within the uncompressed breast.

We assume that we are given the image coordinates of a point of interest

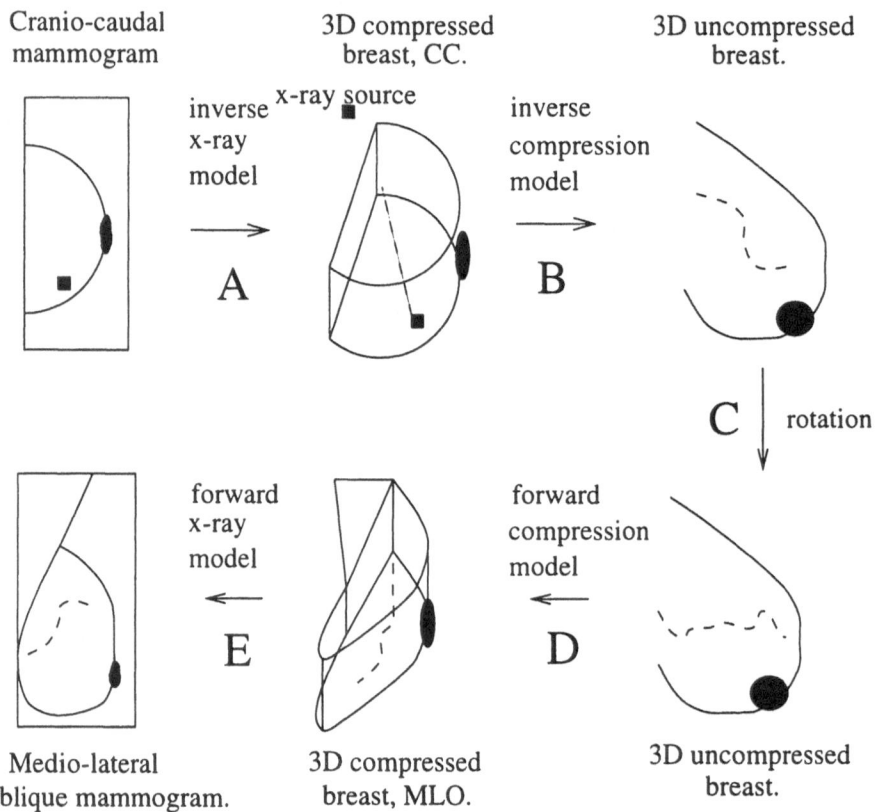

Cranio-caudal mammogram

3D compressed breast, CC.

3D uncompressed breast.

inverse x-ray source

inverse x-ray model

A

inverse compression model

B

C | rotation

forward x-ray model

E

forward compression model

D

Medio-lateral oblique mammogram.

3D compressed breast, MLO.

3D uncompressed breast.

Figure 9.13. The aim of the process is to map from a point in the cranio-caudal image to a curve in the medio-lateral image which represents potential positions. See the text for full descriptions of the five steps A-E.

in the cranio-caudal image, the image coordinates of the nipple in both views as well as the outline of the breasts in the two views. There are five steps in our implemented algorithm which are shown pictorially in Figure 9.13 and explained next:

A The potential 3D positions of the "interesting object" in the CC compressed breast are found by applying perspective geometry to the coordinates of the point of interest. We are particularly interested in the end points and central point of the 3D line of potential positions.

B We attempt to "undo" the CC compression. We assume that when the breast is compressed there is no lateral movement of points and we assume that a side-view of the uncompressed breast is similar to that of the MLO profile. We know the breast thickness and compressed breast shape from the work in Chapter 5. Furthermore, we assume that the plane through the nipple which is parallel to the compression plates does not deform with compression. Using these assumptions we can determine how the two end points and central point of the 3D line from A move when uncompressed; assuming that they lie on a curve allows us to map all the points along the line.

C We rotate the curve about an axis through the nipple to simulate the change of view from CC to MLO; by doing this we are assuming that the 3D coordinates of the nipple do not change between views. Currently, we use a range of angles from 30 to 60 degrees since the angle at which the MLO image is performed is not yet routinely noted down.

D We now need to simulate medio-lateral oblique compression. We assume that the side-view of the breast is a similar shape to the MLO outline. Since the compressed shape and size of the breast is known from our calibration data we can again map the end points and central points for each cross-section and assuming a quadratic curve we can determine how each point on our curve of potential positions moves.

E We now have a curve representing potential 3D positions in the compressed MLO breast. Simple perspective projection gives us the potential positions in the MLO image.

In one of Novak's [187] experiments, vertical lines were marked onto the breast skin while the breast was under CC-compression and then observed on the latero-medially compressed breast. The experiments showed that the lines inclined towards the nipple by 20 to 30 degrees. We attempted to emulate this experiment by simulating marks on a CC breast and where they move to. Simulation using our compression model showed an inclination of 25 degrees.

We have a database of 32 CC and MLO images, which have obvious matching features: usually a circumscribed mass or calcification. We presented to two radiologists outlines of the CC images with objects of interest marked and asked them to mark a line in the outline of the MLO image where they would expect that object to appear (the outlines are similar to those shown in Figure 9.12). Figures 9.14 and 9.15 show examples of the results from the radiologists and from our technique. Overall, the average minimum distance from the radiologist's lines to the actual position was 9.46mm and 11.04mm, respectively, whereas our method had an average minimum distance of 6.48mm. With a pixel resolution of 0.3mm an improvement of 2.98mm represents a reduction in one of search space dimensions of 10 pixels which would give a substantial time-saving.

MATCHING CC AND MLO

Marked mass in CC image   Estimated positions in the MLO image

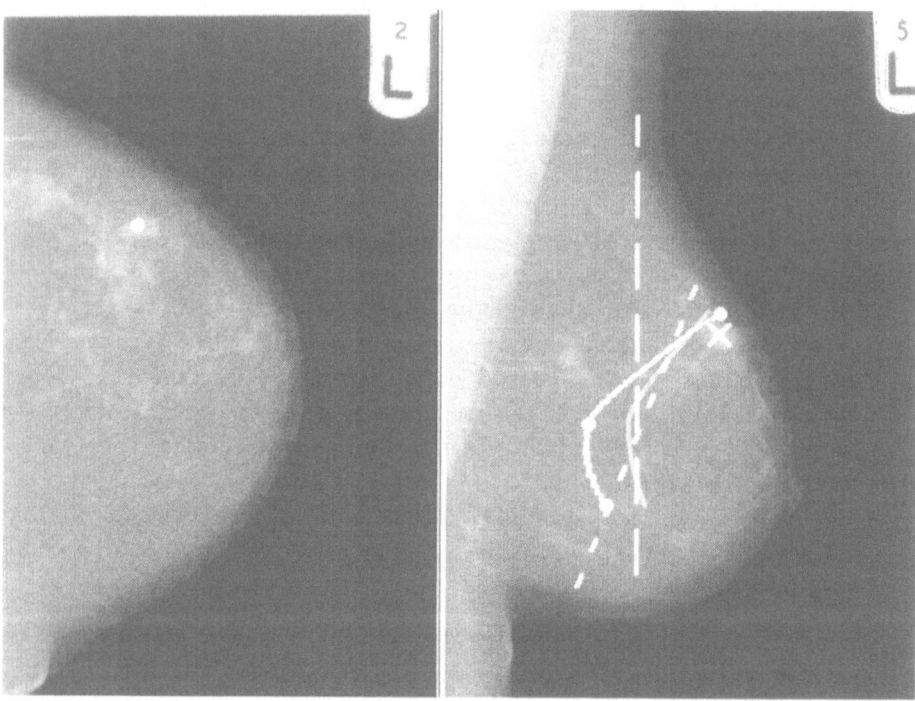

Figure 9.14. This figure shows a cranio-caudal and medio-lateral oblique mammogram of the same breast. Two radiologists were shown outlines of the mammograms (including the nipple and pectoral muscle) and the position of an object in the cranio-caudal image. They were asked to mark a line in the medio-lateral oblique image showing where they felt the object might be. The radiologists attempts are shown by the two dashed white lines. Our method predicts a curve as depicted in white, the other curve (in grey) shows the prediction if we had ignored the medio-lateral oblique compression. The dot in the left image and the cross in the right marks the actual position of the mass.

The work explained in this section is explained in greater detail in [151, 121]. Further work will concentrate on developing a finite element model of the breast and using image features to refine that model within an iterative framework.

MATCHING CC AND MLO

Marked mass in CC image   Estimated positions in the MLO image

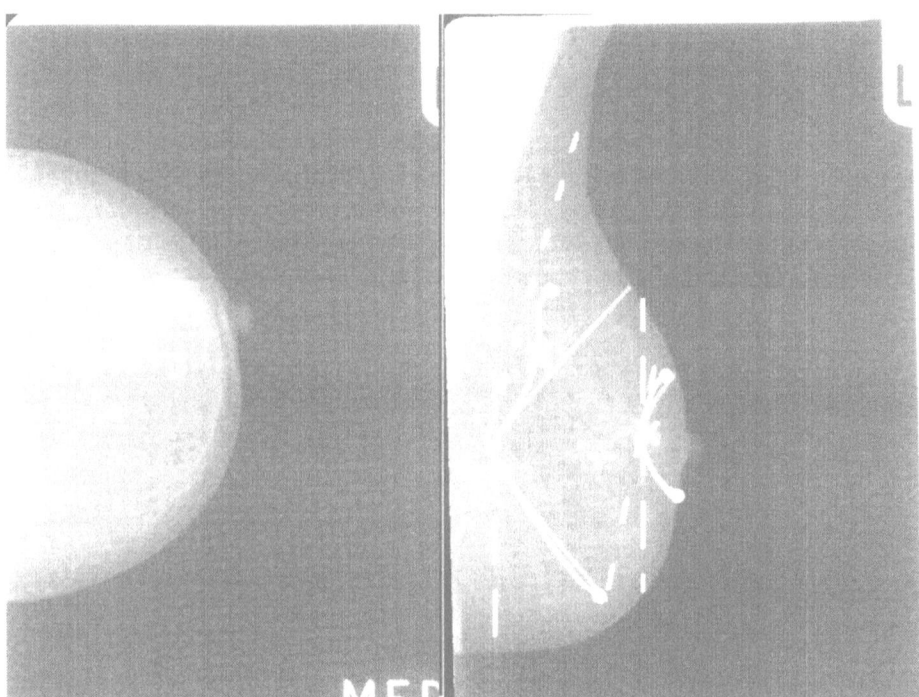

Figure 9.15.   This figure shows a cranio-caudal and medio-lateral oblique mammogram of the same breast. In this example there are two masses which are matchable between the views shown by a dot in the left image and a cross in the right image. The radiologist's attempts to find the mass are shown by dashed lines in the right image with the white curve being our prediction. The other curve (in grey) shows the prediction had we ignored the medio-lateral oblique compression.

9.6. Summary: Breast compression

In the first part of the chapter we showed that breast compression produces large movement and deformation of tissue within the breast. This implies that there are large forces at work and that some internal breast tissues are deformable. The movement seen is restricted by the internal structures and connections of the breast. We have further shown that taking mammograms at two different compressions is a promising way of determining the physical properties of the internal breast tissues, and of determining the breast structure. These results are not surprising since the breast is a flexible, deformable part of the body.

The middle part of the chapter showed that use of the h_{int} representation allows better visualisation of differential compression mammography and might well lead to more robust image analysis systems especially because it allows us to deal with the projective nature of mammography in a logical and systematic way. The chapter ended with yet another example of successful modelling, this time of the movement due to compression.

The major problem with further research into the effects of breast compression using differential compression mammography is the doubling of the radiation dose required. The next chapter develops a technique based on software image enhancement that shows how we can halve the radiation dose and still obtain a good quality mammographic image.

CHAPTER 10

REMOVING THE ANTI-SCATTER GRID

10.1. Introduction

The use of an anti-scatter grid in mammography greatly improves image quality but necessitates an approximate doubling of the radiation dose and increased equipment cost. In this chapter, a software image enhancement technique is developed to achieve similar levels of performance to an anti-scatter grid with just half the radiation dose. We investigate removing the effects of scatter from mammograms taken without a grid using the scatter model defined in Chapter 3. Figure 10.1 shows an example of the results. A major benefit of the use of models is that it allows an enhanced image to be generated in a clearly-defined manner: there is no need to experimentally refine thresholds, mask sizes, or contrast measures for each image. The work in this chapter is vital to the work in Chapter 9 which was about a technique called differential compression mammography that requires an increase of radiation dose; combining this work with that technique should allow differential compression mammography at the same dosage levels as currently used.

We start by developing an analytical model that is used to investigate the signal content of an image taken with and without an anti-scatter grid. In particular, we seek to:

- Compare the primary signal with and without the grid;
- Calculate what time of exposure is required to retain the same primary signal when a grid is not used;

This is followed by an explanation of a trial we conducted which was based upon removing scatter using image processing. Practical examples of mammograms performed with and without the grid and then digitally enhanced are shown. A previous version of this chapter appeared in [119].

10.2. Theoretical analysis

Basic theory

A useful result, used several times as the analytic model is developed, is that the total energy imparted to the intensifying screen is directly proportional

EXAMPLE OF SOFTWARE REMOVAL OF SCATTER
With grid   Without grid   Without grid enhanced

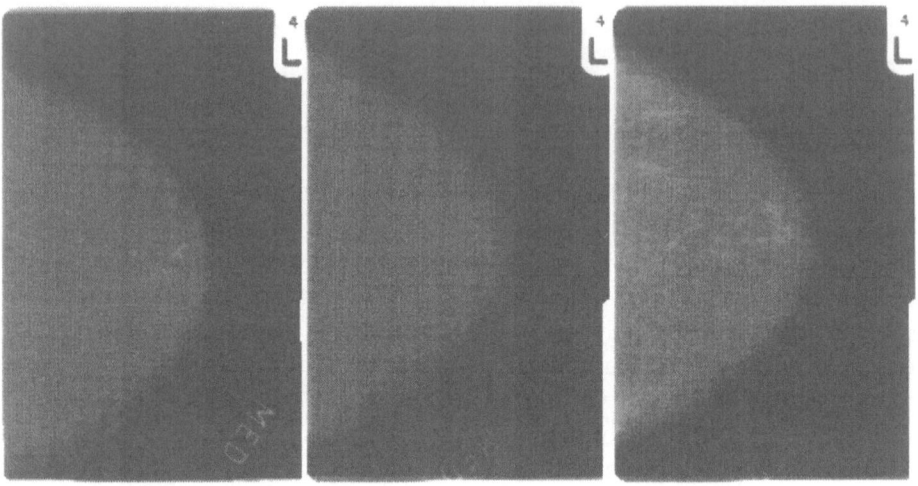

Figure 10.1. The image on the left was taken with an anti-scatter grid. The middle image was taken without an anti-scatter grid, this was enhanced to appear as if a grid had been used which is the image on the right. The image on the right was thus obtained with just half the radiation dose of the image on the left.

to the time of exposure. So, for example, if the exposure time doubles then the energy imparted at all points in the image is also expected to double, as shown mathematically in Box 10.1.

As in previous chapters, the mathematics of our model is simplified in order to make analysis tractable though our conclusions are verified numerically on the full model. We start with several assumptions. The first is that the extra-focal component is ignored, recalling that the intensity of extra-focal radiation is minimal for most of the diagnostically useful breast area. The second assumption is that the use of the grid increases the radiation dose, and thus the time of exposure, by a factor ϕ (the so-called "Bucky factor"):

$$t_s^{\mathrm{grid}} = \phi t_s^{\mathrm{no\ grid}} \tag{10.1}$$

In practice, the time of exposure varies since it is determined by the automatic exposure control, and that is prone to variations due to beam hardening. Table 10.1 shows the times of exposure that were recorded in a trial with and without the grid. For the data shown, the sample mean of ϕ is 2.02 and its sample variance is 0.31. For the following analysis, ϕ is taken to be 2.0.

BOX 10.1: Total energy imparted to screen and time of exposure

The primary component of the x-ray signal is clearly directly proportional to the time of exposure, E_p^{nd} is used to represent that part of the energy imparted not related to time of exposure (the nd stands for not-dependent). In this chapter the superfix imp is dropped from energies. The interested reader can refer to Boxes 2.4 and 2.9 for details of E_p^{nd}. In this chapter, such details are not important. In practice, E_p^{nd} is the energy imparted per unit time. We then multiply that by time of exposure to get total primary energy imparted:

$$E_p(x, y, t_s) = t_s E_p^{\mathrm{nd}}(x, y) \tag{10.2}$$

It also follows from the models developed in Chapters 3 and 4 that the scatter component at the pixel (x, y), $E_s(x, y, t_s)$, and extra-focal component, $E_e(x, y, t_s)$, are also directly proportional to the time of exposure:

$$E_s(x, y, t_s) = t_s E_s^{\mathrm{nd}}(x, y) \tag{10.3}$$

$$E_e(x, y, t_s) = t_s E_e^{\mathrm{nd}}(x, y) \tag{10.4}$$

Using Equations 10.2, 10.3 and 10.4 in the equation for total energy imparted gives:

$$
\begin{aligned}
E_{pse}(x, y, t_s) &= E_p(x, y, t_s) + E_s(x, y, t_s) + E_e(x, y, t_s) \\
&= t_s(E_p^{\mathrm{nd}}(x, y) + E_s^{\mathrm{nd}}(x, y) + E_e^{\mathrm{nd}}(x, y))
\end{aligned}
$$

If the time of exposure is changed, say from t_s to t_s' then the new total energy imparted is thus:

$$E_{pse}(x, y, t_s') = \frac{t_s'}{t_s} E_{pse}(x, y, t_s)$$

As the primary radiation passes through the breast, it is attenuated by the breast tissue and, unfortunately, also by the anti-scatter grid. Thus, if the anti-scatter grid is not present, the primary radiation reaching the film-screen combination actually increases if the same time of exposure is used. Let the increase in the primary be noted by α:

$$E_p^{\mathrm{no\ grid}}(x, y, t_s) = \alpha E_p^{\mathrm{grid}}(x, y, t_s) \tag{10.5}$$

Based upon the typical primary transmission rate of the Philip's grid at 18keV reported by Dance [50], we assume $\alpha = \frac{4}{3}$.

The final assumption is that the scatter component for the same block of tissue without the grid, but at the same time of exposure as with the

Image	Left			Right		
	t_s^{grid}	$t_s^{\text{no grid}}$	ϕ	t_s^{grid}	$t_s^{\text{no grid}}$	ϕ
oxGRID001	0.98	0.46	2.13	0.84	0.38	2.21
oxGRID002	1.19	0.75	1.59	1.08	0.56	1.93
oxGRID003	1.21	0.63	1.92	1.17	0.66	1.77
oxGRID004	0.47	0.19	2.47	0.52	0.26	2.00
oxGRID005	0.90	0.42	2.14	0.66	0.36	1.83
oxGRID006	2.73	0.99	2.76	2.10	1.13	1.86
oxGRID007	0.42	0.22	1.91	0.45	0.25	1.80

TABLE 10.1. These values show the time of exposure for each of the mammograms in our trial (in seconds). The time of exposure is roughly double (ϕ) when the grid is used. The variations from this are due to the performance of the automatic exposure control varying due to beam hardening and differences in compressed breast thickness.

grid, increases by λ:

$$E_s^{\text{no grid}}(x, y, t_s) = \lambda E_s^{\text{grid}}(x, y, t_s) \qquad (10.6)$$

Based upon the increase in the scatter-to-primary ratios with and without the grid reported by Carlsson et al. [32] we use $\lambda = 5.0$. The arguments that follow are relatively insensitive to small variations in the parameters ϕ, α, λ about their nominal values.

The primary signal with and without grid

The primary signal contains explicit information about the breast tissue and we use the initial level of the primary signal as our idealised case. Consequently, we now seek to compare the strength of the primary signal with and without the anti-scatter grid. Recall that the strength of the primary signal is affected by the time of exposure and the presence of the grid. From the work in the previous section, the primary radiation without the grid is approximately two-thirds of what it is with the grid and the scatter-to-primary ratio increases by a factor of 3.75 (the mathematical proofs are shown in Box 10.2). Figure 10.2 shows the primary component for a typical mammogram, with and without the grid, and varying times of exposure. The graphs in that figure come from a polyenergetic simulation. Figure 10.3 shows the total energy component. A typical value for the

---

BOX 10.2: Scatter and primary with and without grid

Combining Equations 10.2, 10.1, 10.5:

$$E_p^{\text{no grid}}(x, y, t_s^{\text{no grid}}) = \frac{\alpha}{\phi} E_p^{\text{grid}}(x, y, t_s^{\text{grid}}) \qquad (10.7)$$

Similarly, the scatter components can be compared:

$$E_s^{\text{no grid}}(x, y, t_s^{\text{no grid}}) = \frac{\lambda}{\phi} E_s^{\text{grid}}(x, y, t_s^{\text{grid}})$$

Using the values in the text for λ, ϕ, α and substituting them in to these equations gives us:

$$E_p^{\text{no grid}}(x, y, t_s^{\text{no grid}}) = \frac{2}{3} E_p^{\text{grid}}(x, y, t_s^{\text{grid}})$$

$$E_s^{\text{no grid}}(x, y, t_s^{\text{no grid}}) = \frac{5}{2} E_s^{\text{grid}}(x, y, t_s^{\text{grid}})$$

and thus:

$$\frac{E_s^{\text{no grid}}(x, y, t_s^{\text{no grid}})}{E_p^{\text{no grid}}(x, y, t_s^{\text{no grid}})} = \frac{15}{4} \frac{E_s^{\text{grid}}(x, y, t_s^{\text{grid}})}{E_p^{\text{grid}}(x, y, t_s^{\text{grid}})}$$

---

scatter-to-primary ratio with the grid for a mix of interesting tissue and fat is 0.1, so our theory predicts a scatter-to-primary ratio of 0.375 without the grid, which is slightly lower than expected from Carlsson et al. [32] but reasonable given the simplified analytical model that we are using.

If a calcification is 0.3mm thick in a breast of thickness 4cm with equal proportions of fat and "interesting tissue", then the expected scatter-to-primary ratio for the calcification is in the region of 8, with the grid. From the expected rise in the scatter-to-primary this would indicate a scatter-to-primary ratio of 30 without the grid which suggests that calcification is much more difficult to see. This is addressed later.

If one considers the signal-to-noise ratio (SNR) in a mammogram in a classical manner then it appears that performing a mammogram without an anti-scatter grid and then digitally enhancing appears infeasible. Conventionally, the SNR might be taken as the ratio of primary radiation to scattered radiation so that:

$$\text{SNR}^{\text{no grid}} = \frac{E_p^{\text{no grid}}}{E_s^{\text{no grid}}} \approx 0.267 \times \text{SNR}^{\text{grid}}$$

However, this analysis hides the fact that the noise, in this case scatter, is far more uniform when the grid is not used and is therefore easier to model

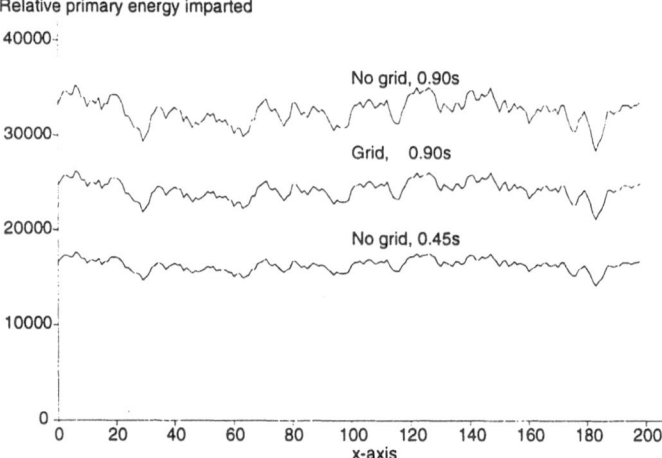

Figure 10.2. This graph shows profiles across the relative primary energy imparted to show the effect of when a grid is used and when not, at varying times of exposure. The middle profile (marked with Grid) is real. The lower and higher profiles are from a polyenergetic simulation using the model presented in Chapter 2. They show that when the grid is not used, but we keep the same time of exposure (i.e. 0.90s in this case), the primary component increases. However, in practice the time of exposure decreases so that the primary is, in fact, reduced and that is represented by the bottom line.

and remove (see Figure 3.7). The important factor in our work is how much information there is in the image. The noise that is important is not scatter but film and digitisation noise.

Retaining the primary signal without the grid

In this section we try to ensure that the primary signal without the grid is the same level as with the grid by choosing ϕ (the Bucky factor) appropriately. Effectively, we choose $E_p^{\text{grid}}(x, y, t_s^{\text{grid}})$ as the ideal case for comparison purposes. Now, suppose we choose $\phi = \dfrac{t_s^{\text{grid}}}{t_s^{\text{no grid}}}$ so that:

$$E_p^{\text{grid}}(x, y, t_s^{\text{grid}}) = E_p^{\text{no grid}}(x, y, t_s^{\text{no grid}});$$

that is, so that the film receives the same amount of primary energy. From Equation 10.7 which explains the relationship between the primary components, it seems we can retain the primary component by setting $\phi = \frac{4}{3}$,

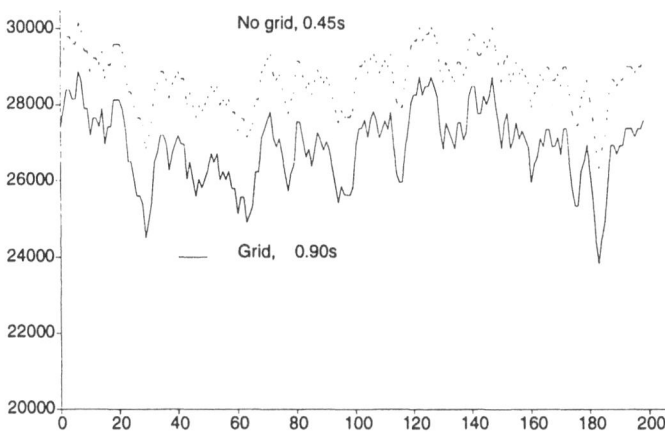

Figure 10.3. This graph shows the total imparted energy when a grid is used and when not. It shows that when the grid is not used the total signal level is similar which is expected given that the automatic exposure control is functioning. However, whereas with the grid the primary is high and the scatter is low, without the grid the primary is lower and the scatter is much higher meaning that there is much poorer contrast in the final image. This can be seen in these graphs by noting how much sharper and deeper the edges are for the case with the grid.

i.e. with only 75% of the time of exposure :

$$t_s^{\text{no grid}} = \frac{3}{4} t_s^{\text{grid}}$$

This shows that we can get the same primary signal with a reduction in radiation dose of 25%. But how would such an image appear on a mammogram? The mathematics is shown in Box 10.3. Assuming a linear film-screen characteristic curve, and taking typical values for the film-screen gradient and scatter-to-primary ratio, means that it is expected that the film densities will rise by 0.291 in the image without the grid but with the same primary radiation. Figure 10.4 shows this graphically.

To summarise, the analysis predicts that to retain as much diagnostically important information as when an anti-scatter grid is used, the time of exposure can only be reduced by 25% when the grid is not used and the film will become markedly darker. This might mean that the film becomes too dark for visual inspection. However, given that mammographic film can record film densities up to 3.7 it appears likely that if the film digitisation is of a high enough quality (in itself a major research area), then it should

---

BOX 10.3: Effect on film of retaining primary signal without grid

Assuming a linear film-screen curve (and remember this is merely for analytical purposes) the film density can be related to total energy imparted:

$$D^{\text{grid}}(x,y) \;=\; \gamma \log \beta E_{ps}^{\text{grid}}(x,y,t_s^{\text{grid}})$$

$$=\; \gamma \log \beta E_p^{\text{grid}}(x,y,t_s^{\text{grid}})(1 + \frac{E_s^{\text{grid}}}{E_p^{\text{grid}}}),$$

where γ is the film-screen gradient and β is the other linear term and is related to system speed. For the case with no grid, and a decrease in exposure of 25%, we have:

$$D^{\text{no grid}}(x,y) \;=\; \gamma \log \beta E_{ps}^{\text{no grid}}(x,y,t_s^{\text{no grid}})$$

$$=\; \gamma \log \beta (E_p^{\text{no grid}}(x,y,t_s^{\text{no grid}}) + E_s^{\text{no grid}}(x,y,t_s^{\text{no grid}}))$$

$$=\; \gamma \log \beta \left(E_p^{\text{grid}}(x,y,t_s^{\text{grid}}) + \frac{15}{4} E_s^{\text{grid}}(x,y,t_s^{\text{grid}}) \right)$$

$$=\; \gamma \log \beta \left(E_p^{\text{grid}}(x,y,t_s^{\text{grid}})(1 + \frac{15}{4} \frac{E_s^{\text{grid}}}{E_p^{\text{grid}}}) \right)$$

$$=\; D^{\text{grid}}(x,y) + \gamma \log \frac{1 + \frac{15}{4} \frac{E_s^{\text{grid}}}{E_p^{\text{grid}}}}{1 + \frac{E_s^{\text{grid}}}{E_p^{\text{grid}}}}$$

If we take typical values, $\gamma = 3.0$ and the scatter-to-primary ratio as 0.1 with the grid, then:

$$D^{\text{no grid}}(x,y) = D^{\text{grid}}(x,y) + 0.291$$

---

be possible to reduce the radiation dose by 25%. We note though that the darker the film, the higher the digitisation noise.

For the case of the same calcification used earlier, the scatter-to-primary ratio is approaching 8 with the grid and 30 without it. This suggests that the film density will increase by 1.6. However, the analysis required that the film curve be linear. Often calcifications are in the non-linear part of the film-screen characteristic curve. If the calcification has a film density of 0.5 with the grid, then, retaining the primary signal a film density of about 1.0 in the film without the grid is expected. Practical results confirm this.

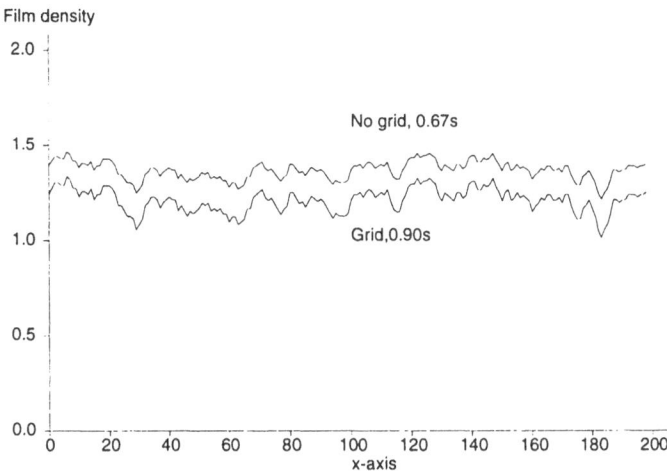

Figure 10.4. This figure shows the film densities when the level of the primary component is preserved between when a grid is used and when a grid is not used. As predicted in the text, the film is darker.

10.3. "Soft" removal of scattered radiation

From the theory, it appears that using software to remove the effects of scattered radiation rather than using hardware to prevent the scatter reaching the intensifying screen is a viable option if the loss of primary is not crucial. As an initial attempt to investigate this we carried out a study on women being recalled to the assessment clinic at the Breast Care Unit in Oxford. Mammograms of the same breast, with and without an anti-scatter grid, were taken. The women were all informed volunteers and the exercise was performed with ethical committee approval. The films were digitised by Philips Laboratories using a Lumisys scanner.

We took the images performed without an anti-scatter grid and then used a modified version of the scatter model from Chapter 3 and the extra-focal model from Chapter 4 to generate the h_{int} representation. These models are actually simpler than the originals since they do not consider the anti-scatter grid. From the h_{int} representation a mammogram was simulated to appear as if an anti-scatter grid had been used.

Figure 10.5 shows an original mammogram with and without the anti-scatter grid. Figure 10.6 shows the mammogram taken without the grid, digitally enhanced to appear as it would if the grid had been used. Figure 10.7 shows the image with the grid and the simulated one side-by-side.

Figure 10.8 shows another image taken with the grid next to another image without the grid after a monoenergetic simulation.

Figure 10.9 shows images of calcifications, digitised to 100 microns, taken with and without the grid and then digitally enhanced to appear as if with the grid. Figure 10.10 shows the image without the grid enhanced to appear as if with no scatter.

Two experienced radiologists were asked to compare the images taken with the grid (and subsequently digitised) to those taken without the grid after they had been digitally enhanced (e.g. Figure 10.7). They were incapable of distinguishing which was which. We also presented the radiologists with the images from a simulation of a monoenergetic examination (e.g. Figure 10.8). They felt that these were of equal, if not greater, quality than the images taken with a grid.

10.4. Summary: Removing the anti-scatter grid

The process of converting an image taken without a grid to look as if a grid had been used can be summarised as in Box 10.4. Although the results are extremely promising, there is a problem with the definition of "quality" since it is obvious, and been shown theoretically, that an image taken with half the radiation dose must contain less information than that at the full dose. The question is: what and how much information is required by the radiologists? This remains an open question.

BOX 10.4: Mapping from an image taken without a grid to one with

(1) Compute the h_{int} values for the mammogram taken without the anti-scatter grid.

(2) Simulate an x-ray examination as if a grid were used.

IMAGES WITH AND WITHOUT ANTI-SCATTER GRID

With grid   Without grid

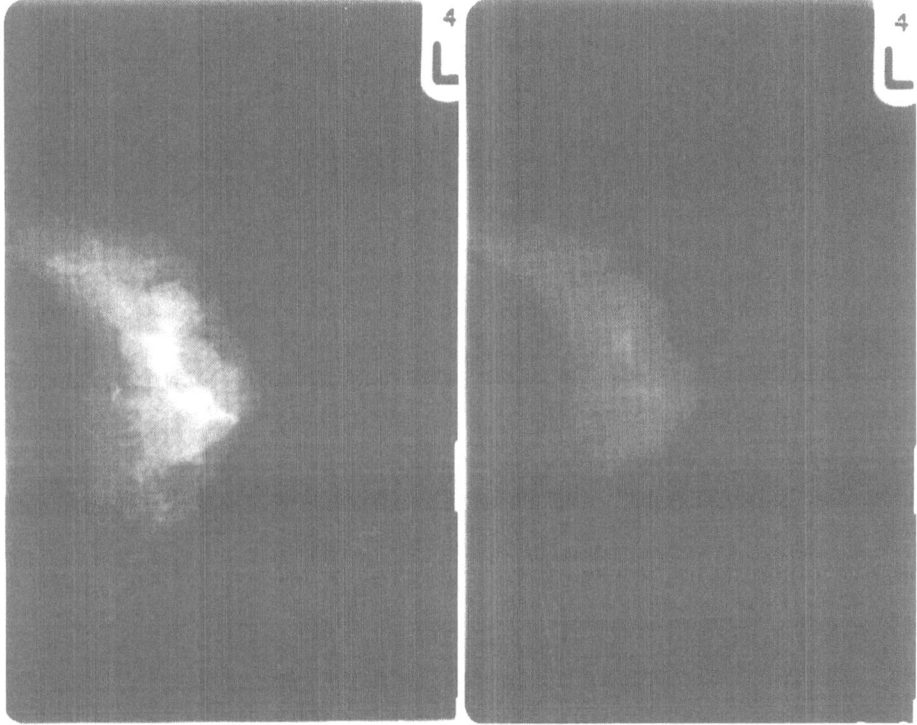

Figure 10.5. The image on the left was taken with an anti-scatter grid and the mAs value was 98mAs. The image on the right is of the same breast and was taken without a grid. This time the mAs value was 46mAs. The breast thickness was approximately 4.5cm in each case.

IMAGE WITHOUT GRID ENHANCED

Original   Enhanced

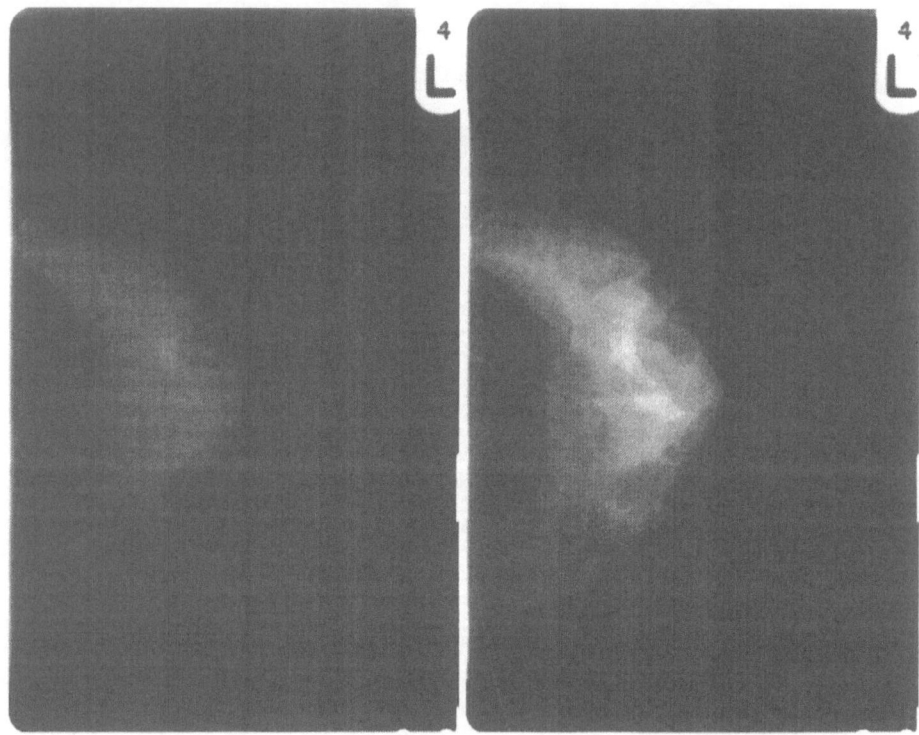

Figure 10.6.   The image on the left was taken without an anti-scatter grid. The image on the right is a digitally enhanced version of the image on the left. The image has been processed to make it look as it would if a grid had been used.

WITH GRID AND WITHOUT GRID ENHANCED

With grid   Without grid enhanced

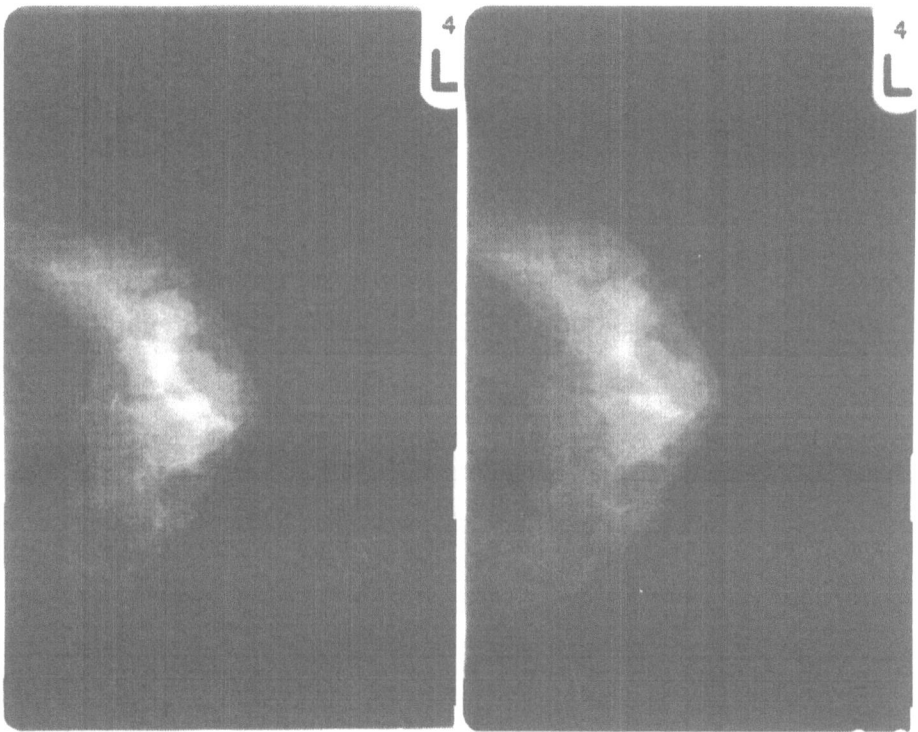

Figure 10.7.   The image on the left was taken with an anti-scatter grid. The image on the right was taken without a grid and then a polyenergetic x-ray examination was simulated as if a grid was present.

WITH GRID AND WITHOUT GRID ENHANCED

With grid   Without grid enhanced

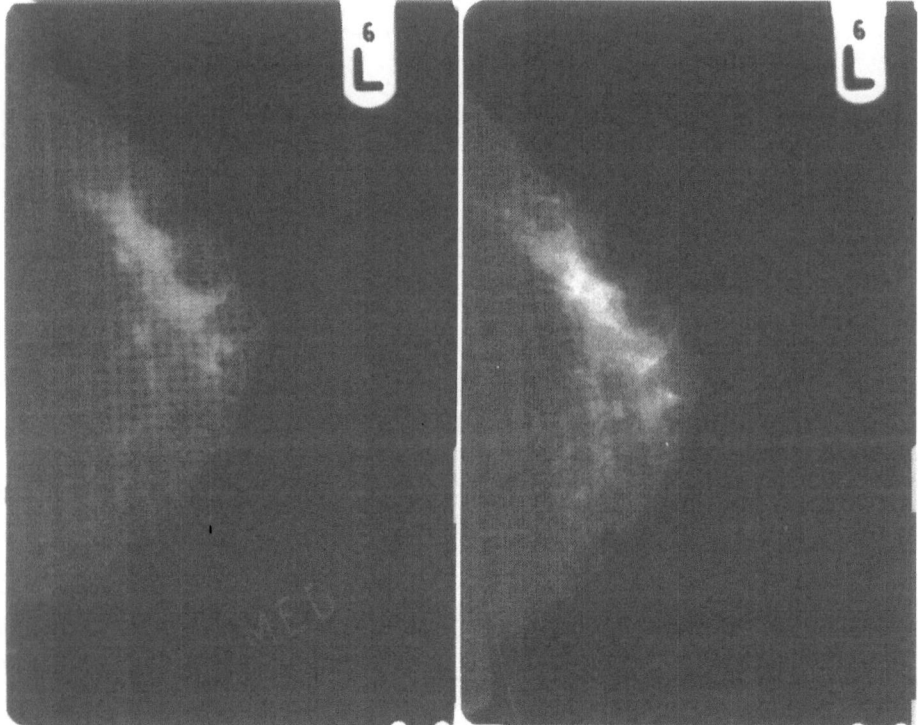

Figure 10.8.   The image on the left was taken with an anti-scatter grid. The image on the right was taken without an anti-scatter grid and then digitally enhanced to simulate a monoenergetic x-ray simulation at 18keV.

WITH GRID AND WITHOUT GRID ENHANCED

With grid   Without grid enhanced

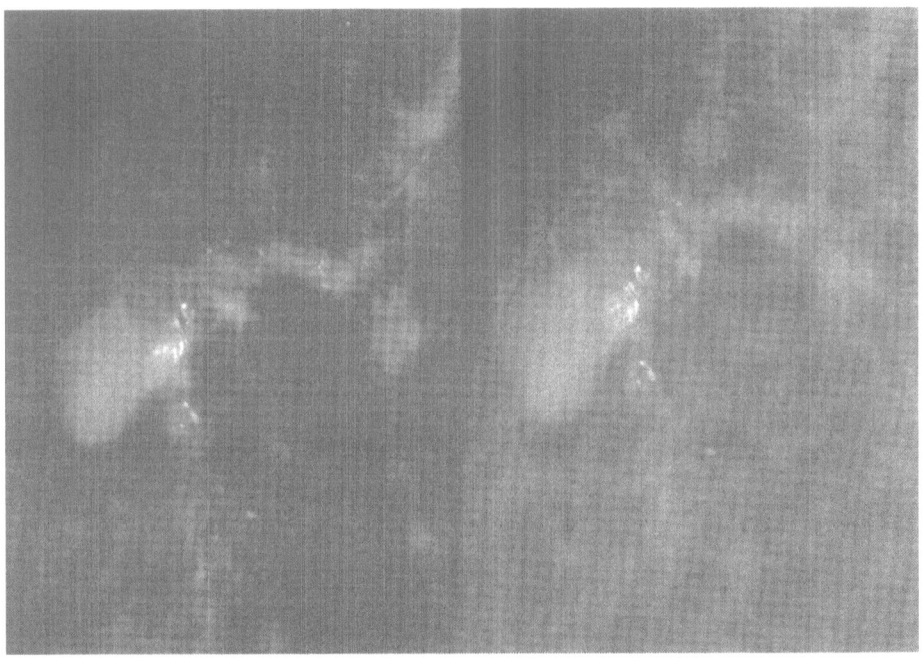

Figure 10.9.   The image on the left was taken with an anti-scatter grid and digitised to 100 micron resolution. The image on the right was taken without a grid and then enhanced to make it appear as it would with a grid.

WITH GRID AND WITHOUT GRID ENHANCED

With grid   Without grid enhanced

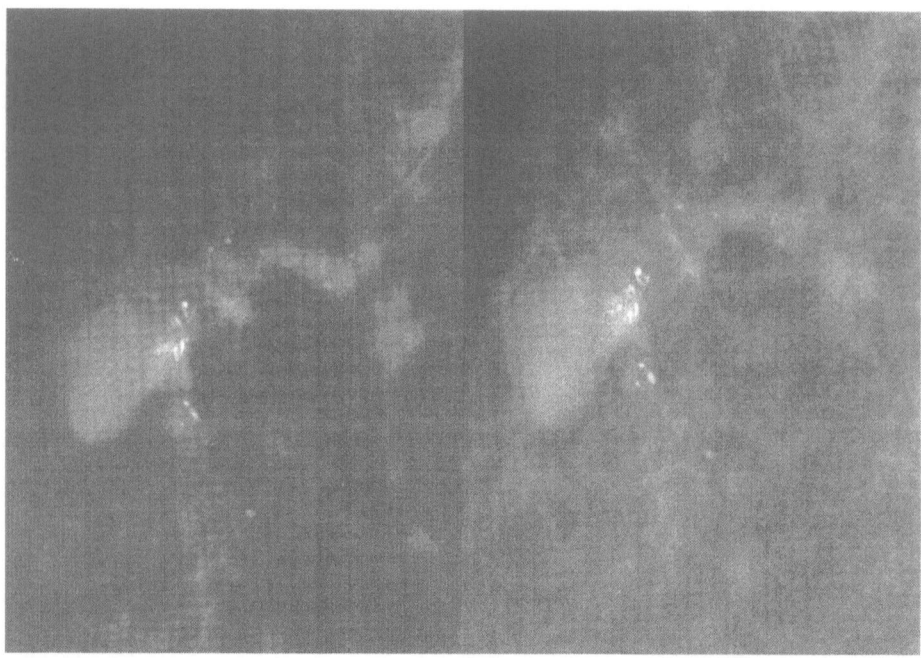

Figure 10.10. The image on the left was taken with an anti-scatter grid and digitised to 100 micron resolution. The image on the right was taken without a grid and then enhanced to make it appear as it would if there had been no scattered radiation at all.

CHAPTER 11

CALCIFICATIONS

11.1. Introduction

One of the fundamental assumptions that underpins the h_{int} representation is that we can ignore calcifications and assume that the breast consists either of fat or of non-fat "interesting tissue". In practice, small regions of calcification appear quite regularly in normal and abnormal mammograms, Figure 11.1 shows examples. Microcalcifications can be the *only* mammographic sign of non-palpable breast disease. For this reason, the computer-aided detection and classification of (micro)calcifications continues to be one of the major goals of mammographic image processing. However, despite the relatively large amount of effort expended toward the goal of assisting radiologists to detect and interpret calcifications, it is only recently that algorithms appear to have achieved a level of performance where they could be used in routine clinical practice. This chapter aims to show how the h_{int} representation can contribute significantly to this goal, since it can be used to:

- Detect film-screen "shot" noise which can be confused with calcifications, and thus is a major source of the false positives that downgrade the performance of algorithms for detecting microcalcifications;
- Estimate the thickness of calcifications, further contributing to the *quantitative* information that can be provided to the clinician;
- Improve the detection of calcifications by removing the effects of variations in the background and imaging parameters.

In addition, recall the two earlier applications of the h_{int} representation vis-à-vis calcifications: in Chapter 7 we showed how to enhance images safely to improve the visualisation of calcifications; and in Chapter 8 we showed how to simulate micro- and macrocalcifications.

The chapter begins by recalling some salient facts about microcalcifications: what and how big they are, how often they appear in mammograms, what they look like, and why not every microcalcification is indicative of breast disease. We then review the differential diagnosis of microcalcifications in radiological practice, *not* for ascertaining whether or not the calcifications in a mammogram have a benign or malignant interpretation,

EXAMPLES OF MICROCALCIFICATIONS

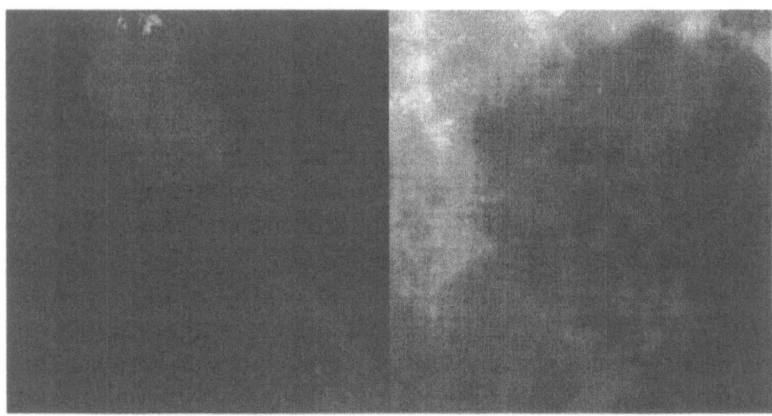

Figure 11.1. This shows two sections from mammograms with real microcalcifications.

but rather to assess whether the risk of malignancy warrants further investigation.

In Section 11.4 we summarise the algorithms that have been developed to date for the difficult image processing problem of computer-aided detection of microcalcifications. We note that the earliest stage of noise filtering is critical to achieving clinically-acceptable levels of performance, and we list a number of previous approaches in Section 11.5. The best performing system developed to date appears to be that developed by Karssemeijer [141], and its main features are recalled in Section 11.6. We then review the sources of image blur in the mammographic image process, since blur is crucial in determining the appearance of calcifications in mammograms. We show how we can detect film-screen noise by generating the h_{int} values and noting where the algorithm breaks down - points that show high x-ray attenuation but little evidence of blur. This leads to substantially reduced numbers of false positives that are typically found by algorithms for the detection of microcalcifications, as we demonstrate. We then show how we can estimate the thickness of the calcifications using the generated h_{int} values and knowledge of the x-ray attenuation coefficients of calcifications. Finally, we look at the differences in appearance of calcifications according to where they are positioned in the breast. From this we argue that a representation invariant to the imaging process with well-chosen feature measurements is fundamental to the reliable detection and classification of calcifications.

11.2. Microcalcifications

Microcalcifications account for over 50% of all the non-palpable lesions detected using mammography [43]. Indeed, Patnick [194] notes that an assessment of the appearance of microcalcifications was most often a primary consideration in the recall of 63,925 women (of 1,207,316 taking part) in the UK N.H.S. screening programme in 1994/5. Fandos-Morera et. al. [69] show that calcifications are typically salts of calcium or magnesium (e.g. calcite, calcium oxalate, and aragonite) or phosphorus (apatite). Calcifications occur in the breast as a result of secretions within structures that have become thickened and dried (inspissated).

Tabar and Dean [233] proposed analysing calcifications by determining the pathological processes that give rise to their development. They note that calcifications tend to take the shape of the cavity in which they are produced, so that analysis of their form and size can help determine their patho-anatomical location, hence reflecting the nature of the lesion. They suggested classifying calcifications according to form, density, size and distribution, in order to categorise them as one of *ductal* or "malignant type", *lobular*, or *miscellaneous*. As an example, what they call the lobular type are caused by a variety of processes. They note that such calcifications are usually associated with an extensive fibrosis (thickening and scarring) of connective tissue) throughout the breast. They propose that this may partly explain the stagnation of fluid in the cystically dilated lobules. The fluid contains many calcium particles (milk of calcium) and, if the cavity is small, the entire contents may calcify. In larger cystic dilations, the milk of calcium settles to the dependent portion of the cavity, giving rise to the so-called tea-cup calcifications. To date, no image processing system has realised Tabar and Dean's programme of relating microcalcification appearance to pathological process, hence diagnosis.

There are, on average, calcifications in 25% of mammograms. When microcalcifications indicate breast cancer, they most often present in clusters. This may be because they locate in the parenchymal structures such as ducts or lobules from where the tumour grows, or because they locate in the blood vessels generated by angiogenesis. The reverse, that clusters of microcalcifications always indicate breast cancer is not true: on average, clustered microcalcifications appear in 1 in every 14 mammograms, but only 7% of presented clusters mark ductal carcinomas (the most common type of carcinomas found using microcalcifications).

The distinction between microcalcifications and (macro)calcifications on the basis of size is somewhat arbitrary. For example, Dilhuydy [61] sets the upper limit of microcalcifications at 0.5mm, whereas Vanel [248] puts it at 1mm. At the other end of the digital imaging process, the resolution of most current scanners is typically either 50 or 100 microns so that some microcalcifications present as single pixels.

We have noted several times throughout this monograph that calcium strongly attenuates x-rays, so that microcalcifications *ideally* appear in a mammogram as localised bright "spots", small regions, or clusters of such small regions. As we shall see, this observation forms the starting point of most detection algorithms. In practice, things are not quite so simple, for at least three reasons:

- The relatively low image contrast of a mammogram, so that the signal-to-noise ratio of a microcalcification, as defined by its local image contrast, can be low in many cases of interest.
- The enormous variability of mammograms, reflecting the variability of breast anatomy, which implies equally large variations in contrast between calcifications and their background. If the background is almost entirely composed of fatty tissue, then detecting microcalcifications is relatively straightforward. If the background is a dense parenchymal pattern, the microcalcifications may be very difficult to discriminate or even be invisible.
- The blurring processes, such as intensifying screen glare, that locally smooth the ideally sharp transition from a bright microcalcification to the background, further lowering local image contrast.

Clearly, the detection and classification of microcalcifications in mammograms is a challenging perceptual task, even for experts. As with all such perceptual tasks, it is extremely difficult to determine what knowledge is mobilised and how. It seems clear, for example, that medical knowledge of anatomy, physiology, and pathology are mobilised, since radiologists perform better at the task than non-experts (though there is some evidence that radiographers can learn to discriminate reliably the "easy" cases). Nevertheless, our human ability to introspect about perception is notoriously poor, and in this regard experts fare no better than non-experts. Radiologists may be able to classify, with high accuracy, whether a microcalcification cluster is benign or malignant, or at least that it warrants further investigation. That does *not* mean, however, that they are able to say what image "features" or clinical knowledge they mobilise in reaching such a decision.

Indeed, Simpson [224] recounts a study which identified 17 terms used to characterise microcalcifications. The aim was to use this set as the basis of a standardised reporting scheme that would be of value for clinical audit. The study found low levels of agreement between the radiologists. More precisely, a statistic known as weighted κ that measures inter-rater agreement was computed for comparisons between pairs of radiologists. Let p_a be the proportion of cases on which two raters agree, and let p_e be the proportion of agreements expected by chance, then κ is defined as:

$$\kappa = \frac{p_a - p_e}{1 - p_e}$$

A zero value for weighted κ indicates agreement no better than chance, whereas perfect agreement corresponds to a value of 1. In Simpson's study, the κ values found for pairs of radiologists varied between the remarkably low figures of 0.05 and 0.43! Simpson concludes: "Skilled radiologists learn to recognise the appearance of cancer on a mammogram, and analysis of individual features may form a part of this, but even this is usually based on previous experience of seeing similar features, not textbook description". That is, radiologists *can* agree on whether or not an abnormality is indicative of cancer; but they cannot agree about the physical characteristics on which it might be thought that they are basing their judgement.

Since it is difficult to discover precisely what medical knowledge and which image features are used by radiologists to detect and classify microcalcifications, and since they have the same limited powers of introspection as the rest of mankind, it is difficult to build pattern recognition systems to carry out the same task! Not surprisingly, some authors have concluded that the best approach is to develop a system that can learn how to detect and classify microcalcifications, for example using neural networks (see, for example, [219, 268, 267]). However, if a neural network is applied directly to images, it has to contend *both* with the variation of interest (in this case microcalcification clusters) *and* the variability due to image formation (exposure time, AEC position, film type, etc.). The most successful applications of neural networks have been on *normalised* images [234], which is precisely one of the key attributes of the h_{int} representation that we have emphasised throughout this monograph.

11.3. Radiological assessment of microcalcifications

The diagnostic importance of microcalcifications was realised as soon as mammography became available. Equally, it was noticed that microcalcifications assumed many different forms, and that there was often a correlation between the form and distribution of microcalcifications and a diagnosis of breast cancer. So, even in the early 1970s, attempts were made to devise guidelines that related the morphology of microcalcifications to diagnosis. One of the first of these, that is still in widespread use in France,

TYPES OF MICROCALCIFICATION

Type I   Type II   Type III   Type IV   Type V

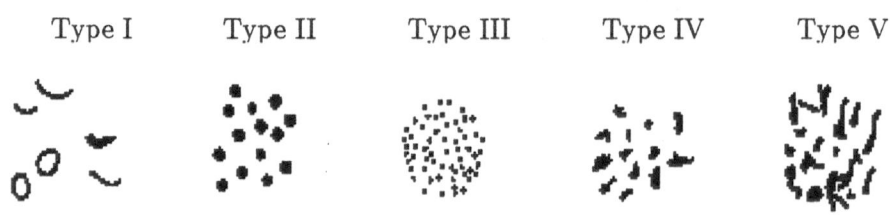

Figure 11.2. The five types of microcalcifications identified by Le Gal. (See text.)

was due to Le Gal [83, 84]. She and her colleagues distinguished five differ-ent morphological types, sketched in cartoon form in Figure 11.2. Each is associated with a different degree of risk:

> Type I: crescent shapes, or round, regular disks with clear centres (Le Gal found that there was 0% risk with this type of microcalcification);
> Type II: round, with regular outline and similar sizes, but without clear centres (19% risk of cancer);
> Type III: very fine microcalcifications, each of which is too small to have an identifiable shape (39% risk of cancer);
> Type IV: polyhedral, irregular shapes, similar to grains of salt (59% risk of cancer); and
> Type V: elongated or branching microcalcifications (96% risk of cancer).

In a recent technical report summarising the clinical diagnosis of breast cancer, Dilhuydy [60] suggests that neither of the distinctions: (i) between Types I and II, both of which are relatively benign, and where a decision to continue surveillance is most likely; and (ii) that between the more serious Types IV and V, for which a biopsy is immediately required, can be made consistently between observers. However, although it is hard to discriminate between Types I and II (or between IV and V), the classification of a cluster as either Type I *or* II or Type IV *or* V can be made quite reliably. Type III is the most problematical in practice. This point concurs with the two-stage process proposed by Sickles [223] (and summarized below), and the protocol proposed by Monsees [175].

In a similar heuristic fashion, Caseldine et al. [34] suggest the following rules for interpretation/diagnosis:

– Large (> 1mm diameter), coarse calcifications are likely to be benign;

Criteria	Tendency to be benign	Tendency to be malignant
Calcifications in any cm^2	1 - 10	11 upwards
Shape of cluster	Generally spherical Ductal streaming	Grossly irregular Whorled
Majority calcification size	1mm upwards	Punctate; 0.5mm or smaller
Uniformity of calcification size	Very uniform Moderately uniform	Mostly non-uniform Grossly non-uniform
Average distance between the calcifications in cluster	1.1mm upwards	1.0mm or smaller
More than one quadrant involved	Yes	No

TABLE 11.1. Freundlich's [82] criteria for malignancy.

- Single calcifications are likely to be benign;
- Rounded calcifications of equal size are likely to be benign;
- Calcifications scattered through both breasts are more likely to be associated with benign disease;
- Groups of calcifications of mixed size with irregular shapes are more likely to signify malignant than benign disease;
- Clusters of fine calcifications are likely to signify malignancy;
- Rows of fine calcifications (in the ducts) are likely to signify malignancy; and
- Short rods of calcification, particularly if they branch, are highly likely to signify malignancy.

Note the close similarity between these rules and the classification proposed by Le Gal. In both cases, the rules are qualitative, intended for human judgement, and would be difficult (though not impossible) to translate into a classification algorithm. In a more quantitative fashion, Freundlich [82] compiled the information shown in Table 11.1.

Lanyi [158] has developed a scheme for the differential diagnosis of microcalcifications, based, in the first instance, on their place of origin, then by assessing the likely process that caused them. He stresses that the goal is not simply to classify a microcalcification cluster as benign versus

malignant, rather to interpret the anatomical site of the cluster as lobular
or ductal, then condition the diagnosis on this interpretation. This echoes
the distinction made by Tabar and Dean (see the previous section). Lanyi
stresses two properties of microcalcification clusters, namely "septation"
and cluster shape. Septation means "separated by fine lines", which he observes to hold for benign clusters caused by microcystic adenosis. Lanyi's
analysis of cluster shape shows that in 97% of breast carcinomas at least
one of the following is evident: triangular or trapezoidal; square or rectangular; bottle or club shaped; propellor or butterfly shaped; rhomboid or
kite shaped; and linear or branched. He deduces that cluster shape is a key
sign in distinguishing ductal from lobular calcifications.

Sickles [223] has suggested a two-stage strategy similar to Dilhuydy
above, following the discussion of Le Gal's classification of microcalcification
morphology:

1. Where possible to base a benign interpretation on distinctive characteristics of benign causes of calcifications of which he enumerated
   six.
2. Then, characteristics of suspicious microcalcifications are used to determine whether an immediate biopsy is necessary, or whether continued
   surveillance suffices.

In summary, a great deal has been learnt over the past thirty years about
the differential diagnosis of non-palpable breast disease from an analysis of
microcalcification clusters. This knowledge has contributed greatly to the
success of the screening programmes around the world. However, there is
much scope for improvement. The low incidence of breast cancer in the
screening population is problematical for the screener, who has to remain
continuously vigilant for subtle signs such as microcalcifications. This mo-
tivates the computer-aided detection of microcalcifications, to which we
now turn, recognising that most of the radiological literature is, from the
standpoint of image processing, quite qualitative and even on occasions
vague.

11.4. Computer-aided detection and classification of microcalci-
fications

Many algorithms for the detection and classification of microcalcifications
have been proposed. Unfortunately, as is almost always the case in pattern recognition, published algorithms are very hard to compare, not least
because: (i) the results reported are based on different datasets; (ii) different sizes of training sets are used; (iii) different criteria to judge success
are used; (iv) the results are reported in different ways; (v) different preprocessing steps are used and it is hard to apportion credit to the different

---

BOX 11.1: Skeletal structure of an algorithm to detect and classify microcalcifications

(1) Filter the image to remove noise and enhance microcalcifications;

(2) Detect microcalcifications and clusters;

(3) Classify clusters.

---

stages of the algorithm; and (vi) though in most cases several image features are used to form the classification, a sensitivity analysis of the efficacy of individual parameters is rarely performed. Consequently, it is difficult to give a succinct, analytical summary of the current state of the art.

One can conclude however that for any algorithm the false positive (FP) rate associated with a sufficient true positive (TP) rate continues to be high (a discussion of TP, FP and receiver operating characteristics is in Appendix A). Several reasons have been advanced to explain FPs and false negatives (FNs), for example:

- Microcalcifications that are too faint to be detected: the response is to attempt to selectively enhance the microcalcifications in a preprocessing step;
- Film errors that are confused with microcalcifications: the response is to attempt to discriminate between them, for example on the basis of size or clustering;
- Benign microcalcifications, for example those in blood vessels: the response is to attempt to extract curvilinear structures and to interpret the microcalcifications in terms of those structures [36, 193]

We note that most published algorithm comprises the three sequential stages shown in Box 11.1.

A characteristic of any sequential pattern recognition algorithm is that successive stages mobilise increasingly application-specific knowledge. In the present case, the first filtering stage has almost always relied on general image processing techniques, whereas the third classification stage embodies morphological features of individual microcalcifications and of microcalcification clusters. Equally, a fundamental problem with any such sequential algorithm is that errors made early in the process have to be identified and corrected by later, more knowledgeable processes. For this reason, there has been a clear trend in the literature toward increasingly smart algorithms to judge putative microcalcifications in order to reduce the number of FPs to acceptable levels.

Consistent with the theme of this monograph, we propose a completely different approach! More specifically, we aim to reduce the number of errors made in the early stages of the algorithm by developing a filtering step based on the physics of mammogram image formation. We will demonstrate how this can drastically reduce the number of FPs, for example by distinguishing between film errors and microcalcifications. In like manner, we hope to demonstrate that by so doing, better levels of performance can be had with simpler, more robust versions of currently published algorithms.

We conclude this section with two subsections that present a brief overview of previously published schemes for the detection of microcalcifications and for their subsequent classification. We find that the initial stage of processing, image filtering, shown in Box 11.1 is critical and Section 11.5 describes some of the approaches adopted to date. One of the most successful approaches to microcalcification detection and classification has been introduced by Karssemeijer [141]. It is based on an elegant and efficient adaptive image noise estimation process which we describe in Section 11.6. We conclude that Karssemeijer's noise model cannot distinguish between "shot noise" and real microcalcifications, and in Section 11.7 we study the sources of blur in mammography and show how we can use a model-based technique to detect shot noise on the basis of blur. Finally, we show how the h_{int} representation can enable us to estimate the thickness of calcifications.

The detection of microcalcifications

Broadly, one can distinguish two approaches to detecting microcalcifications after image filtering: (i) local, adaptive thresholding; and (ii) local contrast. Both approaches rely on the observation that, ideally, a microcalcification should be brighter than its surrounds and should be relatively small. Nishikawa [184] exemplifies the thresholding approach: first, a global grey-level threshold is applied, chosen so that 98% of all breast pixels are set to the background level, then morphological erosion is applied to eliminate regions that are too small (area less than $0.03mm^2$), finally local adaptive thresholding is applied. A similar technique can be found in [41].

Davies et. al. [55] define five overlapping windows $W_1, \ldots, W_5$ surrounding each pixel. A histogram is defined for each window and, if the distribution of brightnesses is bimodal then a threshold is set at the valley of the distribution and those pixels whose brightness is above the threshold are declared to be putative microcalcifications. This is the adaptive local thresholding step. If, on the other hand, the histogram is unimodal, the threshold is linearly interpolated from the surrounding region and again pixels whose brightnesses are above threshold are marked. A pixel is finally

---

BOX 11.2: Estimating the local brightness contrast

Several algorithms have been proposed, of which the following are representative. The names are those suggested by Kegelmeyer and Allmen [146]:

W: Denote the image brightness at pixel (x, y) by $I(x, y)$. Let $\delta_{(x,y)}$ be a neighbourhood of size N centred on, but excluding, the point (x, y). Typically the neighbourhood is square, of odd size, and comprises 8, 24, or even 80 [141] pixels. Then the local brightness contrast at (x, y) is defined to be:

$$c(x, y) = I(x, y) - \frac{1}{N} \sum_{(u,v) \in \delta_{(x,y)}} I(u, v)$$

Kegelmeyer and Allmen [146] attribute this measure to Woods, though it can be found in most standard textbooks on Image Processing.

O: A related idea is to compute the mean brightness in the neighbourhood of the central pixel, then to mark a pixel as a putative microcalcification point if its brightness is more than three (say) standard deviations above the mean. Kegelmeyer and Allmen [146] call this the Outlier algorithm.

B: Apply an edge detector to the image, then morphologically dilate and erode the resulting edge image. Edge points lost after dilation followed by erosion are then restored and the enclosed regions considered as "objects". Kegelmeyer and Allmen [146] call this the Boundary algorithm.

---

declared to be a microcalcification if it is labelled as such in at least three of the five windows. Local contrast in an image is defined as the difference between the value of a parameter at a pixel and the average in the neighbourhood of the pixel. Three algorithms to estimate the local brightness contrast are shown in Box 11.2.

Kegelmeyer and Allmen [146] develop a detection algorithm that combines the results from six different algorithms, including three local thresholding algorithms and the three algorithms to estimate image contrast shown in Box 11.2. They report that the W measure of local contrast gives the best approximation to the outlines of microcalcifications, a result confirmed by Taylor [238]. Taylor applied a version of the Kegelmeyer and Allmen algorithm to the Mammographic Image Analysis Society (MIAS) database [231] and also found that the W algorithm gave the highest number of TPs, the least number of FNs, but by far the highest number of FPs. It seems that the main effect of combining the six different algorithms is to reduce sharply the number of FPs. Unfortunately, it also decreases the number of TPs.

Finally, we note that the problem of detection of subtle signs such as microcalcifications in low contrast, noisy images arises in many applications of image processing. Over the past twenty years a number of techniques have been developed to enhance such images, and one based upon an optimization technique called simulated annealing [86] (sometimes called stochastic relaxation) is perhaps the best known. The idea is to iteratively enhance an image by assigning a value to each pixel by propagating values from surrounding pixels and using Bayes' rule. Sometimes the value to be assigned is a number (for example a depth value in a motion estimation algorithm or depth in a stereovision algorithm), but most often it is one of a discrete set of "labels" that constitute an interpretation of the pixel.

The initial labelling of the image derives from a classification of each pixel on the basis of its local surrounds. Then, as the iterations proceed, this initial labelling can be changed, even in cases where, *a priori*, it seemed to be quite certain. This ability to take back what seemed to be a near certain classification is a major advantage of simulated annealing (known technically as the ability to escape local minima), and is the property that enables such an algorithm to overcome the effects of noise without excessively smoothing an image (which would remove small image features such as microcalcifications).

Simulated annealing, in conjunction with Markov random fields, has been widely applied, for example in enhancing and classifying land utilisation in noisy satellite images. Indeed, a number of image processing algorithms of this sort have been developed that give remarkable results on very noisy images in tough applications. It has been found in practice, however, that a simulated annealing algorithm works most reliably (and most quickly) when the percentage of initial labels that need to be changed is relatively small, and where the number of parameters that control the operation of the algorithm is also small.

Simulated annealing has been applied successfully to the detection of microcalcifications by Karssemeijer[141]. One of four labels is assigned to each pixel: (1) background; (2) microcalcification; (3) points lying on an edge/line; and (4) film errors. The rule for iteratively updating the labelling of a pixel involves three terms: (i) an external field parameter that biases the detection sensitivity for each class (ie. label); (ii) "short range" interaction parameters between the pixel label and the current labels of its eight immediate neighbours; and (iii) a "long range" interaction parameter that attempts to bias the detection towards clustered microcalcifications instead of isolated microcalcifications. There are 4 parameters of type (i), 10 parameters of type (ii) and 1 parameter of type (iii) with an associated distant neighbourhood function. By the standards of image processing, this is quite a large number; but the performance of the algorithm is very promising indeed. Three image features are computed at each pixel: two measures of brightness contrast (that referred to as W in Box 11.2 and a smoothed version of W) and a measure of the likelihood that the pixel lies on a brightness boundary. Karssemeijer [141] reports a number of experiments which demonstrate that the smoothed contrast value adds little to the other two. The algorithm is shown to give 90% of TPs for a FP rate of one cluster per image.

It is hard to judge the stability of the algorithm to changes in the 15 parameters, which is often a key determiner of usefulness of such algorithms in clinical practice. We conjecture that incorporating our method for removing film errors (Section 11.7) would enable the number of labels to be reduced to three and the number of parameters to be reduced to at most 10. Further incorporating a reliable edge/line detector would further reduce the number to 5.

Classification of microcalcifications

Returning to the algorithm outline shown in Box 11.1, after image filtering, and the detection of microcalcifications, an attempt is made to classify the resulting clusters. A number of features are calculated for individual microcalcifications and for the cluster as a whole, then the resulting set of measurements is input either to a conventional pattern recognition system or to a neural network (for the reasons given at the end of the previous section). Taylor's thesis [238] gives a lucid summary of published techniques; his Table 16 showing the range of image measurements used by authors is reproduced as Table 11.2.

Magnin et. al. [167] attempt to classify individual microcalcifications as lobular or ductal. They suggest that compactness, convexity, lengthening rate, and mean ray vector suffice; however, a classifier was not developed. Lefebvre [162] developed a model for simulating clusters of microcalcifications, arguing that the features that enable "convincing" clusters to be simulated should be similar to those used to recognise such clusters. Four clinical features were recorded as well as sixteen image features. A decision tree classifier was developed [63]. The algorithm was able to identify as benign 46% of the benign images on which it was tested. Patrick [195] developed a complex system comprising five expert learning systems, but the learning process is not described in the article. Each expert learning system was provided with a different set of data: (i) individual microcalcification data from a cranio-caudal view; (ii) cluster data from a cranio-caudal view; (iii) individual microcalcification data from a medio-lateral view; (iv) cluster data from a medio-lateral view; and (v) clinical data. The most successful of the five systems recognised 9 of 10 malignant clusters and 9/15 benign.

Shen [219] constructed a three-layer back-propagation neural network (see Bishop [15] for a definition) in an attempt to classify individual microcalcifications as malignant or benign. The algorithm was tested on four images containing a total of 58 benign and 241 malignant microcalcifications. The classification rates were 94% for benign and 87% for malignant despite only using three shape features. Six different neural network architectures using a mixture of cluster features and "image structure" features were used by Chitre et. al. [41]. A k-nearest neighbour process identified the best 5 image structure features and the best 5 cluster features (see [63, 15] for a definition). The aim of the work was ambitious: to classify clusters considered to be "difficult to diagnose". The results were rather disappointing, in that the area under the receiver operating characteristic (ROC) curve varied between 0.57 and 0.61 (see Appendix A for details about ROC curves).

Another back-propagation neural network has been developed by Nishikawa and colleagues [184]. It was tested on a database of 100 images containing 107 microcalcification clusters. Every cluster, even those that transpired to be benign, were judged sufficiently problematical as to warrant biopsy. All 19 patients with cancer were correctly classified as having malignant clusters. However, only 16 of the remaining 34 patients with benign disease were correctly classified. The area under the ROC curve was 0.83. Parker et. al. [191] reported a k-nearest neighbour classifier that aimed to distinguish microcalcifications (located manually by a radiologist) arising from ductal carcinoma *in situ* (DCIS). The initial version of the algorithm used 24 different features of microcalcifications and of clusters, together with the range, mean and variance of those features. This large number of features was then pruned to those shown in Table 11.2 by removing redundancies and by eliminating any single measure that did not give a classification significantly better than chance. The resulting discrimination had a reported ROC area of 91%.

Table 11.2 summarises the features used in the representative sample of algorithms described above. It is immediately apparent that a large number have been tried, with remarkably little duplication between systems, further complicating comparisons. Only Magnin and Parker can be said to contribute to the programme set out by Tabar and Dean (and Lanyi) of assessing a microcalcification cluster conditioned by an interpretation of its underlying pathology.

		Mag	Lef	Ptk	Shn	Cht	Nsh	Prk
cluster shape	compactness		X				X	X
	area						X	
	4th invt. moment							X
density	mean grey level						X	
	contrast							X
density varn.	s.d. grey level		X			X	X	
	s.d. edge strength							X
distribution	mean separation		X			X		
	no. per unit area		X					
	mean dist. from centre					X		
	s.d. dist. from centre					X		
	grav.pot.of other mc.			X				
number	number		X	X		X	X	
shape	perimeter	X						
	compactness	X		X	X			
	hull compactness			X				
	ratio compactnesses			X				
	lowest compactness		X					
	convexity	X						
	lengthening rate	X						
	mean ray vector	X						
	moment descriptor				X			
	moment of inertia		X					
	1st invt. moment		X					X
	invt. moments 2-7		X					
	moment w.r.t. axis		X					
	ratio of moments				X			
	2nd highest irregularity						X	
	entropy (texture)							X
	aspect ratio	X		X				X
	eccentricity							X
	mean gyration							X
	Fourier descriptor					X		
	length of major axis			X				
	s.d. of boundary			X				
varn. in shape	s.d. compactness		X					X
	range of gyration							X
	s.d. of aspect ratio			X				
	max. figure value			X				
size	mean grey level x area						X	
	mean area	X					X	
varn. in size	s.d. of area			X				

TABLE 11.2. Measures used in the classification of microcalcifications. From [238], Table 16. Note that Mag=Magnin, Lef=Lefebrve, Ptk=Patrick, Shn=Shen, Cht=Chitre, Nsh=Nishikawa and Prk=Parker, see text.

11.5. Image filtering

We now return to the first of the three stages enumerated in Box 11.1, namely image filtering. First, we note that a number of algorithms have been developed that do not include an explicit filtering step; rather it is supposed that techniques to detect microcalcifications, such as local thresholding or contrast estimation, will be sufficient to suppress noise and the effect of the background. However, most systems include a preliminary stage that attempts to reduce image noise and provide local enhancement of microcalcifications. Most often, this amounts to:

1. *Smooth the background*: this uses a form of low pass filtering;
2. *Enhance putative microcalcifications*: this uses high pass filtering;
3. Subtract the result of step 1 from the result of step 2.

The first example of such an approach seems to have been by Chan and colleagues [37] who proposed a "signal-enhanced" image in step 1 by convolution with a matched filter, and a "signal-suppressed" image in step 2, using either a median filter or a contrast-reversal filter. Subsequently, [183] replaced the filter used in step 2 by a box-rim filter. A fundamental problem with such techniques, or of the direct application of nonlinear filtering techniques based on mathematical morphology, is that fixed size filters take no account of the wide variation in the sizes of the microcalcifications often found in mammograms. A second problem concerns the image noise model intrinsic to the approach, to which we return below. Chan and colleagues [38] subsequently suggested replacing the filtering steps 1 and 2 by a single modulated "visual response" (VRF) log-Gaussian filter. The details of their filter are shown in Box 11.3. It is a bandpass filter defined so that "If D is properly chosen, then the bandpass response of VRF will enhance the microcalcifications and suppress both the background and high frequency noise". The first task is to choose the spatial frequency u_0 most appropriate to viewing mammograms from a distance of 25cm: since the visual response filter is bandpass, this means choosing u_0 so that the smoothly varying background falls outside the low frequency cut-off of the pass band, while the noise lies above the high frequency cut-off. It is not at all obvious that such a passband exists: the differentiation between noise and microcalcifications does not seem to correspond to a difference in spatial frequencies, especially after blurring during the image formation process.

A variation to the idea of subtracting two filtered versions of the image was proposed by Valatx [247]. It is assumed that, considered as a surface, the image is mostly smooth, except at microcalcifications, intensity discontinuities, and points where the noise is large. The image is approximated (in a least squares sense) with a smooth function ([247] suggest using a bicubic B-spline) and the smooth approximation is then subtracted from the origi-

---

BOX 11.3: Visual response filter

The visual response filters were introduced by Chan and colleagues [38] and they are defined for a spatial frequency u by:

$$\text{VRF}(u) = \exp\{-\frac{\ln u - \ln(25u_0/D)}{2(0.973)^2}\}$$

This has the form of a log-Gaussian filter with half power 0.973, centred on a spatial frequency u_1 which, at viewing distance D, is linearly proportional to the spatial frequency u_0 that is most appropriate when viewing a mammogram from a distance of 25cm. That is, $25\,u_0 = D\,u_1$.

---

nal image, ideally leaving a near-zero signal almost everywhere, punctuated by microcalcifications, points where the noise is large, and edges. Finally, a locally adaptive threshold is used to detect microcalcifications. An alternative would be to use an approximation algorithm such as that developed by Blake and Zisserman [16] that can follow extended intensity discontinuities (edges) so that they would not need to be filtered out subsequently. Similarly, an unbiased, structure-preserving, nonlinear image filter, such as the morphological *comoc* [186], might be expected to give equally good results. The comoc is the *mean* of the close-open (*co*) and the open-close (*oc*) idempotent filters.

Implicit in all of the above is the assumption that the image noise is zero-mean independently, identically-distributed Gaussian, see Box 11.4. In this section we show that this assumption does not hold in mammography and thus give poor results. We can demonstrate simply the noise characteristics of our digitiser and the overall image noise by making the reasonable assumption that the noise is not Markovian (i.e. its statistics do not change over time), which is entirely reasonable for the steady-state and images taken in quick succession. Then the difference between two images of the same scene, for example of a calibration wedge, taken in quick succession with a stationary camera, can be assumed to consist solely of noise. The digitiser noise for our scanner, which is based on a photo-multiplier tube is shown in Figures 11.3 and 11.4. Clearly, the digitiser noise obeys the zero-mean independently, identically-distributed Gaussian assumption. However, the overall image noise certainly does not obey this model as shown in Figure 11.5. This is the problem which Karssemeijer [141] tackles and this we cover in the next section.

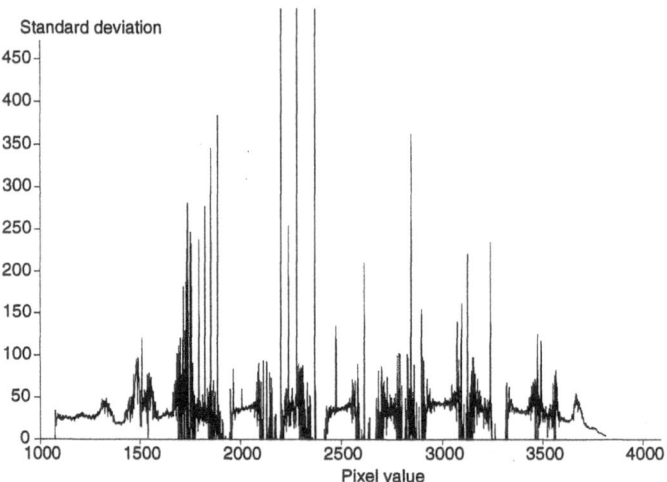

Figure 11.3. Digitiser noise: A mammographic film showing a step-wedge was digitised twice and the two images of the wedge aligned and subtracted to show the noise in the image. The standard deviation in the difference image at each pixel with a set pixel value in the original images was computed and that is what is displayed here. This is effectively noise versus pixel value. The noise is almost constant over the range of pixel values. The high-peaks come from regions in-between the main steps on the wedge image and can be discarded.

11.6. Karssemeijer's adaptive noise estimation process

Karssemeijer [141] has introduced an elegant and efficient adaptive noise estimation process which works directly from the given image and in which intensities are rescaled in order to make the simple "identical" noise model described in Box 11.4 applicable. More precisely, he proposes the rescaling process outlined in Box 11.5.

The first, and key, step in the adaptive noise process introduced by Karssemeijer is to estimate the standard deviation of the noise; the second step is to rescale the image and is standard in image processing (see, for example [91], page 142). Recall that image noise is predominantly high frequency, and so points affected by noise correspond to those where the local intensity contrast is high. For this reason, Karssemeijer estimates the standard deviation $\hat{\sigma}(I)$ of the noise in the given image $I(x, y)$ using the local intensity contrast. For this, he applies the algorithm W shown in Box 11.2.

At this point, Karssemeijer ([141], page 1360) suggests adding a step that improves the statistical reliability of the process to estimate the local

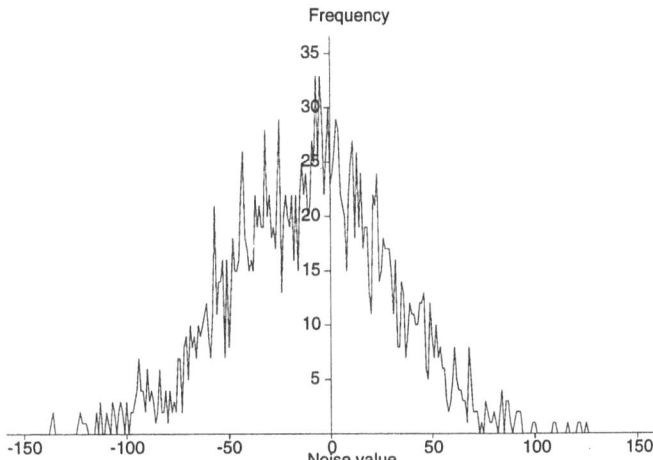

Figure 11.4. Digitiser noise: This is the distribution of noise at a pixel value of 2048 in the original images. The distribution at this and other pixel values is near Gaussian and suggests that the noise for our digitiser is independently identically-distributed.

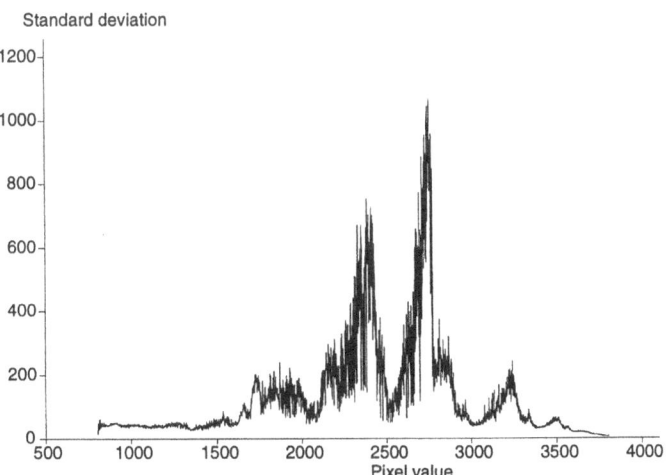

Figure 11.5. Image noise: A mammographic film with a step-wedge was performed twice and the two images of the wedge aligned and subtracted to show the noise in the image. The standard deviation in the difference image at each pixel with a set pixel value in the original images was computed and that is what is displayed here. This is effectively noise versus pixel value. The standard deviation is robust to shifts in the pixel values due to, for example, changes in the time-of-exposure between the wedges. In contrast to the digitiser noise the combined imaging process noise clearly depends on the pixel value.

BOX 11.4: Sensor noise models

Sensor noise is inevitable and for almost all sensors it has been found
that noise is additive, so that:

$$I_{actual}(x,y) = I_{ideal}(x,y) + N(x,y)$$

where I_{actual} is the measured image, I_{ideal} is the (desired) noise-free
image, and $N(x,y)$ is the spatially-varying noise. Several models have
been proposed for N. It is usually assumed that the noise is equally
likely to reduce the intensity as to increase it, that is to say, that it
is zero-mean. It is generally assumed also that the noise process at a
pixel is independently distributed of those at other pixels. Finally, it is
assumed that the noise follows a normal distribution, so that:

$$N(x,y) = \mathcal{N}(0, \sigma(x,y)).$$

The different noise models correspond to different assumptions about
the analytical form of $\sigma(x,y)$. Three models are of interest here:

1. **Identical:** $\sigma(x,y) = \sigma$, that is to say, the noise distribution is constant, independent both of image position and the intensity value
   $I_{ideal}(x,y)$. This is the simplest model, and it has been used with
   success in many applications of image processing and is the model
   that holds for sensors based upon photo-multiplier tubes.
2. **Variance linearly related to intensity:** $\sigma^2(x,y) = \sigma_1^2 + I(x,y)\sigma_2^2$.
   This model is appropriate for sensors based upon charge-coupled de-
   vices (CCDs). The noise in CCD sensors was investigated by Healey
   et. al.[106], who showed that there are several different contributing
   processes. These have different distributions, including Gaussian,
   Poisson and Uniform. They showed, however, that the Gaussian
   component is usually dominant. They also find that the noise is independent of position (x,y) and depends only on the brightness I,
   that is $\sigma(x,y) = \sigma(I(x,y))$.
3. **Application-specific, nonlinear relation:** this is the approach
   proposed by Karssemeijer [141] and described in Section 11.6.

---

noise standard deviation $\hat{\sigma}(I)$. Construct a histogram (a discrete approximation to the intensity probability density function) for the image. In
general, one observes that not all brightness values are equally likely, so
that an estimate $\hat{\sigma}(I)$ calculated directly from the contrast values them-

---

BOX 11.5: Outline version of Karssemeijer's adaptive noise estimation process

1. Estimate the standard deviation $\hat{\sigma}(I)$ of the noise in the given image $I(x, y)$. As noted above, this is a function of the image brightness I, but not image position (x, y);

2. Define a rescaling function $L : I \longrightarrow I_r$, where I_r is the rescaled intensity value and where

$$I_r(x, y) = L(I(x, y); \hat{\sigma}(I))$$

3. The standard deviation $\sigma_r(I_r)$ of the rescaled intensities should satisfy:

$$\sigma_r(I_r) \approx \sigma_r,$$

where σ_r is a constant to be chosen by the user.

---

selves would be biased. Instead, Karssemeijer suggests that the intensity scale is divided into a sequence of intervals (called "bins") so that each bin contains roughly the same number of brightness values, that is, is equally likely. Then the standard deviation of the noise is estimated via the bins as shown in Box 11.6.

We have implemented Karssemeijer's noise estimation technique. We find that our film scanner (a Lumisys scanning microdensitometer) can sense a larger range of optical densities ($0.0 - 4.0$) than that reported in [141] ($0.18 - 2.5$). Similarly, we find that the standard deviation of the noise is significantly lower for our scanner (1.7 times) than that reported by Karssemeijer. However, Karssemeijer's noise model is of no use in differentiating between "shot noise" and real microcalcifications. In the next section we study the sources of blur in mammography and show how we can use a model-based technique to detect shot noise on the basis of blur.

BOX 11.6: Estimating the noise standard deviation in the image

1. For each bin k, determine the distribution of contrasts c for each pixel contributing to the bin. This gives a sample distribution $\hat{f}(c|k)$ that turns out to be approximately zero-mean Gaussian. Estimate the sample standard deviation of the bin by:

$$\hat{s}_c^2(k) = r(T) \int_{c_{min}}^{c_{max}} c^2\, \hat{f}(c|k)dc,$$

   where: T is a threshold to be chosen by the user; c_{max} is the smallest value of c above zero where $\hat{f}(c_{max}|k) < T$; c_{min} is the value of c below but nearest zero where $\hat{f}(c_{min}|k) < T$; and $r(T)$ is a correction factor that is calculated numerically from a truncated Gaussian.

2. Given the estimated standard deviation $\hat{\sigma}(k)$ for the bins, the desired standard deviation $\hat{\sigma}(I)$ corresponding to brightness I is estimated by polynomial interpolation.

11.7. Blur in mammography

There are four primary sources of blur (or "unsharpness") in a digitised mammogram:

- Patient movement;
- Geometric blur from the finite focal spot size;
- Digitiser blur;
- Intensifying screen glare.

Since the breast is tightly compressed during the brief, typically 1 second, imaging period, it can be assumed that patient movement is minimal.

The focal spot size in mammography can be as large as 0.5mm by 0.5mm and the source-to-film distance is typically 65cm. The blur due to the focal spot size is a function of the relative distance of the object of interest and the film-screen. This distance is not known a priori and for the cases where the object of interest is in contact with the film-screen there are no blur contributions from the focal spot. Dance [49] shows that for a focal-spot size common in mammography, the unsharpness due to a finite focal spot is minimal compared to the unsharpness due to the intensifying screen. Intensifying screen glare is the dominant source of blurring in the image: when an x-ray photon is absorbed in the phosphor, light photons are emitted isotropically and so there is exposure to the film over a small neighbourhood rather than at a precise point as explained on Page 53.

The digitisation process also introduces a significant blurring function into the imaging process. Davies [54] presents the modulation transfer functions for a scanning microdensitometer, CCD camera and a laser scanner similar to the one which we use. We use the modulation transfer function presented by Davies in order to remove the blur due to the digitiser.

11.8. Detecting film-screen "shot" noise

Film-screen "shot" noise can arise from dust and dirt on the intensifying screen or from deficiencies in the film. A major difficulty in detecting microcalcifications is that this noise tends to appear with similar characteristics to the calcification: small, low film density (bright) and high frequency. Consequently, automated detection of microcalcifications as localised bright spots tends to generate many false positives . Although some of these can be eliminated by using the clustering property of real microcalcifications it would be preferable to be able to eliminate them individually. We use the absence of blur from bright spots to mark them as noise. The absence of blur indicates they were introduced into the imaging chain *after* the glare from the intensifying screen.

To remove glare from an image, it is first transformed into an image which represents the energy imparted to the intensifying screen. In this representation calcifications and noise have very low values due to their apparent "high x-ray attenuation". When glare is removed from the image, pixels with low energy values due to noise become negative indicating that the original energy value was not feasible. Figure 11.6 shows two film density profiles with confirmed shot noise in them. Figure 11.7 shows an original energy profile and the energies after glare compensation.

Figure 11.8 shows an example of a physical phantom (TOR-MAX, University of Leeds, Department of Medical Physics, X-ray Test Object) and the noise that our detection scheme finds. The phantom contains physically simulated microcalcifications which are not marked by our noise detection scheme whilst all the noise is detected.

We carried out extensive testing of the film-screen shot noise detection algorithm on real mammograms. On a set of 20 sections of mammograms many of which contained microcalcifications an experienced radiologist marked the points corresponding to film-screen shot noise. She marked 156 points of which our algorithm detected 150. The algorithm also detected 6 more points which the radiologist was unable to state categorically whether they were noise or real microcalcifications, no definite microcalci-

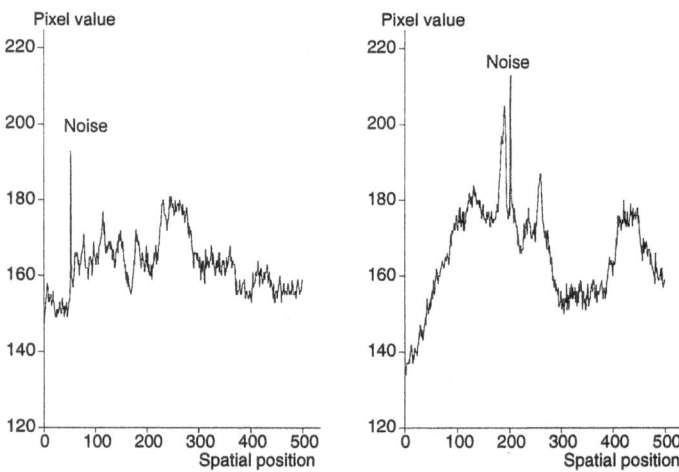

Figure 11.6. This shows two profiles across 100 micron images containing microcalcifi-cations. The pixel value on the y-axis is linearly related to film density, with high pixel value meaning low film density and thus low energy imparted to the intensifying screen. In the left profile our image restoration algorithm for glare picks out $x = 50$ as being film-screen noise, and in the right profile the point at $x = 206$. The peaks at $x = 190$ and $x = 250$ in the right profile are real calcifications.

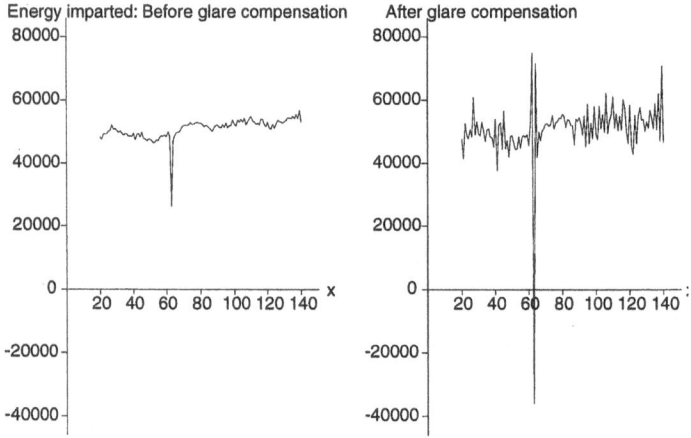

Figure 11.7. This shows two profiles across a 100 micron energy image. The left profile shows the energies imparted before glare compensation. There is a low value at $x = 62$ which is due to noise (low energy means it appears white). The right profile shows the energies after glare compensation, the energy at the noise point is now negative, i.e. it has been introduced to the image after the major blurring stage.

NOISE DETECTION

Phantom image   Detected noise

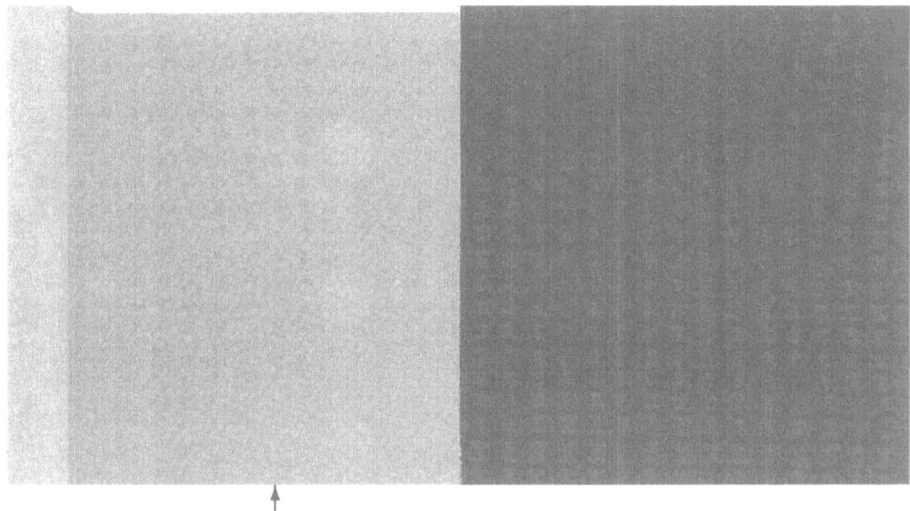

Figure 11.8. The image on the left is of a physical mammographic phantom. The phantom has simulated microcalcifications (pointed at by the arrow), round cylinders of varying densities and, at the far right, patches of texture. Before the mammogram was performed the film-screen combination was opened up and dust and dirt distributed randomly - these show-up as being bright white on the left image. The results of our noise-detection algorithm are shown on the right. All the obvious noise pixels have been detected as well as some far more subtle ones, none of the simulated microcalcifications have been marked as noise.

fications were marked as noise. Figures 11.9 and 11.10 show examples of mammograms and the noise detected.

Although this noise detection scheme works extremely well, there are two considerations which should be noted:

- At points where the film is saturated, that is where it has very high film density, or at very low film density such as in those areas beneath lead markers the estimated energy imparted is inaccurate and that can affect the noise detection. However, this happens only at the very edges of the breast image well away from any likely calcifications. An example of this is in Figure 11.8 where the very low film densities at the top of the image are marked as noise.
- Noise points affect the noise detection at points near to them. The glare removal requires the energies in a local neighbourhood. If one of

NOISE DETECTION: REAL IMAGE

Real image   Detected noise

Figure 11.9. On the left is a section of a real mammogram digitised to 100 microns per pixel. There is a cluster of noise points as confirmed by an experienced radiologist and by our technique as seen on the right which shows in white the noise detected. There is a quite obvious hair in the top right corner and some subtle genuine microcalcifications in the bottom left corner which have not been marked as noise.

the energies is artificially low due to noise then the glare removal might be incorrect and might cause other noise not to be detected. This can be seen in Figure 11.8 where there is a hair which clearly has the end points marked but not the central ones. This might necessitate a two-pass glare removal algorithm or require that any pixels nominated as calcifications within a certain radius of a noise point are also considered noise.

11.9. Improving detection schemes

To show how our noise detection scheme improves automated analysis algorithms our colleague Maud Poissonnier implemented three well-known segmentation methods [201]: the W filter as explained in Box 11.2, the morphological top-hat transform, and graduated non-convexity (GNC) [16]. GNC is based upon detecting intensity discontinuities (i.e. edges). It allows a 'weak' membrane (an elastic surface under weak continuity constraints)

NOISE DETECTION: REAL IMAGE

Real image   Detected noise

Figure 11.10. On the left is a section of a real mammogram digitised to 50 microns per pixel. There is a whole cluster of noise points as confirmed by an experienced radiologists and by our technique as seen on the right which shows in white the noise detected.

to fit the original image whilst breaking at intensity discontinuities. Subtracting a smoothed image from this gives an image with all the salient features. Each of these three algorithms has been used for microcalcification detection. Figure 11.11 shows the results of the three algorithms in the situation where there are known microcalcifications and one noise point. Figure 11.12 shows the result of applying the GNC algorithm to a cluster of noise points and the noise detected using our scheme. Clearly, using our noise detection method can reduce the number of false-positives.

11.10. Estimating thickness of calcifications

From the h_{int} generation stage we have floating point values representing the "interesting tissue" thicknesses. Since calcifications are small it's reasonable to assume that the background tissue onto which they are projected has constant h_{int} and this constant can be estimated from the surrounding neighbourhood, or by performing a morphological operation such as an opening. Subtracting the original from the background gives a thickness of h_{int} which we deem to be from the calcification. Using typical x-ray attenu-

FALSE POSITIVES IN CALCIFICATION DETECTION

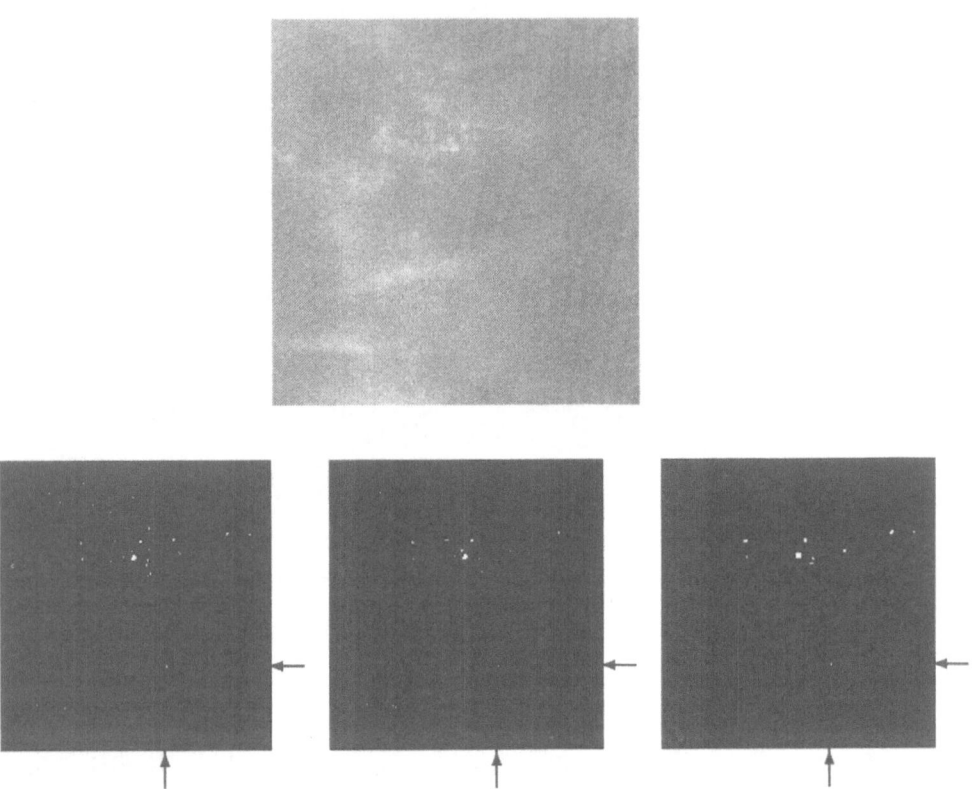

Figure 11.11. The result of three segmentation methods on a 100-micron 12-bit section of digitised mammogram with a cluster. The top image is the original. The three smaller ones show, from left-to-right, segmentation based upon: Woods; morphology (top-hat); GNC algorithm. The arrows on each of the lower images indicates a pixel affected by noise and marked as calcification by all three of the algorithms; our noise detection scheme can remove such pixels.

ation coefficients of calcification as given in Chapter 2 allows us to estimate the thickness of the calcification. The h_{int} values (in cm) from around one microcalcification are as follows, where each pixel has side 100 microns and the asterisks denote a pixel within the calcification:

```
2.99   3.24  *4.21  *4.12  *4.39  *4.13   2.69   2.24
*3.60  *4.11  *4.12  *4.44  *4.91  *4.17  *4.12   3.04
3.04  *3.82  *4.58  *4.51  *4.94  *4.81  *3.97  *3.50
2.70   2.80   3.18  *3.83  *4.17  *4.00  *4.12  *3.95
```

IMPROVING CALCIFICATION DETECTION

Figure 11.12. Comparison between the GNC-based segmentation and the noise map generated by our noise detection algorithm on a 50-micron, 12-bit section of digitised mammogram with no confirmed microcalcification. The left image is the original, the middle is the result of the GNC-based segmentation method and the right is the noise map.

For a simple example, we will take the average h_{int} outside the calcification as the background contribution and then subtract to get the h_{int} attributable to the calcification. Here we write the equations using a monoenergetic simplification, but h_{calc} (the thickness of calcification) can be computed using polyenergetic data. We want the x-ray attenuation measured to be equal to the background attenuation plus attenuation due to the calcification:

$$\mu_{int}h_{int}^{calc}(x,y) + \mu_{fat}h_{fat}^{calc}(x,y) = \mu_{int}h_{int}^{surr} + \mu_{fat}h_{fat}^{surr} + \mu_{calc}h_{calc}(x,y),$$

the left hand side is the measured attenuation and the right hand side has firstly the background contribution and then the calcification. Rearranging this equation and using $H = h_{fat}(x,y) + h_{int}(x,y)$ we get:

$$h_{calc}(x,y) = \frac{(\mu_{int} - \mu_{fat})(h_{int}^{calc}(x,y) - h_{int}^{surr})}{\mu_{calc}}$$

Using the values of the linear attenuation coefficients at 18keV: $\mu_{int} = 1.028$, $\mu_{fat} = 0.558$ and a typical value for μ_{calc} of 26.1, we see that:

$$h_{calc}(x,y) \approx 0.018(h_{int}^{calc}(x,y) - h_{int}^{surr})$$

Applying this to the previously listed h_{int} values we get:

		0.0290	0.0274	0.0322	0.0275		
0.0181	0.0272	0.0274	0.0331	0.0414	0.0283	0.0274	
	0.0220	0.0356	0.0344	0.0421	0.0398	0.0247	0.0162
		0.0221	0.0283	0.0252	0.0274	0.0243	

These values are consistent with the view that this microcalcification is a linear structure of width 400 microns (0.04cm), and if the cross-sectional shape is a circle then we expect a maximum h_{calc} of 0.04cm. We used the h_{calc} values found in this way to simulate calcifications in Chapter 7 and we also use the values in the next section.

11.11. Image analysis

We have consistently argued that image analysis should be carried out on the h_{int} representation that factors out the imaging conditions. In this section we use our simulation model to add the same, realistic cluster of calcifications to five sites across a mammogram. The x-ray process is then simulated and the resulting image, as shown in Figure 11.13 shows the differences in appearance that can be achieved across just one mammogram according to the surrounding tissues and location of the cluster. Taking simple image statistics about each cluster in the h_{int} image and the simulated film density image reveals significant variations between the clusters in the film density image that are not present in the clusters in the h_{int} image. Robust image analysis will need to cope with different surrounding tissues and these are far more reliably and logically dealt with in the h_{int} images as illustrated in Chapter 9.

11.12. A novel detection scheme

It may be recalled that the fundamental assumptions underlying the generation of the h_{int} representation is that the breast consists entirely of fat and "interesting tissue". Since calcifications have an x-ray attenuation coefficient which is about 26 times higher than those tissue types, the attenuation of an x-ray beam through a microcalcification, perhaps of diameter 0.5 mm, is comparable to that through 1.3 mm of interesting tissue. For this reason, we expect the h_{int} value computed for pixels which in fact correspond to calcifications to far exceed those which correspond to non-calcifications.

We are developing an algorithm that exploits this observation. Details of extensive testing and clinical evaluation will be published in future articles. Here we give a brief sketch of our current approach and show sample results. An important quantity used in our algorithm is the interesting tissue

VARYING APPEARANCE WITH LOCATION

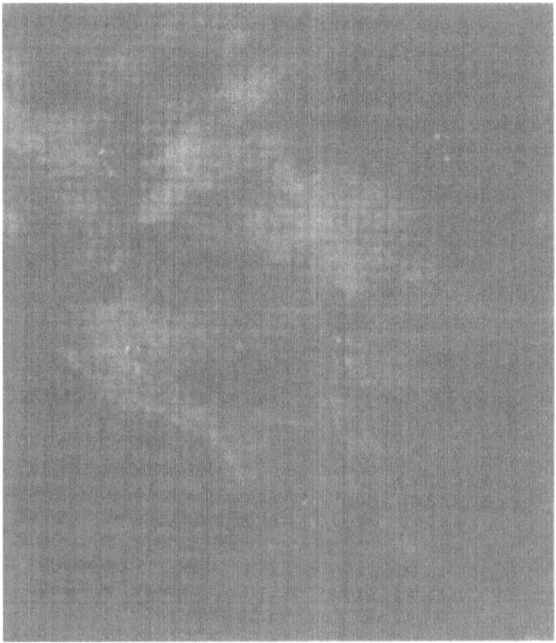

Figure 11.13. This shows the same cluster of simulated microcalcifications implanted into 5 different places in a mammogram digitised to 100 microns. There is clearly a wide variation in the appearance of each cluster due to the surrounding tissues on which they are placed. If the same cluster was implanted into a different breast the differences in the imaging conditions could make the two clusters practically unidentifiable as being fundamentally the same.

volume, denoted by v_{int}, which represents the total amount of interesting tissue present in a mass of breast tissue. v_{int} can be computed from the h_{int} values over the region of interest on the image. Now consider the v_{int} value of a small volume of breast tissue, B, whose actual volume is v_{act}. If no calcification is present in B, v_{int} should be bound above by v_{act}. However, if B is a calcification, the computed v_{int} would exceed v_{act} owing to the violation of the fundamental assumption of the h_{int} model. Thresholding the v_{int} to v_{act} ratio, enables us to differentiate calcifications from other breast tissue. This ratio is subject neither to varying imaging conditions nor to different tissue backgrounds on which a calcification is projected. This is contrary to image contrast, which is what most other calcification detection algorithms use.

We have developed techniques for segmenting candidate regions of the mammogram, namely those that satisfy a weak contrast constraint and which are not too large. We estimate v_{int} for candidate regions by estimating the background h_{int} and subtracting it. The difficulty is to estimate v_{act}, and to do this we currently make the heuristic assumption that the candidate microcalcification has an elliptical cross section, so that its volume can be estimated from its projection in the image.

In an initial experimental study we used a total of 20 image samples taken from 7 different mammograms. The images are digitised to a resolution of $50\mu m$ per pixel. There are altogether 27 microcalcifications in the 20 samples, each of which has at least 1 microcalcification. A 100% TP rate is obtained along with 0 FP per image when the v_{ratio}^{int} threshold is set to 3. Our algorithm detects 4 other regions which the radiologists are unable to make conclusive remarks on whether they correspond to real calcifications or non-calcifications.

We also compared our results with those obtained by simply thresholding the grey level contrast. An ROC analysis shows that our method achieves both higher sensitivity and better specificity, albeit on a small sample. Figure 11.14 shows an example in which a typical contrast-based detector fails to detect a microcalcification. The glare removal process discussed in Section 11.7 enables us to eliminate many FPs that correspond to noise. Figure 11.15 shows this. Algorithms based on contrast measures have difficulty rejecting such FPs. These and other sample initial results obtained are encouraging. However, it now needs to be tested against a larger data set before reliable assessment of the method can be made.

11.13. Summary: Calcifications

Despite the h_{int} representation explicitly **excluding** calcifications it is quite evident that it is useful for detecting them and for differentiating false-positives due to shot noise. However, other false-positives due to normal breast structures and calcification classification have not been studied yet. In the next chapter we examine curvilinear structures and how to automate their detection. We expect that work to provide information as to where the calcifications lie and to reduce the number of false-positives due to overlapping normal breast structures.

DETECTING LOW-CONTRAST MICROCALCIFICATIONS

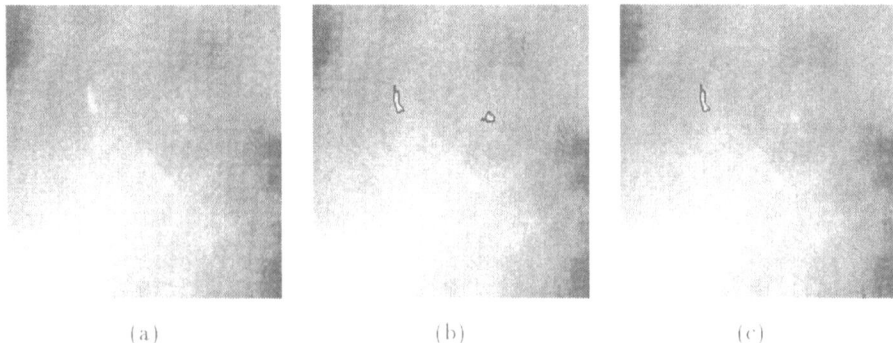

(a)   (b)   (c)

Figure 11.14. Detecting a low-contrast microcalcification: (a) the original image (ox-DATA139RC1c2) with 2 microcalcifications (b) detection result using the volume ratio algorithm: both calcifications are detected successfully; (c) detection result using grey level contrast: the more obscure calcification on the right is missed.

DETECTION OF FALSE POSITIVES

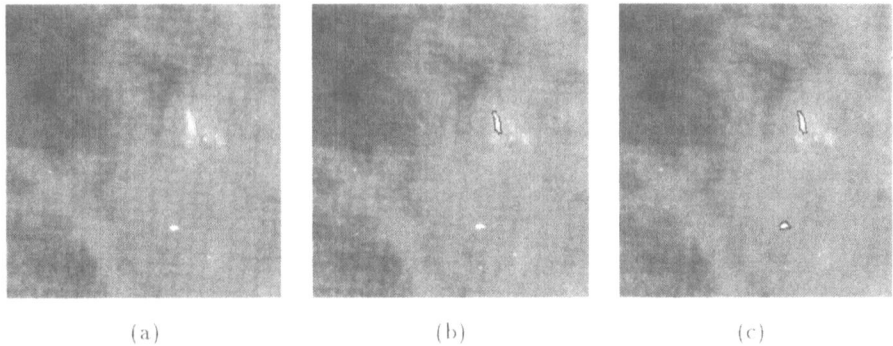

(a)   (b)   (c)

Figure 11.15. An image sample containing image shot noise: (a) the original image (oxCALC010RC1c1) with 1 microcalcification and a number of image shot noise points scattered over the image, of which the one lying horizontally near the bottom of the image is very prominent (b) detection result using the volume ratio algorithm: the region corresponding to shot noise is eliminated and only the real calcification is marked; (c) detection result using grey level contrast: the image shot noise is wrongly marked as a calcification.

CHAPTER 12

CURVILINEAR STRUCTURES

12.1. Introduction

This chapter continues our model-based approach by studying the extraction and, in the next chapter the subsequent use, of what are termed "curvilinear structures" (CLS), which correspond to blood vessels, milk ducts, spiculations, and fibrous tissue. Fundamental to our approach to such an image processing problem is to model the CLS, and the passage of x-rays through them, using the h_{int} representation.

Regions of a mammogram that represent curvilinear structures appear to be those that have (i) a slightly increased intensity relative to the surrounding parenchymal tissue, and (ii) are locally linear; that is to say that they appear locally to be straight and one-dimensional, though of course they are usually curved if one considers them at a larger scale. It is for this reason that these features are commonly referred to by the collective term curvilinear structures (CLS).

Figures 12.6 and 12.7 show typical mammograms and the CLS determined by the algorithms described in this chapter. Notice that the CLS form a complex network of curves, almost as if a pile of hair or spaghetti had been dropped onto the mammogram, disrupting its otherwise slowly-varying intensities. Indeed, Figure 12.11 shows that once the CLS have been found in a mammogram, they can be removed to give an image in which the "blobs" of parenchymal tissue and masses are not only more readily seen but can be found by a computer program both more easily and more reliably. The extraction of masses, as well as techniques for matching and assessing them, will be described in Chapter 13. A preliminary version of this chapter appeared in [36].

Why extract the CLS?

As we discussed in Chapter 11, the shape and arrangement of calcifications is important in assessing the degree of malignancy. However, it is also important to distinguish arterial and ductal calcifications. Indeed, once shot noise has been detected (as in the previous chapter), the common failure to distinguish where calcifications lie is one of the reasons that there are unacceptable numbers of false positives in the vast majority of published algorithms. False positives are why practising radiologists do not have much confidence in using computer prompting systems to help them detect clinically significant calcifications[140, 118]. Consequently, it would be very useful to have a description of the locations of the ducts and blood vessels in an image, allowing for a comparative analysis of calcifications present in an image.

Similarly, when assessing a mammographic mass, a radiologist routinely checks the border surrounding the mass for spiculations or radial fibrous tissue that may be anchored to the mass. Spiculations surrounding a mammographic mass are a strong indicator of malignancy [143]. Similarly the radial spiculations surrounding a radiolucent centre are possibly indicative of malignancy as they are the only signs of radial scar. The detection of radial scar is a difficult problem because of the subtle appearance of these abnormalities in an image. Such mammographic masses (spiculated or circumscribed) appear as spatially slowly-varying patches of higher tissue density. The search for such features is typically complicated by the rapid (textural) variations in image intensity/density due to the fibrous tissue, milk ducts and blood vessels which occur with much smaller spatial extent, which as shown in Figures 12.6 and 12.7 are densely distributed throughout the image. It follows that a description of the high-frequency CLS features enables them to be removed from the images, easing the search for mammographic masses. But for similar reasons removing the CLS makes it easier to match mammograms whether left-right, CC-MLO or temporal.

Clearly, for both classifying calcifications and detecting masses it would be helpful to construct a representation of the milk ducts, blood vessels, mass spiculations and other fibrous tissues and to this end we describe an algorithm developed by our colleague Nick Cerneaz[35]. Consistent with the overall theme of this monograph, the key idea is to base the algorithm and analysis upon a model of the expected CLS cross-sectional profile. We demonstrate that the predicted intensity profile closely matches those found in images, and we argue that this is a necessary contributing factor to the performance of the CLS detection algorithm. Subsequent use of the CLS structures, for finding masses, interpreting calcifications, and matching left-right breasts crucially depends on the CLS image model.

Appearance of the CLS

When imaged mammographically, the extra density of breast tissue that the x-ray beam must traverse when passing through blood vessels and milk ducts causes it to be attenuated slightly more than when it does not pass through such a vessel. Consequently the film is less exposed in these regions and therefore has lower film density. We will show that we can quantify the rise in intensity: for typical breast tissues, the attenuation of the beam due to the CLS feature results in an image intensity increase of approximately 1 grey-level per 180 microns of CLS thickness in an 8-bit grey-scale quantisation and with a typical film-screen system.

In a breast, one expects to find CLS features of thickness greater than 180 microns and, in fact, due to image noise the CLS thickness needs to be substantially greater than 180 microns if it is to be detected. Considering that blood capillaries are 7–10 microns in diameter, this explains why both the capillaries and the majority of the blood vessel network are not visible in mammograms, leaving only the larger vessels to be resolved. An analogous argument can be developed for the milk ducts and fibrous tissues.

It follows that the mammographic footprint of the vessels that are resolved is locally linear, with slightly increased image brightness compared with the surroundings. The situation is analogous for the case of fibrous sheets, which form part of the breast stroma. The strands of the sheets are long, thin and strong, and support the functional material of the parenchymal tissue of the breast. The extra tissue density of the fibrous strands over that of the ducts and vessels attenuates the beam even further; hence they often appear on a film.

The CLS system

The blood vessels and milk ducts comprise systems that are both continuous and connected. The individual segments are necessarily connected, and they are of similar sizes (allowing for natural reduction at junctions as the fluid flow is split between the diverging branches — conversely the diameter increases as the flow converges, e.g. the venous return). In contrast, the fibrous tissues do not need to be connected in any special order/pattern, provided each end of the tissue can be anchored. Consequently, one can mobilise the constraints of connectivity and continuity to delineate the vessels from the fibres. Further, the milk duct network converges at the nipple while the blood vessel networks diverge from the posterior arterial and venous supplies. This difference can also be used to differentiate the blood vessels/milk ducts.

It follows that for the task of describing the milk duct, blood vessel and fibrous tissue networks in an image, their respective mammographic features are quite similar at a local scale, though subtly different at a more global scale. For many of the radiological applications to which it is required to apply the description of CLS features, it is not necessary to be able to distinguish between them. Rather, simply being able to identify those areas of an image that are the milk ducts, blood vessels and fibrous tissues collectively suffices. Of course, if a method could be found to distinguish extremely reliably the different types of CLS structures, this would be a significant contribution, one that would combine effectively with techniques described here. To this end, Parr and colleagues [193] have recently reported encouraging progress by modelling intensity profiles of CLS features and training a recognition system for the different types. That work provides an elegant counterpart to the work presented here.

The image processing task

In its most naïve conception, the image processing problem of finding the CLS features corresponds to locating two nearby parallel, low contrast, step intensity changes that are of opposite sign (dark-to-light followed by light-to-dark). Complicating the issue is that although the CLS features are generally of slightly higher intensity than the surrounding 'background', the images are very noisy and so the signal-to-noise ratio (SNR) of the required features is typically small. Additionally, two different CLS features can lie adjacent and closely parallel to each other, yet they are quite distinct and must be resolved individually. It is well-known that edge detection algorithms that incorporate a prior smoothing step (e.g. the Canny edge detector) confound two nearby steps whenever their spatial separation is less than the scale of the smoothing filter. One may confidently predict, therefore, that attempting to extract the CLS by the application of edge detection algorithms that incorporate a prior smoothing step, will give very poor results. This is what is found in practice, as can be seen in [35] and [236].

An alternative technique, developed in computer vision, is to treat a pair of nearby intensity changes having opposite gradient signs as a primitive, called a ridge. Considerable effort has been expended on techniques to find ridges at different spatial scales (see Haralick and Shapiro [100] for a comprehensive account). We have implemented several of what appear to be the best published techniques, particularly those by Haralick, and by Sha'ashua and Ullman [35], however we find that they give poor results on mammograms. There is a fundamental reason for this, namely that general-purpose ridge finders were developed for visual images, not for x-ray images, and they are invariably based on the assumption that the ridge is delimited on either side by a sharp intensity change of large contrast. This is not characteristic of the kinds of intensity changes that correspond to CLS, whose edges tend to have small contrast relative to the

---

BOX 12.1: The CLS extraction algorithm

(1) *Filter the image.* The output from this first stage is a representation of the set of pixels in the image that are candidates for being considered part of the CLS. This step is the key to the algorithm and it is based on the model of the expected CLS profile developed in Section 12.3.

(2) *Create a binary image that contains the "backbone" of the CLS pixels.* This step is based on slight variants to well-known techniques for thinning the pixel sets found in step 1, then joining them together to form a representation of the CLS network.

(3) *Extract the CLS.* The final step gathers together the CLS pixels starting from the backbone extracted in step 2.

---

surrounding tissue, and have a curved profile rather than a pair of steps of opposing sign, so that the intensity gradient across both sides of the CLS is quite low. It follows that tuning a general purpose ridge finder so that it will pick up the low ridges characteristic of CLS, i.e. guaranteeing that it finds all the true positives, inevitably leads to it finding a massive number of false positives.

Both of the above considerations about spatial frequency and low SNR, argue the need for a model-based ridge finder such as we develop in the next section.

12.2. The CLS detector algorithm

We now summarise briefly the CLS extraction algorithm, to establish the context for the ideas presented in the rest of the chapter. The three main steps stated informally are shown in Box 12.1. First, the CLS features are modelled in Section 12.3 as having an elliptical cross-section. We use a simplified imaging model assuming that there is no scatter and that the x-ray beam is monoenergetic though the simulations later in the chapter use the full x-ray model. Also, the analysis is developed using continuous mathematics and so Section 12.4 discusses in more detail the transformation to the discrete image. Results typical of the many dozens that we have achieved using the implemented algorithm are presented in Section 12.6. In Section 12.7, we show how to remove CLS features prior to searching for masses and for matching mammograms, which are the subjects of the next chapter.

BOX 12.2: Step 1, Image Filtering

Let T be a negative threshold. Apply to the image I the directional filters Δ_i'' defined in Figure 12.1 in the directions i. More precisely, denote the convolution $\Delta_i'' * I$ of the filter Δ_i'' with the image $I(x, y)$ by $I_i''(x, y)$, which is the second-difference value at pixel (x, y) in the i-direction. Then a pixel (x, y) is judged to have strong negative second difference response if:

$$\min\left(I_1'', I_2'', \ldots, I_n''\right) < T \quad \text{and} \quad \max\left(I_1'', I_2'', \ldots, I_n''\right) \approx 0 \qquad (12.1)$$

or:

$$\min\left(I_1'', I_2'', \ldots, I_n''\right) + \max\left(I_1'', I_2'', \ldots, I_n''\right) \approx 0^- \quad \text{and}$$

$$\min\left(I_1'', I_2'', \ldots, I_n''\right) \ll 0 \qquad (12.2)$$

Equation 12.2 identifies instances of the saddle points of interest, while Equation 12.1 identifies other simpler cases such as points near a part of the CLS feature that are locally quite straight.

Image filtering

The candidate pixels to be returned at step 1 of the algorithm are those where there is an increase in intensity (surrounding tissue to CLS) quickly followed by a decrease. Mathematically, this can be stated succinctly: those pixels that have negative image surface curvature, with no prior smoothing of the image. While we often work at a spatial resolution of 100 microns, we show that the algorithm works effectively even at a resolution of 300 microns, though in that case CLS features are often only a single pixel in width. Working at 300 microns has the advantage of speed (only 1/9th as many pixels need to be considered) but the disadvantage of lowered sampling.

Our approach to estimating the (negative) image surface curvature was inspired by Fleck's *Spectre* edge detector [75], and, like her, we apply second difference filters Δ_i'' at n (currently 4) orientations α_i, where $i = 1, \ldots, n$. We combine the n outputs of these filters at each pixel to decide whether or not a pixel should be labelled putatively as a CLS feature. The algorithm for combining the filter responses is given in Box 12.2. The choice of the (negative) threshold T turns out to be justifiable, and the results are not overly sensitive to the choice (see Nick Cerneaz's thesis [35]).

To complete the discussion of step 1 of the algorithm, we note the following four points. First, for simplicity of description and implementation, we restrict attention in this monograph to a single spatial scale. Over the past decade, it has become well established in image processing to develop and implement filters at multiple spatial scales, since the objects of interest (here CLS features) have a range of different sizes and it has been found better to have a set of filters spanning the different sizes than to try to design a single filter to cater for all. The extension of the single scale treatment developed in this chapter to a multi-scale version is quite straightforward. Interestingly, the results that we have obtained with a single scale implementation of the CLS feature detector are considerably better than one might initially have supposed, or, in other words, the results appear robust against changes of scale. We consider that this is further evidence in support of the power of the model-based approach to image processing that we advocate in this monograph.

Second, because the CLS features are low contrast and low signal-to-noise ratio, we avoid prior smoothing, preferring instead to base our approach on the directional, finite-difference filtering technique[76][1]. A consequence is that we need to decide in how many directions i the image should be filtered. We conducted a number of experiments to evaluate whether 4 or 8 directions gave significantly different results. In fact, very little difference was observed, and so for simplicity of implementation, we set the number of directions to 4.

The third point concerns the choice of convolution filter Δ_i'' to estimate the negative directional second differences of the image I. Consistent with the approach of Fleck, we use the simplest possible filters of size 5 pixels, as shown in Figure 12.1.

The fourth and final point concerns how to set a value for the threshold T. To do this, we computed histograms (discrete approximations to probability density functions) of the second-difference values returned by the kernels shown in Figure 12.1. By far the vast majority of responses are at values close to zero reflecting the smoothness of the majority of the image, that is the 'background' regions surrounding the CLS features. The responses at the CLS pixels lie in the tails of this distribution, and so we set the threshold T to be a function of the distribution width. By adopting this approach, we incorporate a self-tuning feature into the selection of CLS pixels, allowing for instance, a lower threshold in images of particularly fatty breasts showing little breast structure for instance. Rather simplistically, we set T to be a fraction of the standard deviation σ of the second-difference distribution, that is $T = -t\sigma$. Using empirical methods

---

[1] We note that Fleck's technique operates at multiple scales, further reinforcing our first point.

$$\begin{bmatrix} 1 \\ 0 \\ -2 \\ 0 \\ 1 \end{bmatrix}^{T} \qquad \begin{bmatrix} \sqrt{2}-1 & 0 & 0 & 0 & 0 \\ 0 & 2-\sqrt{2} & 0 & 0 & 0 \\ 0 & 0 & -2 & 0 & 0 \\ 0 & 0 & 0 & 2-\sqrt{2} & 0 \\ 0 & 0 & 0 & 0 & \sqrt{2}-1 \end{bmatrix}$$

$$\Delta_N'' \qquad\qquad\qquad\qquad \Delta_{NE}''$$

$$\begin{bmatrix} 1 \\ 0 \\ -2 \\ 0 \\ 1 \end{bmatrix} \qquad \begin{bmatrix} 0 & 0 & 0 & 0 & \sqrt{2}-1 \\ 0 & 0 & 0 & 2-\sqrt{2} & 0 \\ 0 & 0 & -2 & 0 & 0 \\ 0 & 2-\sqrt{2} & 0 & 0 & 0 \\ \sqrt{2}-1 & 0 & 0 & 0 & 0 \end{bmatrix}$$

$$\Delta_E'' \qquad\qquad\qquad\qquad \Delta_{SE}''$$

Figure 12.1. The second difference directional convolution kernels for estimating the second derivative of the image surface.

we have seen that a value of $t = 0.7$ gives a good compromise between sensitivity and specificity.

We now elaborate, though only slightly, steps 2 and 3 of the CLS algorithm (full details in [35]). Steps 2 and 3 deal with continuous curves in binary digital images. Characteristically, a binary image is segmented into foreground and background regions. The CLS pixels and the backbone pixel-wide curves that represent them constitute the foreground. A key property of the CLS features is their connectedness. In general in image processing, a pixel has four horizontal and vertical neighbours (N, E, W, and S), and four diagonal (NE, NW, SE, SW). In digital image processing, a crucial choice in determining connectedness is whether the foreground should be 4-connected (horizontal and vertical), in which case the background has to be 8-connected (all 8 compass points), or vice versa. Since the CLS are not restricted to being horizontal and vertical, and since we seek feature points by computing second differences in the horizontal, vertical and the two diagonal directions, we choose to make the foreground 8-connected, so that the background is 4-connected [211]. With this choice, steps 2 and 3 may be described as in Box 12.3.

The algorithm has evolved through analysis and extensive experimentation. It is justified since it succeeds at the task it was formulated to deal with, since the resulting CLS features seem to accord well with what radiologists perceive, and they support subsequent processing such as the identification and description of potential masses and the matching of a left-right breast pair. We emphasise that the model-based step 1 and the careful implementations in steps 2 and 3 contribute to the algorithm's success.

BOX 12.3: Steps 2 and 3 in more detail

(2a) Thin the regions of the set generated at Step 1, call it **N**, retaining in a new set **S** the pixels that comprise the simply-connected skeletons of **N**'s regions. There are many published algorithms appropriate for this step; the one we use for this returns a simply-connected topologically equivalent skeleton lying at most a single pixel from the medial-axis of the region under consideration [35].

(2b) Break the skeleton into its segments s_i by scanning the set **S**, collecting into linear portions l_i those 8-connected pixels that collectively share a common global heading/direction. At each branch (or junction) in the skeleton initiate another linear portion. Form the set **L** of all linear portions l_i that result from classifying all $s_i \in $ **S**.

(2c) Scan the set **L**, merging into wires w_i those linear portions with both a (nearly) common endpoint and a sufficiently similar heading. Scan the wires w_i searching for merges involving a short intermediate linear portion joining two dissimilar linear portions. Exclude the least convincing of the two merges, returning a junction at this location. At the completion of this phase, those linear portions that are not merged with others to form wires are transcribed directly to the set **W** creating a new wire for each such linear portion.

(2d) Search the set **W** for small and/or disconnected branches of the skeleton and reject them.

(3a) Search the set **N** in the region surrounding each wire $w_i \in $ **W**, collecting the 8-connected neighbourhood pixels in the new set cls_i associated with w_i.

(3b) Declare the set **CLS** of all cls_i (with corresponding wires w_i) to be the curvilinear structures of the original image I.

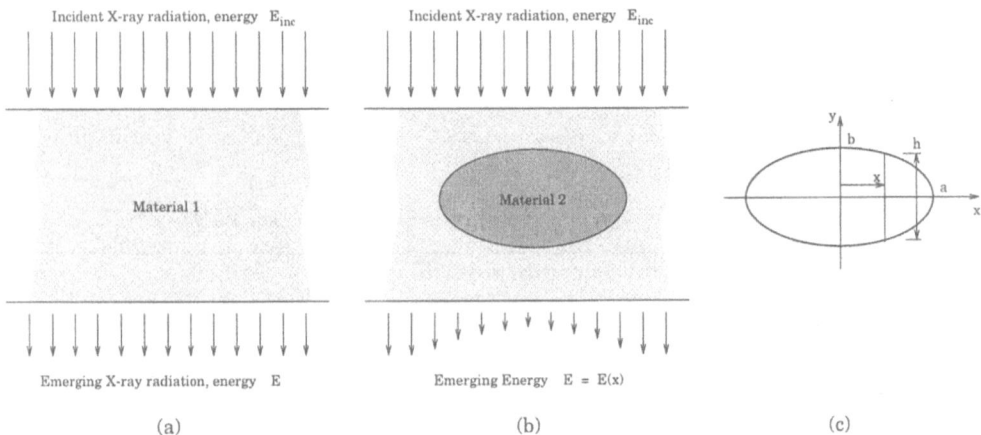

Figure 12.2. h_{int} model of the cross section of a CLS feature. (a) A one-dimensional slice through the h_{int} surface without the CLS feature. The height $h_{surr}(x)$ is assumed to vary slowly and smoothly. (b) A compressed elliptical CLS feature is added to the h_{int} surface. (c) detail of the CLS feature added.

12.3. Modelling the expected CLS profile

To model the expected profile of a CLS feature, recall that it is expected to be locally linear. We assume also that a CLS feature has a circular cross-section in the uncompressed state and that the compression is in the direction of the photon flux making an ellipse an appropriate model of the cross-section. After compression, it is unlikely for CLS features to be vertically thicker than they are horizontally wide so that the major axis of the ellipse is orthogonal to the incident x-ray beam rather than parallel to it. We consider it in profile, "end on", thereby reducing the analysis to one dimension, which we denote x. Figure 12.2(a) shows a portion of the h_{int} surface surrounding the CLS feature in the direction x. Figure 12.2(b) adds a CLS feature, whose analytical shape is shown in Figure 12.2(c). The shape of CLS can be seen in the h_{int} surface depicted in Figure 12.3.

For mathematical convenience, the origin of the coordinate x is set at the centre of the CLS feature. Eventually, we will need to remove the surrounding h_{int} and to do this we will exploit the assumption that (locally) its height $h_{int}^{surr}(x)$ varies slowly and smoothly. In fact, we will assume that the second derivative $h_{int}^{surr\prime\prime}(x)$ is negligible. Box 12.4 gives more detail. Recall that in Chapter 6 it was suggested that, except in the case of careful calibration, it is necessary to work with changes in h_{int} rather than absolute values, since its estimation is normally only available up to an image-wide shift in values up or down.

AN h_{int} SURFACE

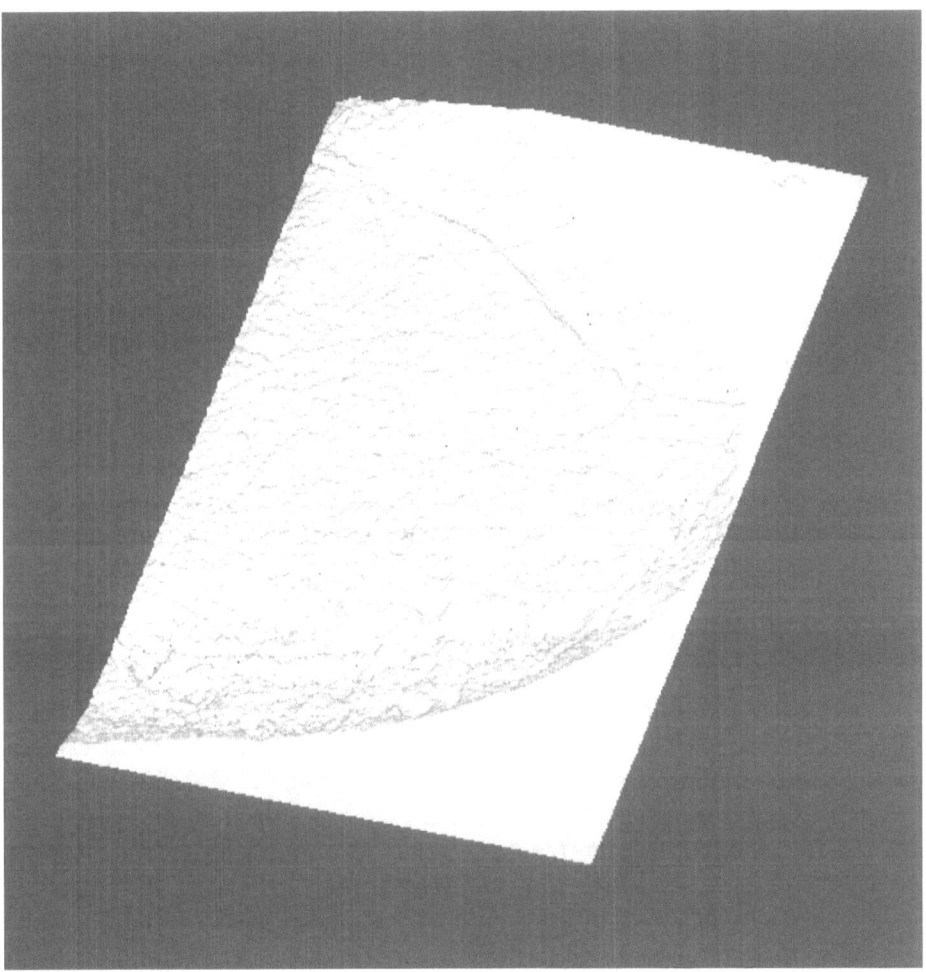

Figure 12.3.   Depiction of the h_{int} surface of a breast. The height corresponds to the amount of non-fatty tissue. In this way, anatomical features correspond to topographic features of h_{int} surfaces. There are many curvilinear structures evident and we model the cross-sections of these structures as ellipses.

BOX 12.4: Interesting tissue model of a CLS feature

$$h_{int}(x) = \begin{cases} h_{int}^{surr}(x) + h_{int}^{cls}(x) & -a \leq x \leq a, \\ h_{int}^{surr}(x) & otherwise. \end{cases} \qquad (12.3)$$

where

$$h_{int}^{cls}(x) = \frac{2b}{a} \sqrt[t]{(a^2 - x^2)}, -a \leq x \leq a. \qquad (12.4)$$

The assumption that $h_{int}^{surr}(x)$ varies slowly and smoothly is so that:

$$\begin{aligned} h_{int}^{surr''}(x) &\approx 0 \\ h_{int}''(x) &\approx h_{int}^{cls''}(x) & -a \leq x \leq a, \\ &= -2ba(a^2 - x^2)^{-\frac{3}{2}} & -a \leq x \leq a \end{aligned} \qquad (12.5)$$

The relation between this h_{int} model of a CLS feature and the energy E^{imp} imparted to the intensifying screen can now be developed. Then we will be able to develop a representation of the film density D. We aim to show that significant changes in the negative second difference of h_{int} correspond to significant changes in the negative second difference of D. As we noted earlier, the analysis that follows is carried out for the idealised case of a monoenergetic incident beam and assuming that there is no scattered radiation. Both of these restrictions have been lifted in numerical simulations using the programs described in earlier chapters. Box 12.5 gives the energy imparted.

As noted in earlier chapters, once the beam has been attenuated during its travel through the breast (or in this case, the cross-sectional sample), there are a number of processing stages before the digitised image is available. Each of these must be considered so that the absolute pixel intensities of the image can be estimated. To estimate the image intensities resulting from the digitisation of the film, we need to model the digitisation process. There are several ways to do this, however, they generally can be classed as those that quantise the film density D, and those that quantise the light transmitted through the film T_l for a given back illumination. The direct digitisation of the film density (for example by a scanning microdensitometer) returns image intensity values $P_d(x)$ in an approximately linear relationship with D, while digitisation of the transmitted light (for example using a CCD camera and a film back lit on a light-box) corresponds to a linear relationship between the image intensity $P_l(x)$ and T_l. Box 12.6 develops the quantised film density representation $P_d(x)$ and we note that the analysis of transmitted light image intensities $P_l(x)$ can be carried out in exactly the same way. Box 12.7 models the digitisation of the film densities.

BOX 12.5: From h_{int} to monoenergetic energy

For the surrounding tissue, $h_{int}^{surr}(x)$ is the amount of interesting tissue, so that $H - h_{int}^{surr}(x)$ is fat. It follows from the assumption of a monoenergetic beam with no scatter and an ideal x-ray detection scheme that the energy imparted is:

$$
\begin{aligned}
E^{imp}(x) &= E^{inc}e^{-\mu_{fat}[H-h_{int}^{surr}(x)]}e^{-\mu_{int}h_{int}^{surr}(x)} \\
&= E^{inc}e^{-\mu_{fat}H}e^{-(\mu_{int}-\mu_{fat})h_{int}^{surr}(x)} \\
&= E^{inc}e^{-\mu_{fat}H}e^{-\mu_1 h_{int}^{surr}(x)}
\end{aligned}
$$

where $\mu_1 = \mu_{int} - \mu_{fat}$ is the difference between the attenuation coefficients of interesting tissue and fat and E^{inc} is the incident radiation. Similarly, within the CLS feature, there is $h_{int}^{surr}(x)$ of interesting tissue and $h_{int}^{cls}(x)$ of CLS tissue. In practice we use $\mu_{cls} \approx \mu_{int}$ and it follows that:

$$
\begin{aligned}
E^{imp}(x) &= E^{inc}e^{-(\mu_{int}h_{int}^{surr}(x)+\mu_{int}h_{int}^{cls}(x))}e^{-\mu_{fat}(H-(h_{int}^{surr}(x)+h_{int}^{cls}(x)))} \\
&= E^{inc}e^{-\mu_{fat}H}e^{-(\mu_{int}-\mu_{fat})h_{int}^{surr}(x)}e^{-(\mu_{int}-\mu_{fat})h_{int}^{cls}(x)} \\
&= E^{inc}e^{-\mu_{fat}H}e^{-\mu_1 h_{int}^{surr}(x)}e^{-\mu_1 h_{int}^{cls}(x)}
\end{aligned}
$$

Thus, the energy imparted that we expect for a situation such as shown in Figure 12.2(b) is:

$$
E^{imp}(x) = \begin{cases} E^{inc}e^{-\mu_{fat}H}e^{-\mu_1 h_{int}^{surr}(x)}e^{-\mu_1 h_{int}^{cls}(x)} & -a \le x \le a, \\ E^{inc}e^{-\mu_{fat}H}e^{-\mu_1 h_{int}^{surr}(x)} & \text{otherwise.} \end{cases} \tag{12.6}
$$

BOX 12.6: From energy imparted to the screen to film density

Assuming a linear film-screen curve:

$$
D(x) = \gamma \log_{10}\left(\beta E^{imp}(x)\right). \tag{12.7}
$$

$$
= \frac{\gamma \ln \beta}{\ln 10} + \frac{\gamma}{\ln 10}\ln E^{imp}(x) \tag{12.8}
$$

where D is the film density, γ the film-screen gradient, and β is related to the film-screen speed. Inserting $E^{imp}(x)$ from Equation 12.6, the predicted film density of the modeled feature, for the CLS feature of interest, that is for $-a \le x \le a$, is:

$$
\begin{aligned}
D(x) &= \frac{\gamma \ln \beta}{\ln 10} + \frac{\gamma}{\ln 10}[\ln E^{inc}-\mu_{fat}H-\mu_1 h_{int}^{surr}(x)-\mu_1 h_{int}^{cls}(x)] \\
&= A - B\mu_1 h_{int}^{surr}(x) - B\mu_1 h_{int}^{cls}(x) \tag{12.9}
\end{aligned}
$$

where A and B are constant factors. We'll state B explicitly since it turns out to be important: $B = \gamma/\ln 10$.

BOX 12.7: From film density to image intensity

The film scanner is modeled as a linear function of film density:

$$P_d(x, y) = q + mD(x, y) \qquad (12.10)$$

where m and q are digitisation calibration constants. From Equation 12.9:

$$P_d(x, y) = (q + mA) - mB\mu_1 h_{int}^{surr}(x) - mB\mu_1 h_{int}^{cls}(x) \qquad (12.11)$$

BOX 12.8: Relating negative second derivatives of image intensity and of h_{int}

$$
\begin{aligned}
-P_d''(x) &= mB\mu_1 h_{int}^{surr''}(x) + mB\mu_1 h_{int}^{cls''}(x) \\
&\approx mB\mu_1 h_{int}^{cls''}(x) & (12.12) \\
&= mB\mu_1 \times (-2ba)(a^2 - x^2)^{-\frac{3}{2}} & (12.13)
\end{aligned}
$$

where B is as in Box 12.6.

Having derived the relationship between the pixel value from a film scanner and the h_{int} surface of a CLS feature, we can finally compare their negative second derivatives as shown in Box 12.8.

In order to analyse the typical response from these equations, typical values are inserted for the constants as given in Table 12.1. The digitisation constants m and q can be measured by solving the set of two simultaneous equations resulting from substitution of known (film density, digitised value) data pairs obtained from calibration data. With these values we deduce the second derivative of the CLS feature is closely related to the pixel value with the monoenergetic assumptions, more specifically:

$$h_{int}^{cls''}(x) \approx \frac{P_d''(x)}{55.767} \qquad (12.14)$$

Evaluation of Equations 12.11 and 12.13 gives the second-derivative curves shown in Figure 12.4.

The above analysis can be used to compute an estimate of the spatial extent of a CLS feature in an image in order to select both an appropriate image resolution and second difference kernel size. From Equation 12.11, the difference ΔP between the intensity of the surrounding tissue and the CLS feature peak tissue intensity is given by:

$$\Delta P = -mB\mu_1 h_{cls}^{int}(0) = -mB\mu_1 2b. \qquad (12.15)$$

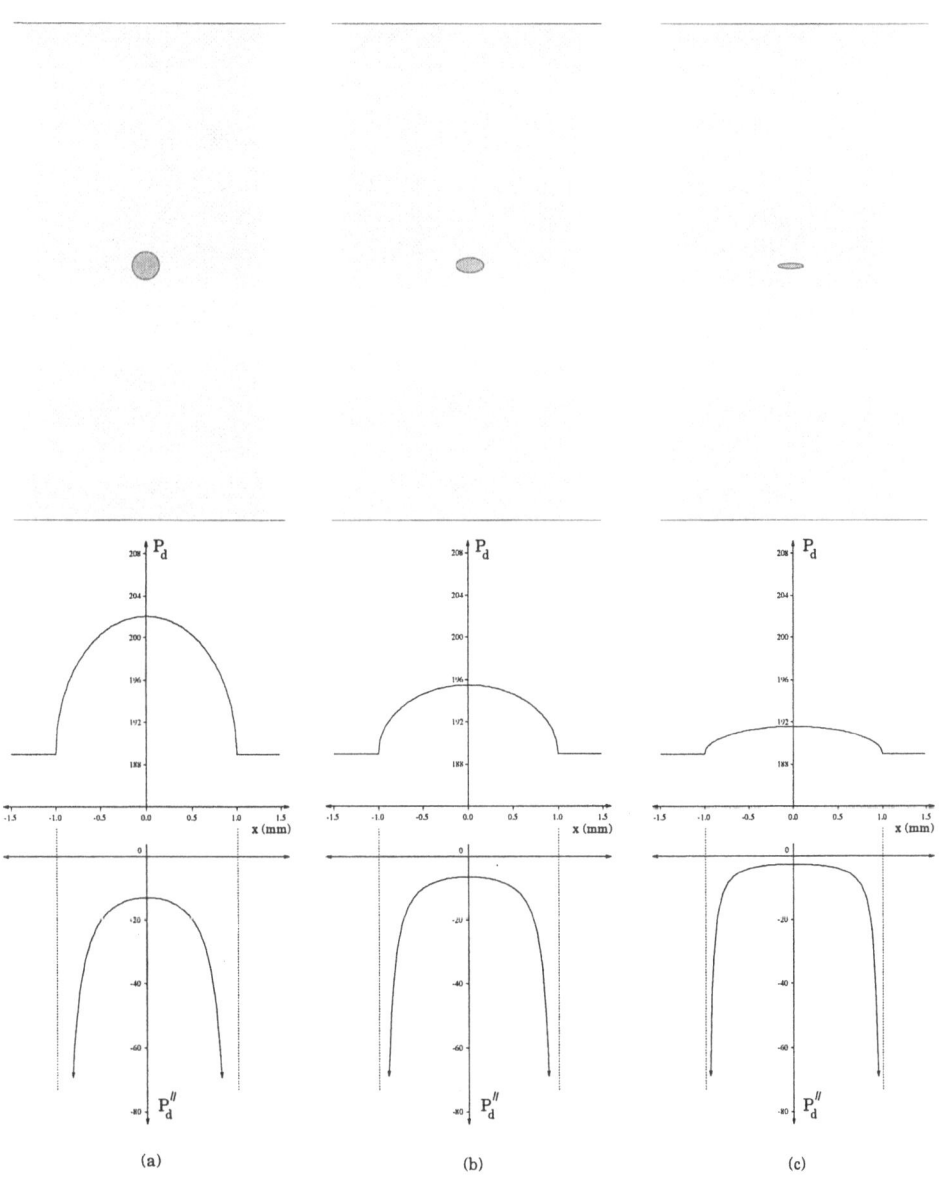

Figure 12.4. The object and second-derivative curves for idealised elliptical CLS features where pixel value represents film density. In all cases the major radius of the ellipse is $a = 1$mm, however the minor radius is (a) $b = 1$mm, (b) $b = 0.5$mm and (c) $b = 0.2$mm. The top row of each column shows the cross-sectional proportion of feature to breast-tissue, the middle row shows the image pixel intensity values expected across the feature, and the bottom row shows the second-derivative of the intensity curve above it.

Constants	Value
Film density range	$0.2 \leq D \leq 3.0$
Image intensity range (8-bit)	$0 \leq P \leq 255$
Film gradient	$\gamma = 3$
Beam energy (keV)	$\mathcal{E} = 17.4$
Attenuation coefficients (cm^{-1})	$\mu_{fat} = 0.558, \mu_{int} = 1.028$
Breast thickness (cm)	3.5
Size of feature (cm)	$a = 0.10, b = 0.02$

TABLE 12.1. Parameters for calculation of the CLS image.

Inserting the same values for the constants, we can relate the smallest intensity change $\Delta P = 1$ to the (compressed) height b of a CLS feature. Recall that the units of attenuation coefficients, e.g. μ_1 are cm^{-1}. It follows that when $\Delta P = 1$, $b = 0.0179\text{cm}$, so that the minimum possible CLS thickness capable of producing a detectable change in the image surface (assuming the absence of noise) is 179 microns. In practice, a CLS feature needs to be thicker in the noisy/polyenergetic/scattered case compared to the noiseless/monoenergetic/scatterless case. This means that the value of 179 microns should be considered as a lower limit for the thickness of CLS features which simply cannot be successfully imaged.

12.4. From continuous to discrete

For numerical simulations, we use the algorithms described in Chapters 2, 3 and 4. Initially, to verify the analysis of the previous section, the method was applied using a monoenergetic beam, non-scattered radiation and zero noise. The simulation returns the digitised x-ray image that would be obtained if the CLS model described above were added to a homogeneous breast. This allows a direct comparison between the discrete digital results obtained and the results of the continuous analysis of the previous section. Figure 12.5 shows the simulated intensity profile using the values in Table 12.1 for a feature with varying radii at different spatial resolutions.

This digital image surface can be directly compared to the continuous surface (Figure 12.4) given by Equations 12.9 and 12.10. To facilitate this comparison, Figure 12.5 includes the respective continuous curve (the dotted curve) for each case.

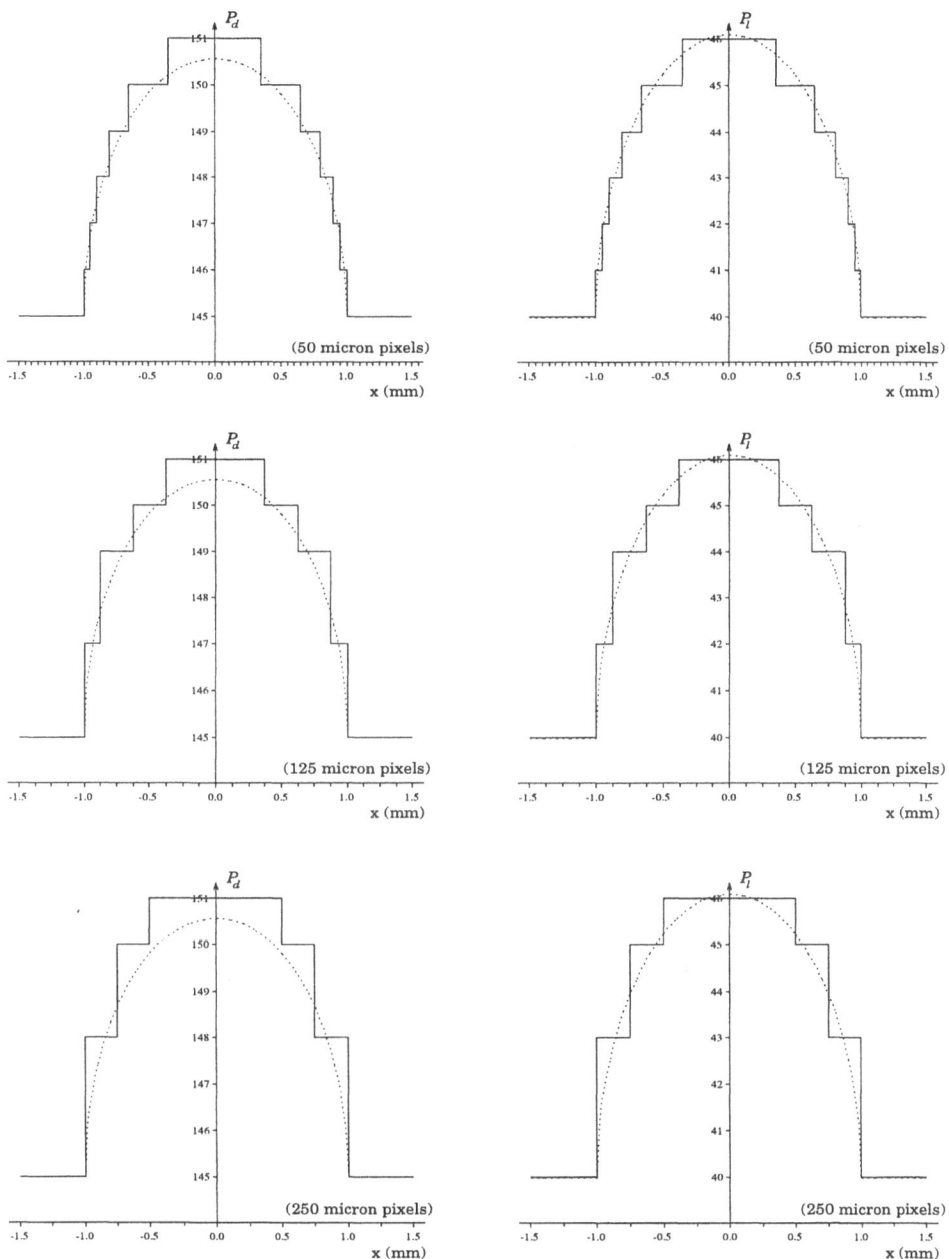

Figure 12.5. Comparison between the analytical (continuous) expected image intensities (dotted lines) versus the simulated discrete approximation (solid lines) for an elliptical CLS feature with major and minor radii 1mm and 0.5mm respectively. The simulations on the right represent transmitted light as discussed in Chapter 7, the ones on the left are as discussed in the text. The top row shows the simulation at a resolution of 20 pixels/mm (50 micron pixels), middle at 8 pixels/mm (125 micron pixels) and bottom at 4 pixels/mm (250 micron pixels).

12.5. CLS modelling conclusions

By assuming compressed CLS features have approximately elliptical cross-sections, the previous sections have developed a model of the imaged CLS features. The conclusions may be summarised as follows:

- With the assumptions of a monoenergetic incident beam and no scattered radiation, the second derivative of the (analogue) image surface is strongly negative at locations representing CLS features.
- By numerically simulating the effects of polyenergetic beams and scattered radiation, a correspondingly strong negative response is apparent in the second difference of the (digital) image surface at locations representing CLS features.
- The response of CLS features in an image surface to the second difference kernel is strongly dependent upon matching the image spatial resolution, image intensity resolution, kernel size, and the range of CLS feature sizes.
- Under the conservative assumption that one expects a CLS feature to be no thicker than it is wide whilst under compression (relative to the x-ray path), only CLS features wider than some 180 microns can attenuate the incident x-ray beam sufficiently to produce any change in the image intensity surface for an 8-bit intensity quantisation.

For these reasons, step 1 of the CLS feature detection algorithm sketched in Section 12.2 involves searching for pixels with strongly negative second derivative. The analysis is conducted in the film density image representation, looking for features as small as a single pixel in width in images reduced to a resolution of 300 micron/pixel.

12.6. Results

The CLS algorithm has been applied successfully to 350 mammograms. Typical results are displayed in Figures 12.6, 12.7 and 12.8, each of which shows an original mammographic image and a corresponding image displaying the pixels identified as CLS pixels. Note that it is difficult to display the fact that the algorithm has extracted a single CLS feature for the longer curvilinear portions of the CLS pixel-trees and thus no attempt has been made to do so, although for completeness it should be noted that such an extraction has been achieved.

Observe that the CLS pixels identified in each case include the long connected curvilinear features of the image. Although many of the smaller regions of CLS pixels might appear to clutter the image and thus complicate the CLS description they are in fact representations of the less salient CLS features present and therefore their identification and extraction is

DETECTING CURVILINEAR STRUCTURES

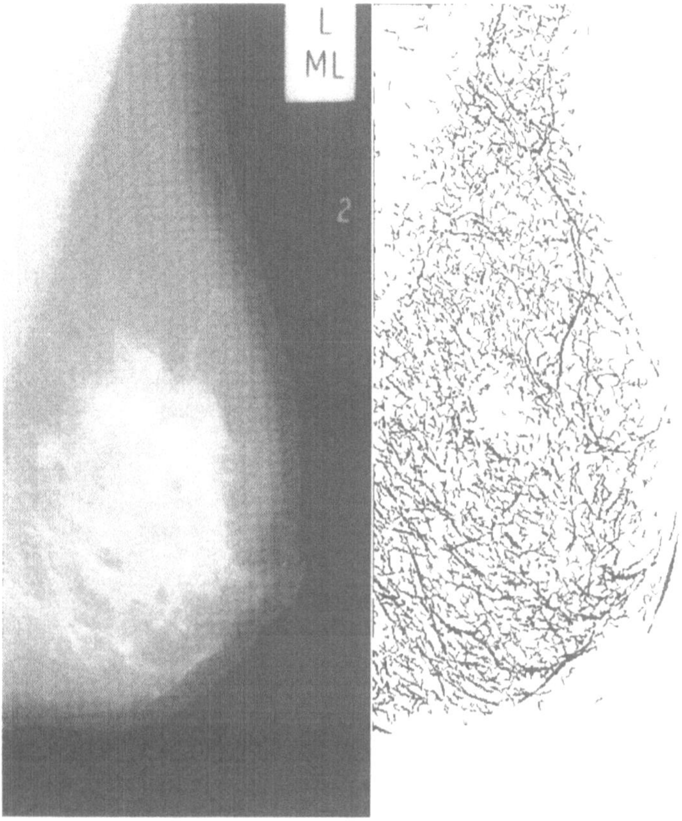

Figure 12.6.   A medio-lateral oblique image and the CLS pixels identified.

warranted. This viewpoint is sustained by the further processing that this feature description supports, including the identification of significant mammographic masses [35].

As as expected from the formulation of the model, the CLS detector algorithm is insensitive to the absolute grey-level in a local region, and is capable of extracting the CLS features at all local image intensities.

As mentioned previously these results are typical of the results obtained from extensive application of the algorithm to many mammographic images, and importantly, the CLS feature description thus obtained has allowed a systematic, logical and model-based development of subsequent higher-level mammographic image processing and analysis tools.

DETECTING CURVILINEAR STRUCTURES

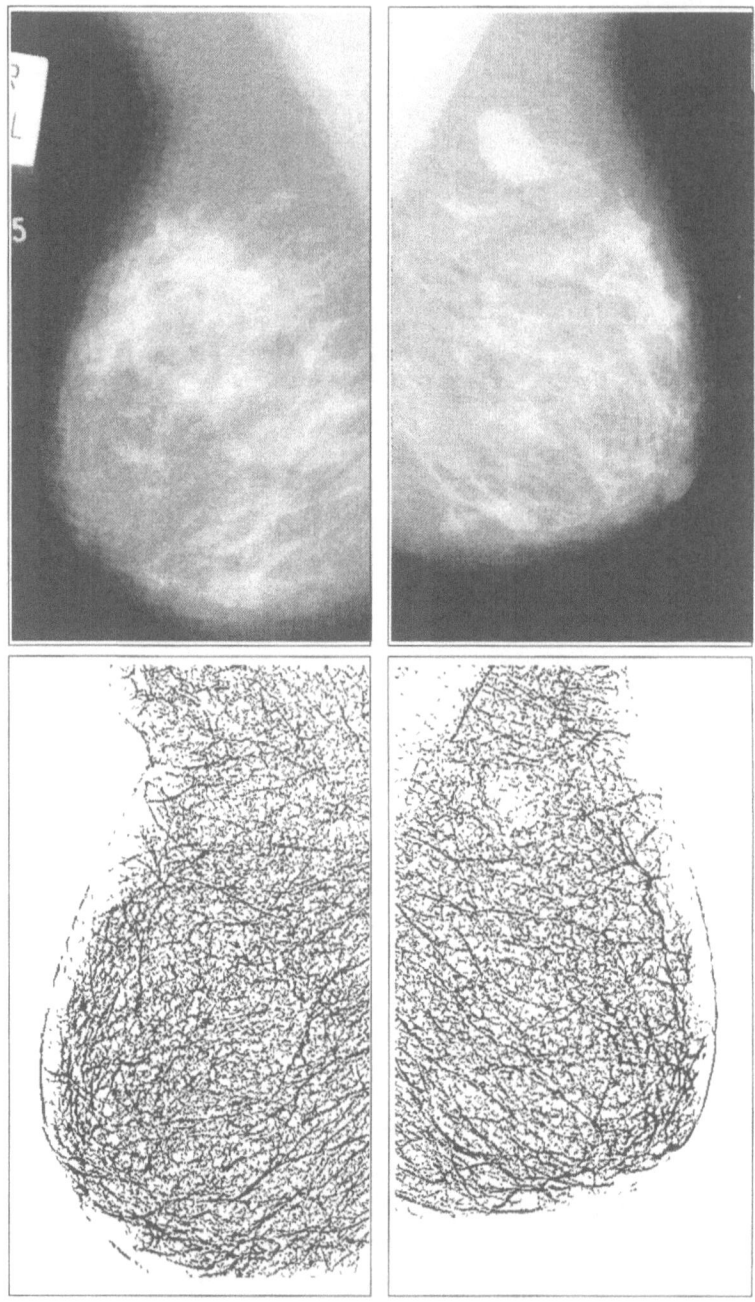

Figure 12.7.   A medio-lateral oblique pair and their corresponding CLS pixels. There have been few CLS features found in the pectoral muscle in the left breast mammogram because the film densities are close to saturation.

DETECTING CURVILINEAR STRUCTURES

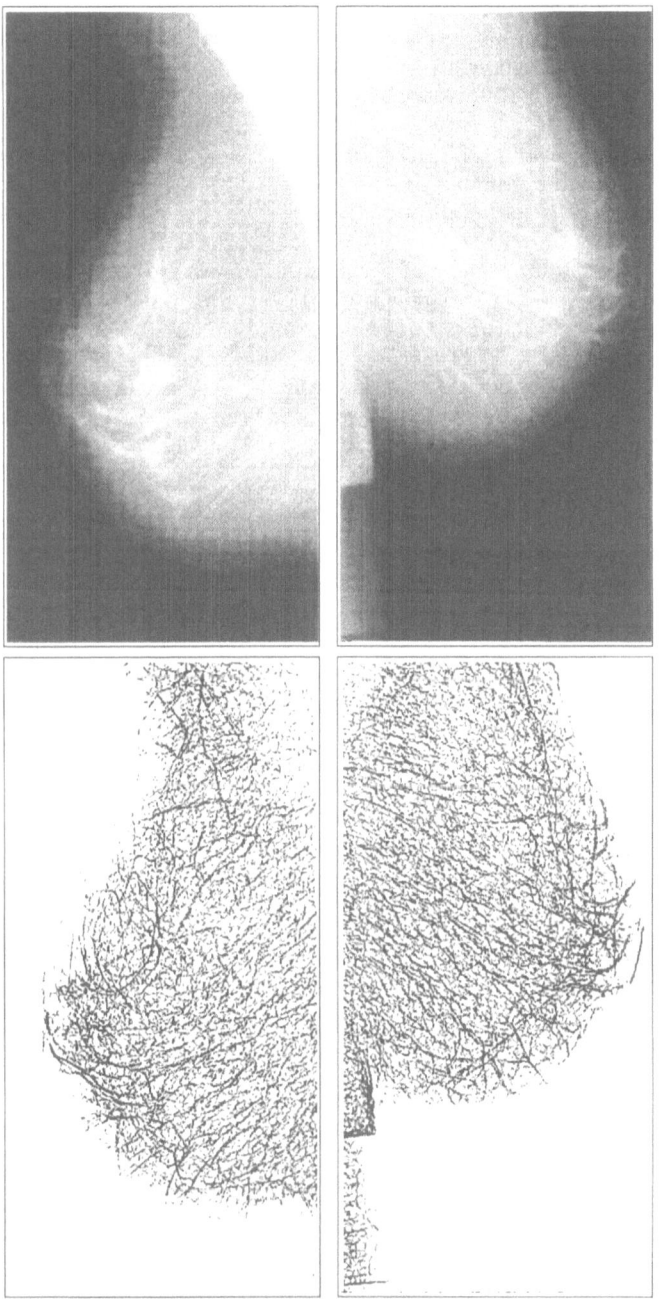

Figure 12.8.   A medio-lateral oblique pair and their corresponding CLS pixels.

BOX 12.9: Algorithm to remove CLS features

(1) Fit a low order polynomial to the pixels of the wire $\mathbf{b}_i$ corresponding to the current CLS. Since polynomials are single-valued functions, in practice the wire pixels are least-squares fit to two polynomials, using respectively the x-axis and the y-axis as the polynomial domain. The fit with the smallest residual fitting error is selected as the best-fit of the data. Typically we use fourth or fifth order polynomials.

(2) At each pixel of the CLS, look in both orthogonal directions for the edge of the CLS and subsequently the pixels defining the local 'background' intensities as discussed above.

(3) If the current CLS pixel and background intensities are suitable we linearly interpolate new intensities for every pixel on the linear path joining the current pixel and the two 'background' pixels. Keep a record of each new value calculated for each pixel by this process.

(4) Assign each pixel the median value of all the new values calculated for it during the previous steps.

12.7. Removing the CLS

In Section 12.1 we motivated the extraction of the CLS, *inter alia*, by suggesting that if the (high frequency) CLS pixels were removed then the search for, and analysis of, masses would be easier and more robust. We return to this in the next chapter; here we describe an algorithm to remove the CLS pixels once they have been found.

The basic idea is straightforward: for each CLS pixel, estimate the direction orthogonal to the CLS at that point and then search backwards and forwards in that direction to find the flanking background pixels. Finally, replace the CLS with intensities interpolated from those background intensities. In practice, there are a number of details that complicate this story, for which the interested reader is referred to [35]. Estimating the local direction of the "wires" of the CLS (recall step 2c of the algorithm presented in Section 12.2) is done using a low-order spline fitted to the wire pixels, see Figure 12.9. The pixel interpolation algorithm is spelled out in Box 12.9 and the principle is illustrated in Figure 12.10. Finally, Figure 12.11 shows the result of removing the CLS features from the mammogram pair shown in Figure 12.7.

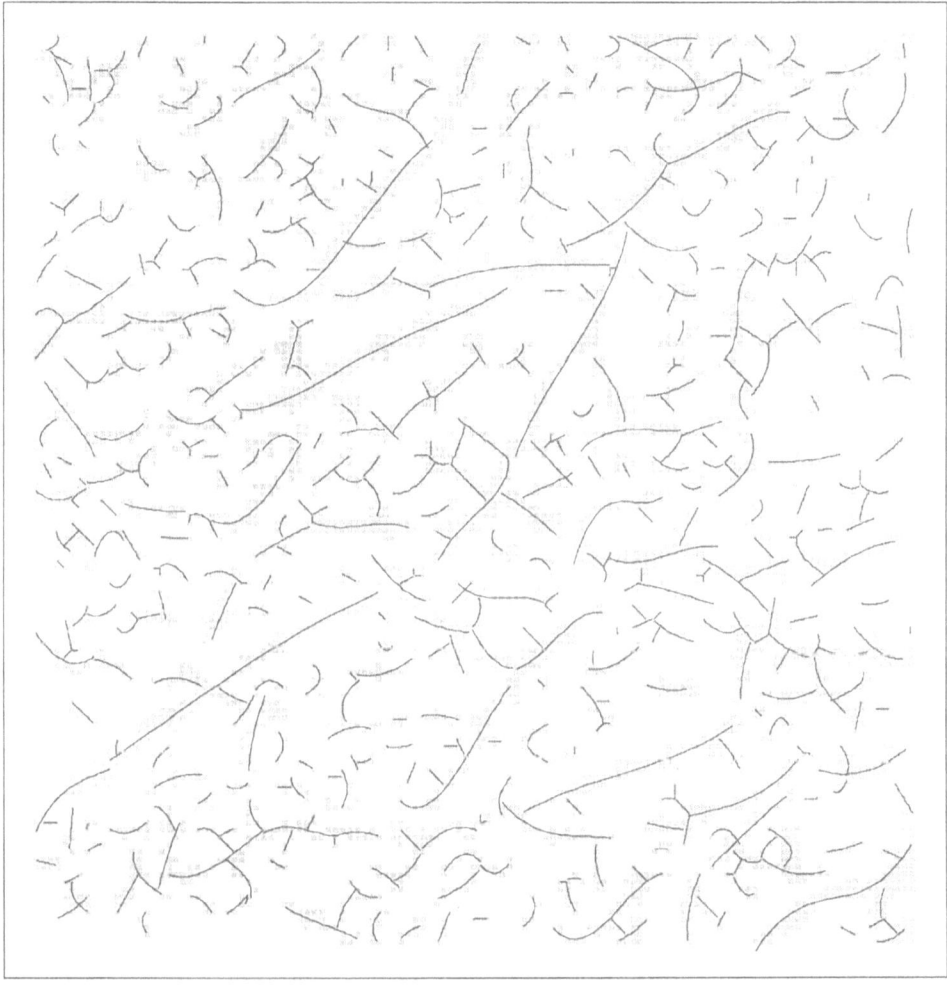

Figure 12.9.   Polynomial curves shown in black are fitted to the CLS features identified from the wires shown in grey. These curves allow the calculation of the local normal direction at each CLS pixel, and subsequently the identification of the background on either side of the CLS.

REMOVING CURVILINEAR STRUCTURES

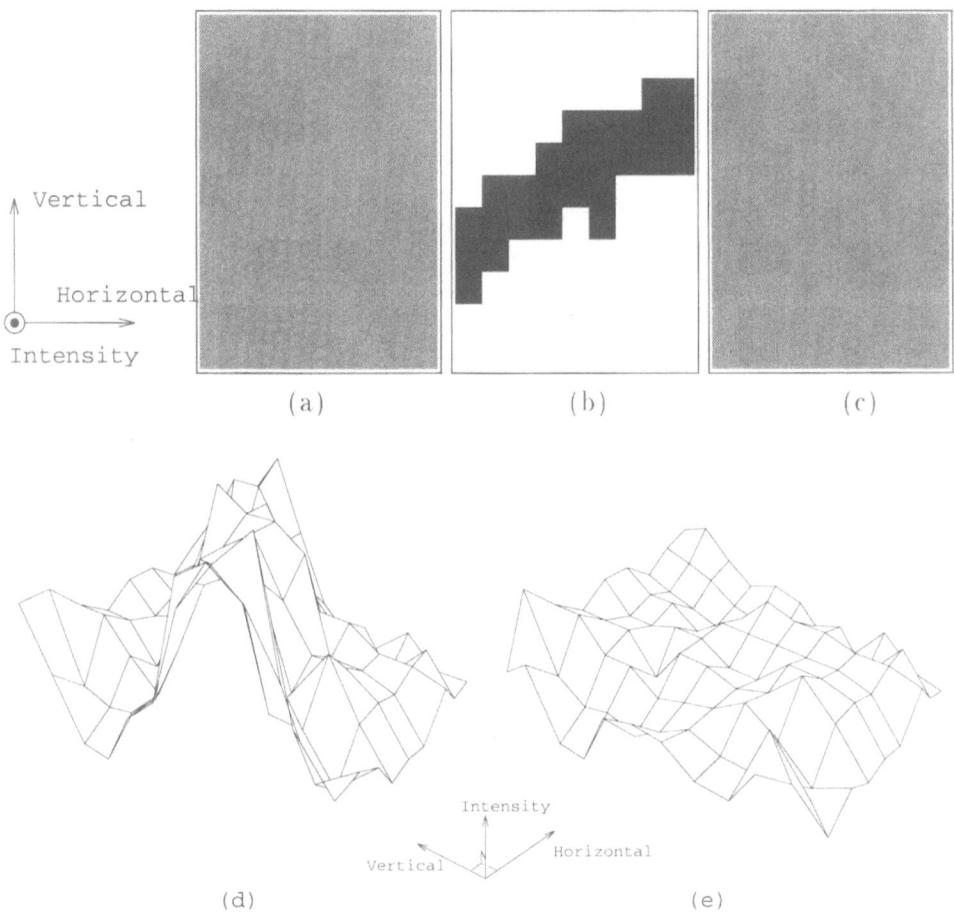

REMOVING CURVILINEAR STRUCTURES

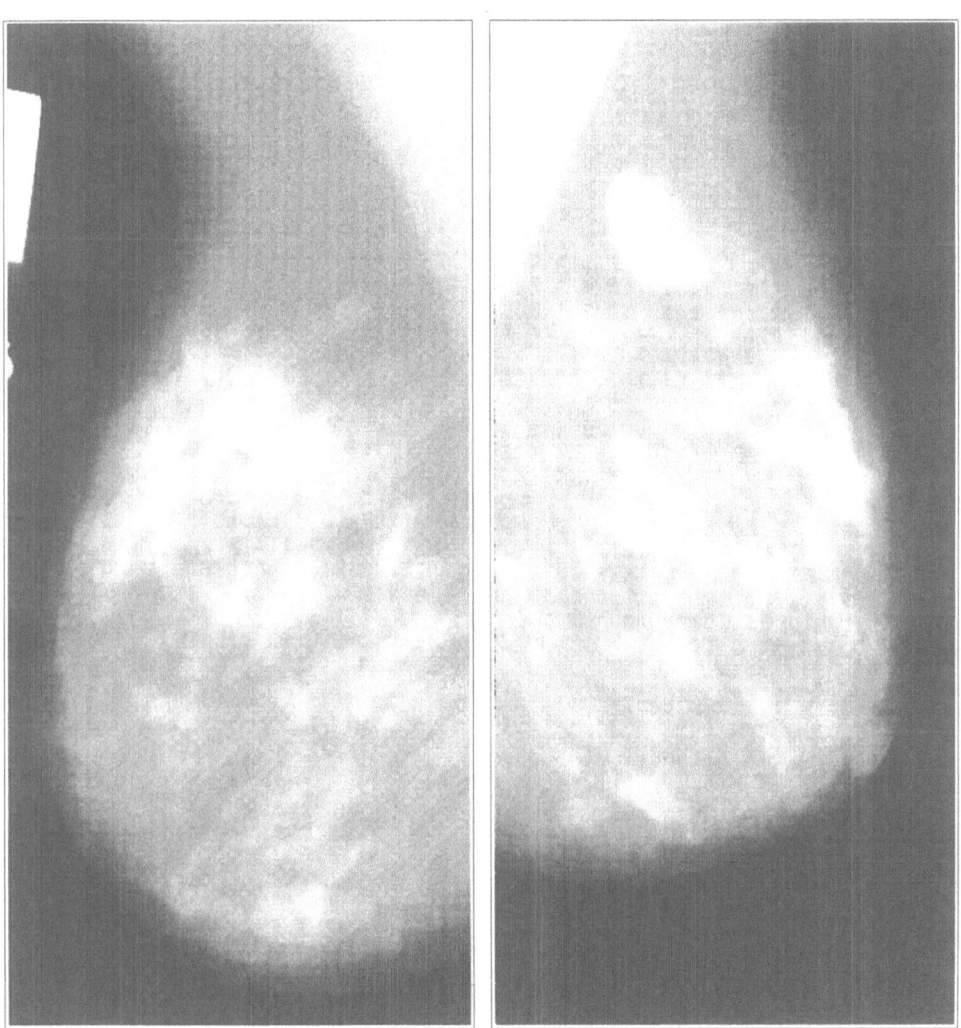

Figure 12.11. CLS-removed images for the original mammograms shown in Figure 12.7.

12.8. Summary: Curvilinear structures

We have developed an algorithm to extract the curvilinear structures in x-ray mammograms, based on an analysis of their anatomy and appearance in x-ray images. The algorithm works well, in the sense that the results accord closely with the CLS structures observed by radiologists. Furthermore, the algorithm supports further processing to identify potential lesions and to match left and right breast x-ray pairs and it works considerably better than conventional ridge following algorithms. Once identified, the CLS features can be removed, which produces a surface comprising parenchymal tissue and masses that can more reliably be matched, as discussed in the next chapter.

CHAPTER 13

MASSES

13.1. Introduction

This chapter presents a number of preliminary explorations of applying automated image analysis to masses, abnormal anatomical structures that often indicate breast pathology. In particular, we present results for three important applications:

- *Matching temporal pairs*: "Salient" regions are extracted independently in two mammograms of the same breast and the same view taken at two different times. The salient regions in the later mammogram are then matched with the isointensity regions in the first, and those that have either appeared in the later mammogram but not in the earlier one, or which have changed significantly between the two mammograms are drawn to the attention of the radiologist.
- *Matching bilateral pairs*: In a similar fashion, salient regions are extracted from the same-view left and right breast mammograms of the same woman, taken at approximately the same time. They are matched by an algorithm that draws the radiologist's attention to those that appear in one breast but not in the other.
- *Locating abnormal regions*: Salient regions are extracted from a breast image and for each a number of features are computed. These features are used to assess the "normality" of the region, as defined by a probabilistic model learned automatically from approximately 5000 bright regions found in the Mammographic Image Analysis Society (MIAS) database [231] of images. If a salient region is determined to be in the tails of the probabilistic model, it is declared to be "abnormal" and is drawn to the attention of the radiologist.

Common to our approach to each of these three applications are representations of bright regions in a mammogram.

We note at the outset that there is a significant difference between the first two applications and the third: the third depends on *interpreting* a bright region as a probable mass, whereas the first two do not attempt interpretation, even if they are based on a model of image formation. We stress, however, that a great deal of further research is needed if masses are to be correctly classified, and that the explorations presented in this chapter should be considered preliminary. Common to all three applications is the need to minimise the number of false positives. It has been found experimentally [129] that a radiologist prompted by too many false positives will lose confidence in the system and stop using it.

Masses typically appear in a mammogram as well-defined, relatively bright regions. The converse is not true, however; by no means do all relatively bright, circumscribed regions correspond to masses. A mammogram is a two-dimensional projection of three-dimensional compressed breast tissue, and so two spatially separated regions of dense fibroglandular tissue can overlap in the image. Since (primary) x-rays have to pass through both, the overlap region can appear as a single bright region of dense tissue. Similarly, the projection of a real mass can overlap a region of dense tissue, complicating the search for the occluded boundary of the mass. In fact, it is often impossible for a radiologist to classify a mammographic density from a single view, either as a mass, or as a dense portion of fibroglandular tissue, or as an overlap of such structures. For this reason, it is normal to take at least two different views of the breast (e.g. cranio-caudal and medio-lateral oblique) and we showed how to determine where to look for correspondences in Chapter 9.

It is advantageous to think of masses in terms of the h_{int} surface representation: a mass corresponds to a quite localised hill surrounded by gently undulating terrain that corresponds to normal fibroglandular tissue. It is easy to deduce from the mathematical development in the previous chapters that:

- Iso-height contours on the h_{int} surface approximately correspond to iso-intensity contours on the film density image.
- Nested contours of increasing height on the h_{int} surface correspond to nested iso-intensity contours of increasing brightness.
- The h_{int} surface factors out image formation effects and encodes only the intrinsic breast tissue.

The first two observations imply that we can perform calculations on the film density image while using a model of a mass developed from the h_{int} surface. The third observation warns us against comparing film density images directly, for example for the temporal pair matching problem, unless the imaging conditions were almost identical when the two views were taken. However, the representation we choose for matching is invariant to imaging conditions and so for convenience we work with film density images rather than with their h_{int} surfaces but we develop the theory based upon h_{int}.

In Sections 13.4 and 13.5 we describe the algorithm we have developed with our colleague Siew-li Kok-Wiles [154, 153] for matching structures between temporal mammogram pairs. Typical results of the matching algorithm are shown in Section 13.5. The approach is extended to bilateral mammogram pairs in Section 13.6. Then, in Sections 13.7 we describe separate developments with several of our colleagues [235] aimed at assessing the "novelty" of a bright region, and estimating the likelihood that it is a mass.

13.2. Preliminary considerations

How might we find the significant new anatomical structures appearing in the second mammogram forming a temporal pair? Clearly, we need to establish some sort of correspondence between the two mammograms and then we need to find significant differences. This raises a number of inter-related problems, the approach to them largely defines our overall technique:

- What entities, computed in the images separately, are matched to form the correspondence?
- How are significant differences between the two images determined?
- How is the correspondence between the two images established?

We discuss these in turn. Note that low signal-to-noise ratio, poor contrast, large inter and intra-image variations, and the presence of numerous subtle mammographic symptoms, all conspire to make the problem of matching a pair of mammograms very difficult. Published papers are typically based on features such as the local "brightness" of sets of connecting points, their "brightness variations"[159, 174], or on more global features such as shape[174, 1], boundary gradients, and line orientations.

The entities to match

Many techniques for matching medical images use "landmark" points [20], computed separately in each image, as match primitives. To date, however, landmarks have not been defined for mammograms, and the visual complexity of a mammogram strongly suggests that to do so would be difficult. Other techniques are based on matching curves; again, the currently poor results obtained by applying conventional edge detection algorithms to mammograms rule out such approaches.

Since candidate masses correspond to bright regions, a promising alternative is to identify and match a suitable set of regions in the mammograms. But which regions? Kimme et al.[149] divided each image into small rectangular regions. Since such regions do not correspond to anatomical structures it is quite unreliable. Furthermore, it is unclear how the method could cope with a large misalignment between the images. Miller and Astley [174] attempted to extract a single non-fat region from each breast using texture measures; but they found this unreliable with uniform densities. They currently use manual extraction. More recently, Vujovic et al.[251] partitioned the breast into circular regions that are homogeneous in intensity, and used the ducts and vessels as landmarks to find similar regions. Circular regions also do not correspond to anatomical structures, while ducts and vessels are not always reliable landmarks, since they may not appear in both images because their appearance depends on compression.

In the approach described in this chapter, we define and match "salient" bright regions of varying sizes, each of which corresponds to an area of mammographically dense tissue, hence is *a priori* a candidate mass. The set of regions is organised into a tree structure that represents the nesting of the salient bright regions in the mammogram. Significant differences between the mammograms correspond to bright regions in the later mammogram that have no match in the earlier one. This is manifested as a structural difference between the trees of salient bright regions computed for each image.

Often, the parameters that determine the image characteristics, such as breast compression, exposure time, and film speed, do not vary much. It follows that a pair of temporal mammograms nearly always present the same nested fibroglandular structures albeit with different intensities and contrasts. Since our representation aims to emphasise that nested structure, it should be essentially invariant over time and to small changes in imaging parameters. An exception to this is involution, the transformation of dense to fatty tissue. Similar observations can also be made about bilateral mammograms, though the relationship between the left and right images is less likely to be exactly similar.

How differences are detected

The simplest technique to find the differences between two images is simply to subtract them. However, this is ineffective for mammograms because it requires both perfect geometric and intensity registration of the images, that is, exactly the same degree of compression of the breast and the same exposure time. These requirements are quite unrealistic.

Since the salient bright regions are organised as a tree structure that makes explicit the nesting of the regions, and since, in general one expects that the changes in the tree structure will be relatively localised and small, it may be expected that an algorithm to match the tree structures will be effective at detecting significant differences. This is the approach that we adopt.

A key assumption of the matching algorithm developed in Section 13.5 is that the intrinsic fibroglandular structures of healthy breast tissue do not change much in the interval between taking a pair of temporal mammograms. Of course, the mammograms can be expected to differ as images, but, as we will argue below, the nested structure of the parenchymal tissue remains relatively invariant. The incorporation of a set of judiciously chosen features for each region makes the match process quite robust.

The correspondence between the images

Although we have chosen to match mammograms by matching tree structures of nested salient bright regions, we mention briefly, for completeness, the techniques developed in computer vision/image processing for establishing a correspondence between a pair of images. Usually, a geometrical transformation is computed, the advantage being that for any point in the first image the corresponding point in the second can be found simply by applying the transformation.

Most previous research assumes a global, rigid transformation [259, 265, 1, 99, 159, 26, 229, 155] that is estimated, for example from the breast boundary. However, the alignment between two mammograms is often poorly approximated by a rigid transformation. An alternative is to use a scheme for non-rigid registration, though these are more difficult to compute robustly. In any case, most such techniques are point-based which is problematical for mammograms, and, being quite general they ignore the available constraints that derive from a model of breast compression. Recently, there has been some work on image unwarping, in which a non-rigid transformation is estimated[269, 22, 216]. However, image unwarping may distort the true breast parenchyma, and requires reliable control points, but this is difficult because of the lack of internal "landmarks" in mammograms. Note that the transformation associated with a tree match between mammograms is intrinsically non-rigid as is the transformation computed by our algorithm. Inaccuracies of registration are finessed by extracting and matching regions in the two mammograms that are significant and similar to each other.

There is not always a tractable mathematical description of the transformation between two images. This is the case for example for two images that are snapshots of a motion field. In such cases, the best that can be done is to compute an approximation to the flow field between the images. Techniques for doing this have been developed recently, but have not yet been applied to mammograms.

13.3. A representation of salient bright regions

The definition, computation, and use of a representation of the nested bright regions in an image has been studied remarkably little in image processing.

BOX 13.1: Guissin-Brady saliency measure for a region

Denote $\dfrac{\sum_S |\nabla I|}{\sum_S 1}$ by μ, a measure of the average image gradient ∇I along the contour S. Then the Guissin-Brady measure $\mathcal{M}_{GB}$ is given by:

$$\mathcal{M}_{GB} = \sum_S |\nabla I| \times \frac{\sum_S |\nabla I|}{\sum_S 1} \times \left[\frac{\sum_S 1}{\sum_S (|\nabla I| - \mu)^2} \right]^{\frac{1}{2}}$$

The third term measures the stability of the region and is the standard deviation of the image gradient along the contour. Iso-intensity contours which mark significant changes in this measure relative to small changes in intensity are dubbed "salient".

A major exception to this is the work of Lindeberg [164] who developed a relevant representation in the context of intensity surfaces. There are, however, a number of limitations to Lindeberg's definition, which limits its usefulness as a representation of breast anatomical structures. Cerneaz [35] gives examples.

Another exception is the work of Guissin and Brady [94] involving image thresholding at every intensity. The resulting set of 'iso-intensity' or 'level' curves include all the salient bright regions that we seek; but much more besides. To reduce the enormous set of level-curves to a manageable number, they develop a measure to assess each contour, retaining only those contours that exceed some adaptive threshold. Although their technique might be acceptable for relatively small images containing large features, the computational cost involved in finding small blobs in large mammogram images is prohibitive.

Guissin and Brady overcome this problem by developing a metric for the significance of a contour that quantifies the saliency of a region relative to its local neighbourhood. Given such a measure of region saliency it is possible to compare the relative saliency of associated regions, and to reject some regions if other more salient regions adequately describe that part of the image. For visual images, the most important aspect is the edge strength at the region's bounding contour. They therefore base the definition of their saliency metric on three aspects of the contour: its length, contrast, and stability. Box 13.1 gives the details.

The Guissin-Brady metric works well for visual images, but it is not suitable for mammography, not least because the magnitude of the measure is linearly related to the contour length, favouring larger regions with longer perimeters. This is clearly at odds with our *a priori* knowledge that mammographic masses can be significant at any size, and although it is important to detect larger masses, it is the smaller masses that allow the early detection of disease processes within a breast, and so they should not be de-emphasised. Furthermore it is conceivable that a large bounding contour enclosing the entire parenchymal tissue of a mammogram, with relatively low, but stable, contrast along the boundary between the fatty tissue background and the parenchymal tissues could have a significance measure equalling or exceeding a small region with high, but less consistent contrast. Clearly this is not desirable for the representation of anatomical structures.

From such considerations, Nick Cerneaz [35] developed a representation that combines the ideas of Lindeberg, and Guissin and Brady. Rather than locating every region (such as the segmentation provided by every iso-intensity contour), he located only the most salient region from each location which adequately describes the given part of the image. By developing a saliency metric, comparative analysis of the saliency of the regions in a given part of the image is used to select the most appropriate region to represent that part.

Cerneaz supposes that for each gradient measure there is a corresponding confidence weighting w. In noisy regions it would be expected that w would be small. Conversely, in regions with low noise and good gradient estimates, we would expect values of w close to one. With such a confidence measure, the first term in the Guissin-Brady saliency metric can be replaced by the average weighted gradient measure over the region boundary. In like manner, Cerneaz based a contrast measure on the weight parameter w to replace the second term in the Guissin-Brady metric.

Our colleague Siew-li Kok-Wiles further developed Cerneaz's representation and saliency metric in order to make it more suitable for matching temporal and bilateral pairs of mammograms [154]. In the case of matching, the set of regions has to include small "abnormal" regions, as well as the largest possible dense region, namely the entire breast. Stable regions that represent the boundaries of dense tissue regions exhibit strong boundary gradients. Kok-Wiles found it useful to incorporate the weighting into the stability, changing the third term in the Guissin-Brady formula. With this final definition, the equation for saliency captures both high and shallow, but flat regions. The resulting metric is given in Box 13.2.

However, even when we restrict attention just to embedded regions of locally maximum saliency, in practice we still find ourselves dealing with a large number of regions. We cut down the number by restricting attention further to the subset of salient regions that correspond to a "significant" change in an associated description that includes the area of the region and the average intensity of the region. We retain only those regions for which the rate of change of the description exceeds a threshold, and call the corresponding iso-intensity contour "salient".

BOX 13.2: The saliency measure developed by Cerneaz and Kok-Wiles for matching temporal and bilateral pairs of mammograms.

$$\mathcal{M}_{KW}(r) = \frac{\sum_S \nabla I(s)w(s)}{\sum_S w(s)} \times \frac{1}{1 + \sum_S(1 - w(s))} \times \left[\frac{\sum_S w(s)}{\sum_S(w(s)\,|\nabla I(s) - \mu|)^2}\right]^{\frac{1}{2}},$$

(13.1)

In this formula, μ denotes the average intensity gradient along the length of the contour, $\dfrac{\sum_s |\nabla I|}{\sum_s 1}$.

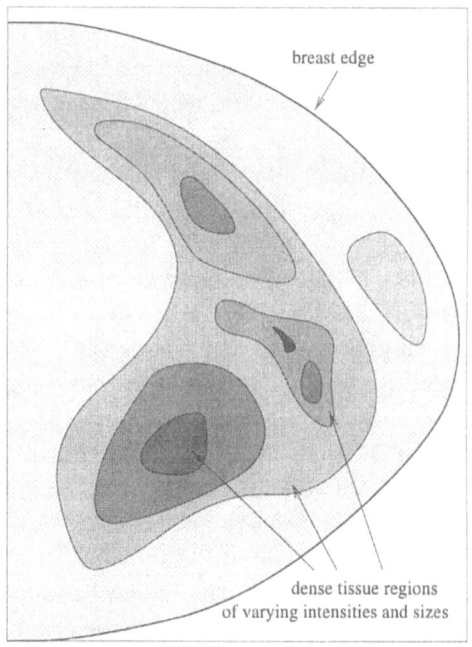

Figure 13.1. This illustrates the dense tissue regions. The grey scale tone of a region indicates the iso-brightness of the corresponding region. Although fibroglandular regions are brighter than their surrounds, for illustrative convenience, the darker a region the higher the corresponding iso-brightness, i.e. the brighter the region. Nested regions correspond to nested contours of iso-brightness, hence to increasingly bright regions.

Two thresholds, one for change in area and the other for the change in grey level intensity, were set empirically to yield regions that correspond to those judged mammographically significant. We have found that a fixed value for the change in area works well, but that the suitable values for the change in intensity fall within a range. After thresholding, about 20–30% of the total iso-intensity contours are retained as putatively significant contours. If the values are set too high, too few regions would be retained, and small abnormal lesions may be excluded; if the values are set low, more contours would be included in the significant contour set. Although it is preferred that more regions are included, rather than risk omitting potential lesions, the smaller the regions, the less confident we are of their matches; this is reflected in their match scores, a measure of confidence for the matched region pairs. Examples of the nested structure of salient regions are shown in schematic form in Figure 13.1 and in the figures in Section 13.5.

Having developed the representation of regions and salient regions, the next few sections put it to work, first for matching both temporal and bilateral pairs of mammograms, and then for the detection of novelty.

13.4. The transformation between a temporal pair

If the bright regions that correspond to essentially unchanging structures such as fibroglandular tissue always appeared in exactly the same locations in both the first and second mammogram of a temporal pair, then novel structures, corresponding to candidate masses, could be detected by subtracting the first image from the second one. However, image subtraction is most often ineffective, for three major reasons:

1. The breast might be positioned differently in the x-ray machine;
2. There might be a change in breast compression;
3. There might be image changes due to differences in the x-ray imaging conditions.

Each of these differences corresponds to a different sort of image transform. These are summarised in Figure 13.2 and are elaborated below. There are two major anatomical changes to consider: (i) the normal process of involution, in which denser (brighter) glandular, fibrous, and supporting tissues transform into less dense (darker) adipose tissue; and (ii) the development of new dense structures, that may be benign or malignant but which are always of interest. Note that the former process corresponds to a loss of brighter areas whereas the latter corresponds to the development of new ones. It follows that the appearance of "significant" brighter regions in the more recent mammogram should be investigated, while their disappearance may be disregarded.

As we noted in the introduction to this chapter, the h_{int} representation effectively eliminates the third transformation factor. Even so, as we noted in the previous chapter and in Chapter 6 we should not trust absolute heights in h_{int} or, if there has been no change in imaging conditions and

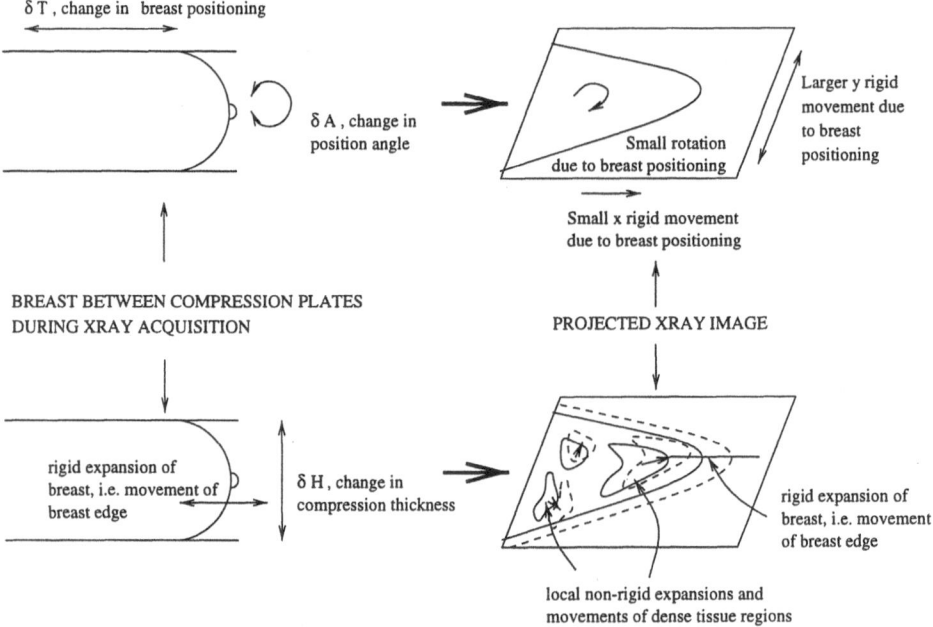

Figure 13.2. Global and local transformations between temporal mammograms.

for convenience we choose to match images, absolute intensity values. That leaves the non-rigidity of the transformation between the two images of a temporal pair, and, mathematically, this would seem to be the most difficult problem. Fortunately, we can identify a number of constraints that make the problem tractable.

In most countries there are agreed standards for good radiographic technique. For most standard views, the woman's posture is manipulated by the radiographer to bring her chest wall as close as possible to the leading plate edge of the x-ray machine, so that the breast is approximately aligned with the longitudinal axis of symmetry of the plates. A consequence of the considerable care taken by the radiographer to position the woman is that for a given posture, the breast is in approximately the same position and orientation relative to the lower plate (before compression). To a very good approximation, therefore, the transformation between the two positions of the uncompressed breast can be regarded as rigid, with a small translation and rotation.

By far the most difficult problems correspond to changes resulting from differential breast compression (see Chapter 9). Generally, an increase in compression causes a global expansion of the imaged surface of the breast, corresponding to a global scaling of the image, away from the chest wall. A consequence is that each mass moves away from the chest wall. Most masses move according to a smooth (essentially divergent) flow field, hence smoothly relative to their neighbours. However, harder tissues (for example tumours) may move differently than those that are softer (for example cysts or fibroglandular tissues) and this is more difficult to model. Also, there are local tissue interactions, for example those involving spicules, and these can cause aberrant motions. This disrupts the smooth flow field, and results in locally non-smooth movements between the masses [114]. Though the change in compression of the same breast may be expected to vary only by a small amount (typically 0.5 cm) between sessions, the relative motions of bright regions can be quite substantial. It follows that the absolute positions of bright regions cannot be relied upon in a matching algorithm. Rather, it is important to represent a bright region in a way that enables it to be matched despite being scaled and moved relative to its neighbours. A key part of this is to make explicit the bright regions in which it is embedded.

Constraints on the transformation

Suppose, for the reasons described earlier in this chapter, we represent and match mammograms in terms of "dense mammographic tissue regions". Such regions are delineated by intensity changes corresponding to a change in tissue density. The mammogram density image can be considered to be three-dimensional, with the coordinates of the mammogram forming the x-y plane and h_{int} or image intensity as the z-axis. Imagine now that we have three perceptual regions in a mammogram, as shown in Figure 13.3 (I). If there were no changes of the sorts described above, then the same three regions would appear in the same positions in the second image, as shown in 13.3 (II), and the relationship between the grey values in the current and previous image would be the identity, as shown in 13.3 (III). In this hopelessly ideal case, there would be no difference between the set of regions in the two mammograms. That is, for every region, in the current image there would be a matching region in the previous image. Figure 13.4 shows a more realistic case and whilst it is more complex the same conclusions apply.

Involution corresponds to a loss of bright regions in the current image relative to the previous one thus we should extract bright regions from the current image, then search for matches in the previous image. Furthermore, since we may reasonably assume that new growths persist and may enlarge, regions should appear for the first time, or increase in size in the current

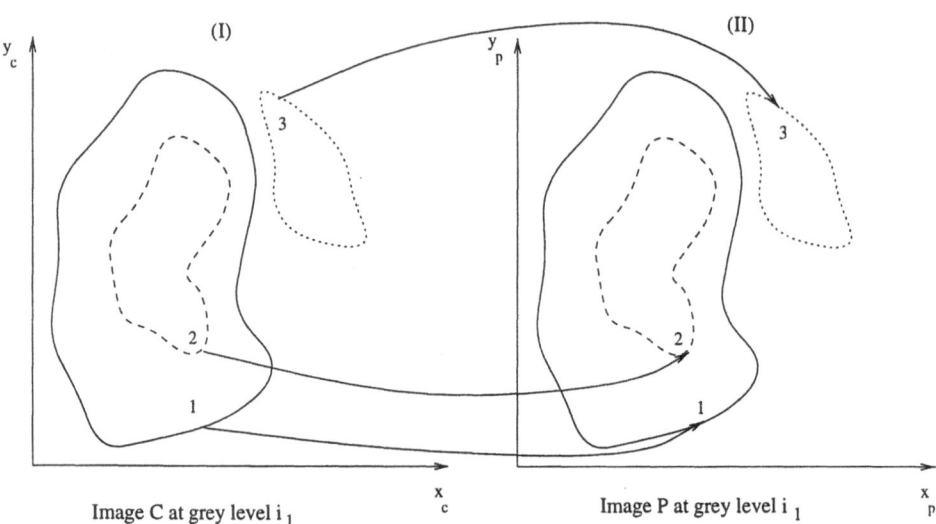

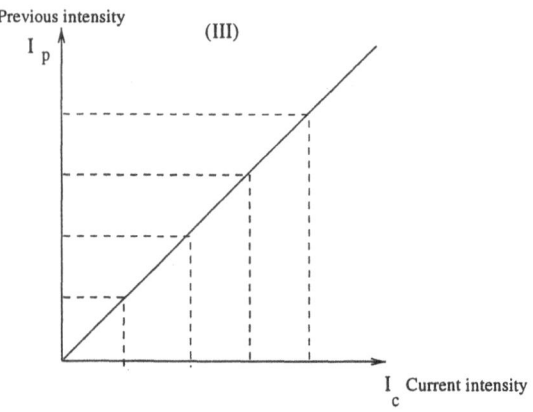

Figure 13.3.   Identical pairs of mammographic regions and the relationship between their intensities. Figure (I) shows three regions in the current image at grey level i_1 and Figure (II) the identical regions in the previous image also at grey level i_1. Figure (III) is the relationship between the intensities in each image, in this case the identity.

image. Similarly, changes in breast positioning correspond to a global rigid transformation of the current image, with small translation and rotation relative to the previous image; but the set of salient regions should be preserved as should their nested structure.

We warned in Chapter 6 against relying on absolute h_{int} heights or absolute image intensities. The transformation between the images can be

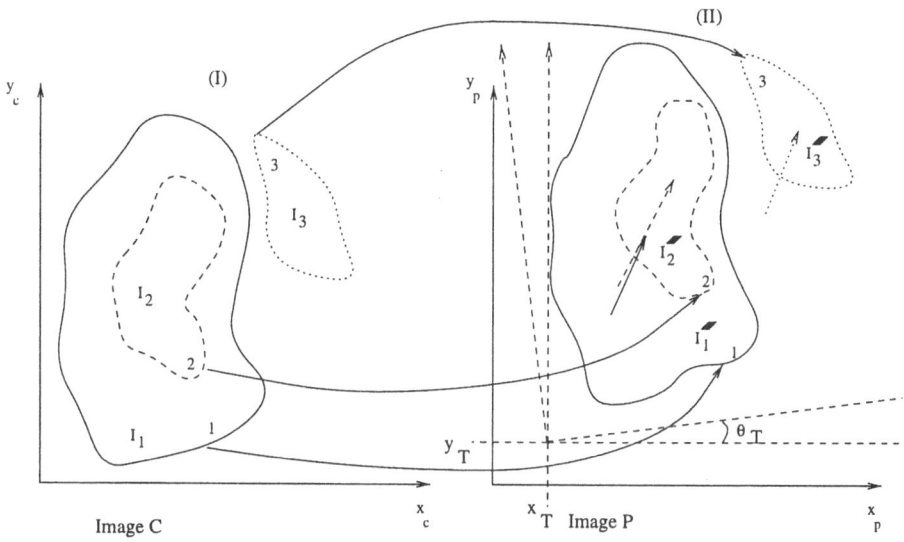

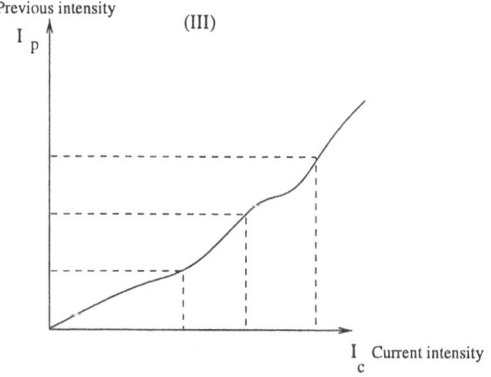

Figure 13.4. Local non-rigid transformation of identical pairs of mammographic regions and the relationship between their intensities. Figure (I) shows three regions in the current image at grey levels I_1, I_2, I_3 and Figure (II) the identical regions in the previous image with local non-rigid transform and new grey levels. Figure (III) is the relationship between the intensities in the images, in this case a non-linear transform.

accompanied by a global transform of the intensity distribution in the two images. A key observation about the height/intensity transform is that it is monotonic. It follows that if the average grey level for one region is greater than that of another in the current image, then the same should apply for the two corresponding regions in the previous image.

Finally, a change in compression not only leads to a global transformation between the two images, but also causes local movements of tissue regions according to their hardness and local tissue interactions. Novak's[187] work on compression, which we used in Chapter 9 on matching medio-lateral oblique and cranio-caudal mammograms, enables us to deduce a number of weak heuristics on the transformation. They are "weak" because they are not guaranteed to hold all of the time, rather they hold mostly. We have embodied them in a program that matches temporal and bilateral pairs of mammograms. The following can be expressed mathematically, but since this is incidental to our present purposes such a treatment is suppressed here. The interested reader is referred to Kok-Wiles' thesis [153].

Smooth motion constraint : the mammogram results from the attenuation of the breast tissues by the x-ray beam. If we consider the image to consist of connecting fatty tissues inlaid with denser fibroglandular tissues, it is reasonable to suppose that relative movements of the tissues during compression are neither sudden nor large, therefore that the differences between local neighbouring transforms for the regions vary slowly and smoothly.

Topological constraint : consider a nested set of progressively brighter and smaller regions in the current image. The topological constraint states that the same nested structure can be found in the previous image. That is, if a region s_2 is enclosed by another s_1 in the current image, then the region corresponding to s_2 in the previous image should also be enclosed by the region corresponding to s_1.

Order constraint : this is so-named because of its similarity to the order constraint of stereo vision [70], where it is also assumed to hold "most of the time" (in that case, it is violated for transparent surfaces, fishing lines, and similar rare events). It is usually the case that if a region s_2 appears to the right of region s_1 in the current image then the region corresponding to s_2 in the previous image will also be to the right of the region corresponding to s_1.

Monotonicity of geometry constraint : it is usually the case that order relationships between geometrical properties of regions are preserved. To date, we have only used the geometrical properties of area, contour length and contour saliency, so, for example, if a region s_2 has smaller area than a region s_1 in the current image then the region corresponding to s_2 in the previous image will have smaller area than the region corresponding to s_1.

13.5. Constraint-based region matching

The goal of the matching algorithm is to find, for each salient region in the current image, that region in the previous image that most closely corresponds to it. We recall that the salient regions in the current image are organised as a nested structure that has the mathematical form of a tree. That is, each salient region has a "parent" which is the unique salient region that it is embedded in. It may have several "children" regions of which it is the unique parent. The ancestral root of the tree is the entire breast region. Because image intensities/h_{int} heights[1] can not be trusted, it may be that the best correspondent of a salient region in the current image is not salient in the previous image[2]; however, it will be bounded by an iso-intensity contour. For this reason, the input to the match algorithm consists of (i) the nested (tree) structure of salient regions for the current image and (ii) the entire set of regions bounded by iso-intensity contours for the previous image.

The match algorithm proceeds from coarse-to-fine. That is, it starts by matching the entire breast regions in the current and previous images. The best global rigid transformation is computed between the entire breast region of the current image and that of the previous image. Then the algorithm tries to establish progressively finer matches, where the local non-rigid movements of the regions dominate. The search for matches is repeated until all the salient regions in the current image are matched (or labelled "unmatched" if no matches exist within the given match score threshold).

While proceeding coarse-to-fine, the match algorithm exploits the match constraints described in the previous section. The tightest of these is the topological constraint. Suppose, recursively, that we have determined the region $r_p = \mathrm{match}(r_c)$ in the previous image that is the best match for a salient region r_c in the current image. Then the matches for the salient regions in the current image that are the "children" of r_c are searched for among the iso-contours embedded within r_p. Clearly, there are two cases where this constraint cannot be used: at initialisation, and when a match cannot be found for the parent region r_c. These will be discussed below. The topological constraint not only dramatically speeds the search; but, equally importantly, it reduces sharply the number of mismatches, in particular for those small regions that are near the "leaves" of the tree. A final advantage in using the constraint is that it allows us to use relatively simple descriptors for feature matching between candidate regions. The descriptors that we

---

[1]For the rest of this section we refer to intensity, but note that it refers either to image intensity or to a h_{int} height, depending on which representation is being used for matching.

[2]Here and in the following, "salient" means both that its saliency score (Box 13.2) is high and that its rate of change of saliency exceeds a threshold (Section 13.3).

use, and which are described in detail below, normally have very poor
discrimination qualities, but used in the framework of the coarse to fine
matching algorithm they are highly effective.

Application of the smooth motion, topological, order, and monotonicity
of geometry constraints, reduces sharply the set of candidate matches for a
salient region r_c in the current image that need to be considered. Suppose
that during the coarse-to-fine match we have already matched the parent
p_c of region r_c. This matched region for the parent will have an iso-intensity
boundary, as will the match for r_c that we seek. The monotonicity in intensity constraint requires that the iso-intensity of r_c's match is greater than
that of p_c's match, but that the difference is within an empirically determined constant, which we set to between ±10 to ±30 intensity levels in our
experiments. If, as happens occasionally, for example with new growths,
there is no match for p_c, we constrain the iso-intensity of r_c's match to be
not too different from that of r_c itself.

There may still remain a (by now small) set of candidate regions in the
previous image to match a region r_c in the current image. Of these, we
choose that one that has the best match score with r_c, so long as it exceeds
a threshold (otherwise we proclaim "no match"). We now sketch briefly the
match score that we have used to date. This has worked surprisingly well,
given its simplicity. We re-emphasise that we believe this to be so because
the score is used only in the context of the constraints set out above. Figure
13.5 summarises the matching strategy.

The match score

The match score evaluates the match between a salient region in the current
image and a putative match for it in the previous image. There is usually
only one putative match with a good score. We find in practice that the
scores of incorrect putative matches are poor, so we can use the match score
as a confidence in the match. The score is a weighted sum of the differences
in the values of a set of features for the two regions being compared. We
find that the results we have obtained are quite insensitive to the precise
choices of the weights [154].

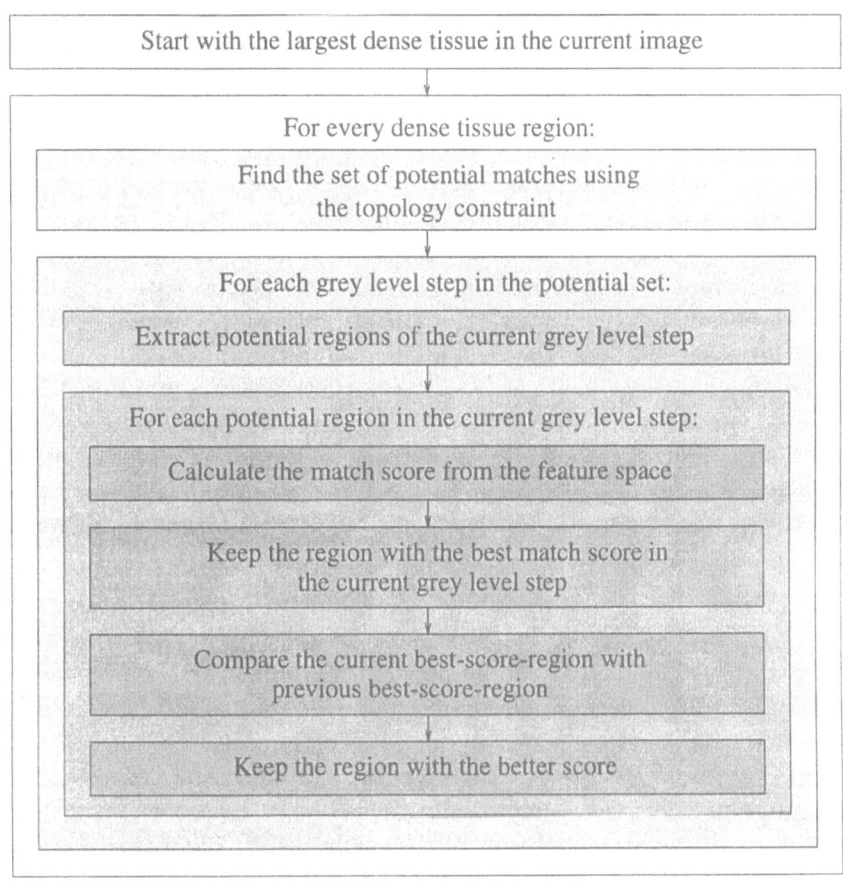

Figure 13.5. Summary of matching strategy.

Currently, we use six features for each region, in three groups as follows:

1. *The centroid of the region.* The difference between the centroids measures the movement of the region between the two images, and this, in turn, embodies the order and smoothness of motion constraints.

2. *The area, contour length and contour saliency.* Taking account of the differences in these features amounts to applying the monotonicity in geometry constraint.

3. *The average intensity and the standard deviation of the intensity within the region.* The differences between these makes further application of the monotonicity in intensity constraint necessary.

Results

The search algorithm outlined above has first been applied to numerous simulated image pairs, in order to establish its robustness to geometric and intensity distortion, and then (to date) to 28 real mammogram pairs. In fact, we currently have available many more bilateral pairs (26) than we have temporal pairs (2); though this situation is rapidly changing as women return for a second screening round. For the experiments, the six weights defined above were "tuned" for good performance on six mammogram pairs (three simulated and three real, bilateral), and the parameters were then fixed for the rest of the experimental period. We found that the difference between the centroids of the regions is the most important weighting parameter, so it was accorded twice the weight of the others, which were all given the same weight.

Simulated mammogram pairs are extremely valuable for investigating the correct operation and robustness of an algorithm, since ground truth is available. Of course, if the simulated "mammogram" pair bears scant similarity to a real mammogram pair, then the results will be of little value in assessing or developing the algorithm. Fortunately, we can build on the system described in Chapter 8, in which simulated masses can be added to a mammogram (via the h_{int} representation). The first set of experiments used an original image and the result of conversion to h_{int} and then back again. This test corresponds to the case of an identity global transformation, and tests the sensitivity of the algorithm to slight intensity changes. Happily, but not surprisingly, the algorithm performs perfectly on this base case!

Secondly, and more interestingly, the mammogram with the simulated masses is then subjected to a known transformation typical of those encountered in practice (for example: a translation of 6mm in the x and y mammogram coordinates, followed by a rotation of 15° about the z axis). We find that the algorithm is essentially invariant to translation, and that, for a fixed mass, as the rotation becomes larger the "new" (i.e. added) mass region is still successfully detected but additionally is accompanied by a small number of false positives. Also, as the size of the added mass is reduced in size, the influence of the displacements on the match scores becomes more significant. This suggests adaptively propagating the difference between the feature vectors for the base regions matched; but we have not yet done this.

Figure 13.6 is a temporal pair of mammograms taken 3 years apart. Both mammograms were taken during routine screening visits. In the current

TEMPORAL MAMMOGRAMS

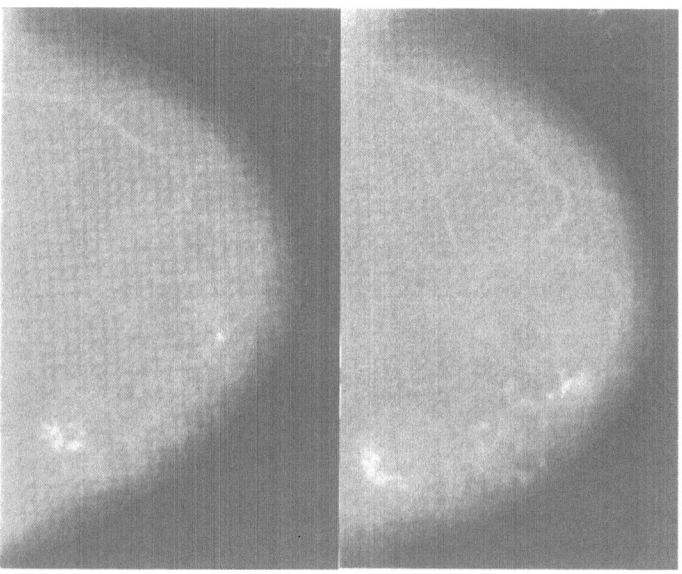

Figure 13.6.   Temporal pair 001: (a) previous image (left); (b) current image (right).

image (Figure 13.6b) an interval cancer has developed (near the bottom right of the breast), at the point where, in the previous image the area contained a cluster of microcalcifications. As can be observed clearly in the images, the position of the breast, the breast compression, and the x-ray settings are different, resulting not only in translation and relative enlargement of the image, but also slight movements of the dense tissue regions relative to one another. The result of matching the two images is presented in Figure 13.7: Figure 13.7(a) shows the significant regions in the current image for which no match has been found in the previous one. Observe that the regions corresponding to the interval cancer have been successfully classified as "no matches". 13.7(b) shows both the "no matches" from 13.7(a) and those regions that have bad match scores. There are in fact relatively few false positives in this case. Finally, 13.7(c) and (d) show the matched regions found for the previous and current mammogram respectively.

MATCHING TEMPORAL MAMMOGRAMS

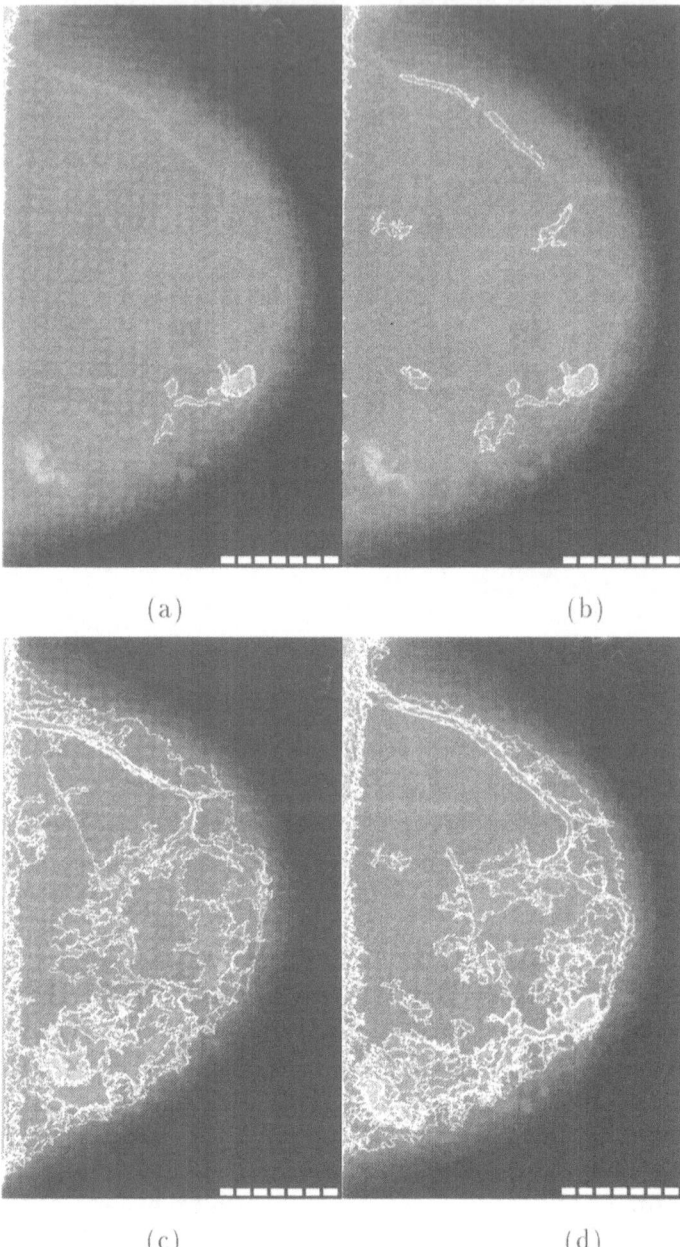

(a)   (b)

(c)   (d)

Figure 13.7. Result for temporal mammogram pair 001:(a) current mammogram showing regions with no matches found (b) current mammogram showing regions with no
matches and bad matches found (c) previous mammogram with all corresponding matches
(d) current mammogram with all significant contours.

The temporal image pair shown in Figure 13.8(a) and (b) were taken a year apart. There is no new growth in the current mammogram; but its appearance is markedly different from the previous mammogram because of substantially different x-ray parameter settings. Figure 13.8(c) shows that the algorithm has correctly determined that there are no "no match" regions in the current image. However, Figure 13.8(d) shows that two regions have been identified as "bad matches", that is, they have above average match scores.

13.6. Matching bilateral pairs

The matching algorithm for temporal pairs is predicated on the fact that the two images are of the same breast that is compressed to roughly the same extent, and whose parenchymal tissue is largely unchanged in the interval between the mammograms being taken. The bilateral case is rather more complex, since there are two images of different breasts involved. The constraints used successfully in the temporal case need to be re-examined for their applicability. Of course, the two breasts belong to the same woman, and this affords considerable constraint. Recall the discussion of asymmetry in Chapter 1:

"The breasts are mirror images; therefore, mammographically the distribution of the glandular tissue should appear the same, with only slight variation from one breast to the other ... Asymmetry is the radiologist's greatest aid in determining abnormalities both benign and malignant" [4] (page 144). However, the use of the word "symmetry" here is more qualitative than mathematical.

Though weaker than the temporal case, we may reasonably assume that the two breasts are similar in size, shape, compressibility properties and parenchymal structures. Assuming that the sizes and compressibilities of the bilateral pair are quite similar leads one to conjecture that the compression applied and the machine settings during the separate image acquisitions would also be very similar. This is indeed supported by Table 13.1, which shows the compression thickness and exposure recorded for a few of the images from one of our databases. Further support comes from the data used in the work described in Chapter 5 which shows that the average difference in compressed thickness between left and right breasts is 0.274cm although we note that such changes in thickness can cause the exposure time to alter dramatically.

Assuming that the nested tree structures of the salient regions in the left and right breasts are closely similar, amounts to assuming that a bilateral pair of breasts is more like each other than either is to a random different woman. This seems to be the case as we have successfully applied the match algorithm described in the previous section to the bilateral pairs currently available to us. In the bilateral case, of course, we run the algorithm twice,

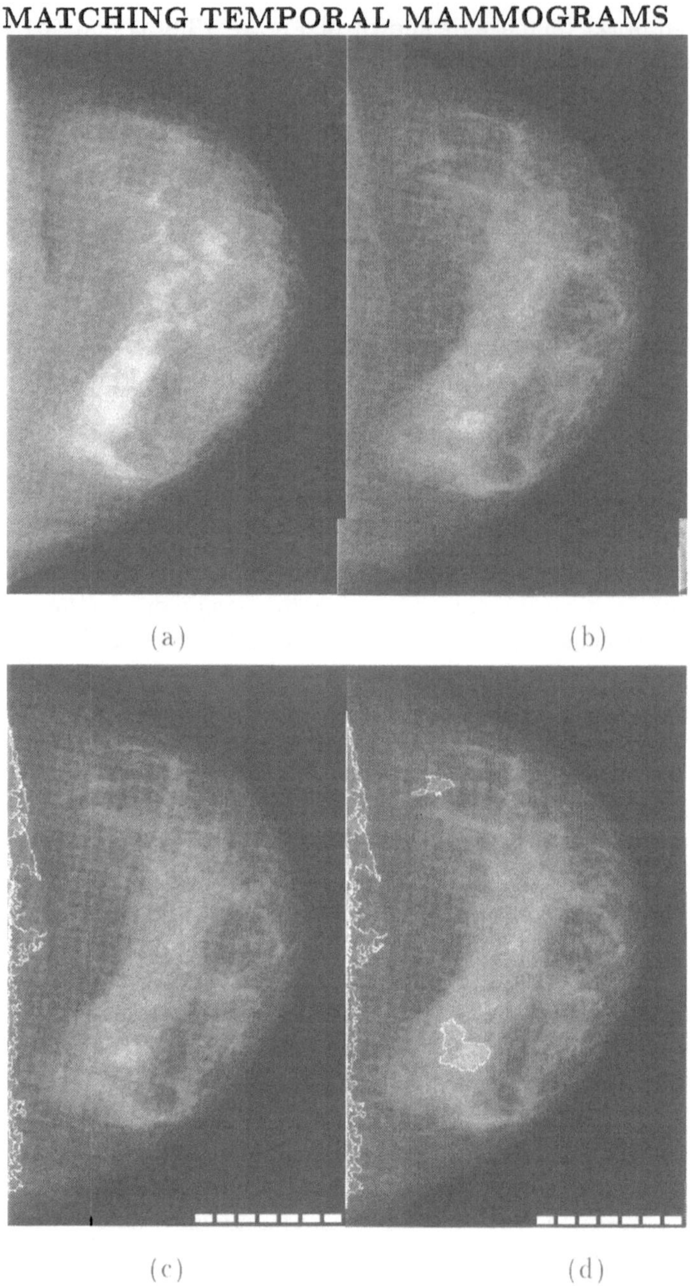

MATCHING TEMPORAL MAMMOGRAMS

(a) (b)

(c) (d)

Figure 13.8. Temporal mammogram pair 002: (a) previous mammogram (b) current mammogram (c) current mammogram showing regions with no matches found (d) current mammogram showing regions with no matches and bad matches found.

Image number	Left image		Right image	
	Thickness (cm)	Exp (mAs)	Thickness (cm)	Exp (mAs)
1	3.8	36	4.3	42
2	5.0	87	4.8	84
3	-	37	3.6	36
4	3.9	44	4.1	46
5	5.0	93	6.1	123

TABLE 13.1. Compression thickness and exposure recorded for bilateral images.

first using the salient regions of the left breast and all the regions defined by iso-intensities in the right image; then second reversing the role of left and right.

The algorithm has been tested on 26 bilateral pairs of mammograms, 14 from the MIAS database, and 12 digitised using a Lumisys scanner. Two typical results are shown here. Figures 13.9(a) and (b) shows a bilateral pair of mammograms taken from the MIAS database. The mammograms are rather dense with feathery fibroglandular streaks permeating both breasts. The parenchymal regions in the two mammograms are ill-defined because of the fibrous texture, but appear approximately symmetrical. There is an abnormal mass in the right image, near the top. This is a very challenging pair of images for most algorithms, not least because of the poorly defined boundaries of the parenchymal structures. Figure 13.9(c) shows the "no matches" found in the right image are a reasonable representation of the true lesion. Figure 13.9(d) shows the "bad matches", which lie in the parenchymal tissue and stem from the considerations noted above.

Finally, Figures 13.10(a) and (b) show another bilateral mammogram pair from the MIAS database, this time one with marked asymmetry. Both images are fairly dense. There is a lesion near the bottom of the left mammogram. Figure 13.10(c) shows the "no match" regions detected by the algorithm, and corresponds closely to the lesion. Figure 13.10(d) shows the "bad match" regions, which in this case flag the same lesion.

MATCHING BILATERAL MAMMOGRAMS

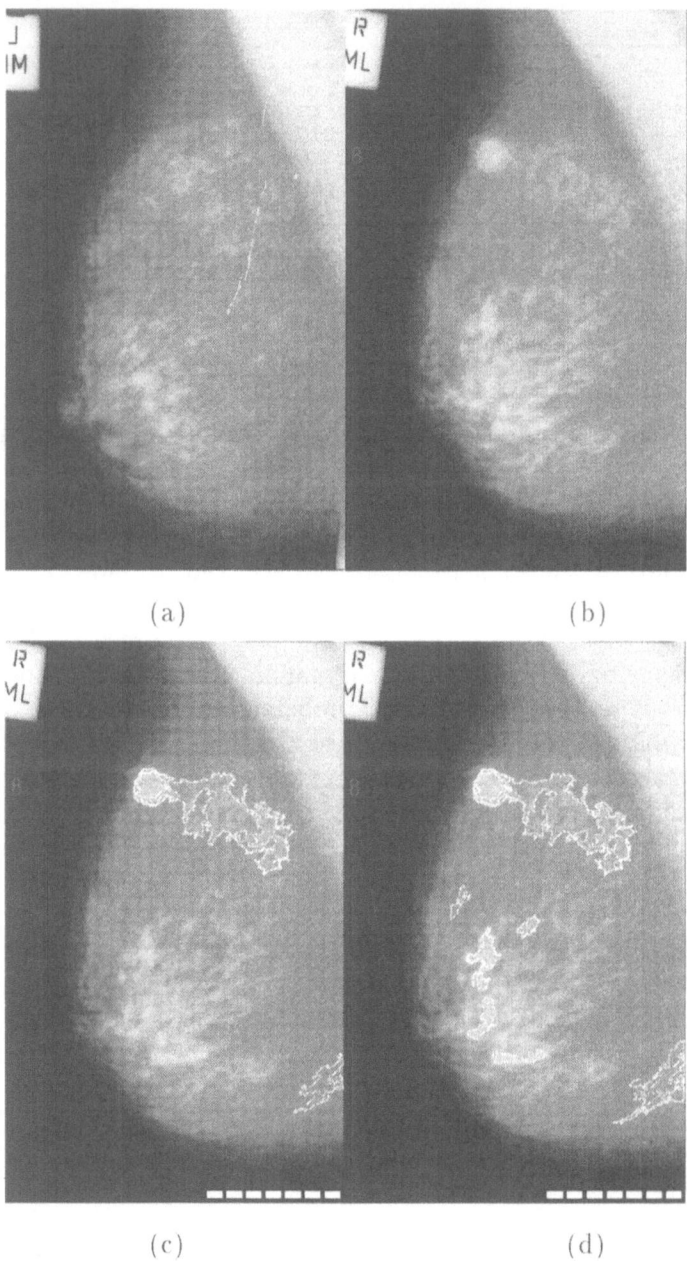

Figure 13.9. MIAS mdb201,202 bilateral pairs and results: (a) mdb201 (left) mammogram (b) mdb202 (right) mammogram (c) mdb202 (right) mammogram showing regions
with no matches found (d) mdb202 (right) mammogram showing regions with no matches
and bad matches found.

MATCHING BILATERAL MAMMOGRAMS

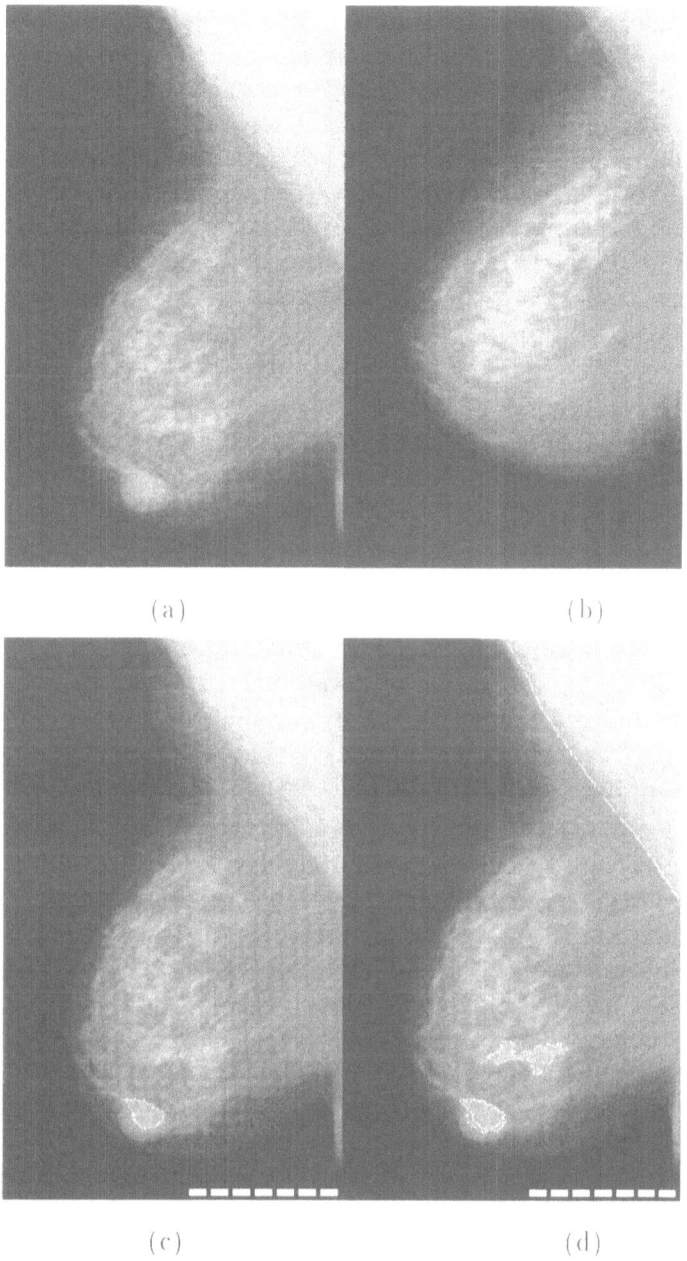

Figure 13.10. MIAS mdb021,022 bilateral pairs and results: (a) mdb021 (left) mammo-gram (b) mdb022 (right) mammogram (c) mdb021 (left) mammogram showing regions with no matches found (d) mdb021 (left) mammogram showing regions with no matches and bad matches found.

13.7. Locating abnormal regions

We turn finally in this chapter to the third of the problems outlined in the
introduction to this chapter: locating abnormal regions in a single mammogram, in an attempt to recognise masses automatically. Primarily, this
is because the ultimate goal is to explain or interpret an iso-brightness region as normal fibroglandular tissue, benign lesion, or as a malignant mass.
This is irrespective of whether or not the region has been highlighted after
comparison with a previous image of the same breast, the corresponding
mammogram in a left-right pair, or even as a result of matching a cranio-
caudal and medio-lateral oblique mammogram.

In the technique that we now describe, prominent regions are extracted
from each breast image in a database. We use the word "prominent" as
opposed to "salient" since although it uses the idea of a saliency measure
like that given in Box 13.2, and insists that to be "prominent" a region
should have both a high measure and high rate of change of the measure,
the measure used in this section differed slightly from that given in Box 13.2.
The difference relates to the expression for stability that is the third term
in that measure. For further detail, the interested reader may consult [35].
For each prominent region a number of features are computed. From a large
training set of feature sets (2,500 used to date), we automatically compute
a probabilistic representation of a "normal", i.e. healthy, region. Finally,
we use the learned representation of normality to estimate the likelihood
that a newly seen region is "abnormal", that is corresponds to a mass that
should be drawn to the attention of a radiologist.

However plausible and intuitively attractive this scheme sounds, we immediately encounter a fundamental problem. The algorithm that extracts
prominent regions generally finds dozens per mammogram. Only a very few
of these correspond to masses. Mammography is typical of many problems
in medicine: masses are grossly under-represented relative to regions of normal tissue in the screening population – for every thousand women who are
screened, only five, on average, go on to develop cancer. A consequence is
that if a neural network classifier is trained in one of the normal ways, the
interesting, but under-represented, class will be ignored! Despite this fundamental observation, most previous work on attempting to classify regions
as malignant masses has concentrated on learning a description of cancer,
though with very limited success.

With our colleagues Lionel Tarassenko, Nick Cerneaz, and Paul Hayton, we have been exploring an alternative approach in which we attempt to
learn a description of normality using the large number of available mammograms which do not show any evidence of mass-like structures. The idea
is then to test for novelty against this description in order to try and iden-

tify candidate masses in previously unseen images. The model of normality which we develop makes as few assumptions as possible about abnormalities, though of course no model is ever free of assumptions. In the following, we note the assumptions being made at different stages of the analysis and interpretation and present a sample of the results obtained on the MIAS database.

The first step in novelty detection requires the extraction of a set of features which has some ability to discriminate between normal and abnormal breast tissue. This leads to the first assumption, namely that an "appropriate" feature is one for which the examples of abnormalities appear in the tails of the probability distributions obtained for all the normal cases. The second assumption is that the abnormalities can be considered to be uniformly distributed outside the boundaries of normality. This latter assumption essentially says that there is no set of feature values that captures all cancers, rather it is a very heterogeneous class; this has worked well in practice. In order to determine these boundaries, we need to settle on a representation of normality: the best description, in the statistical sense, is the unconditional probability density function $p(\mathbf{x})$, where $\mathbf{x}$ is the feature vector, for the normal data. If, subsequently, a test data vector $\mathbf{x}$, corresponding to a region in a newly seen mammogram, is such that $p(\mathbf{x})$ is below a pre-determined threshold, then that vector is deemed to be novel or "abnormal".

Approximately 120 images from the MIAS Database were analysed. The curvilinear structures were found in each mammogram, using the algorithm developed in Chapter 12, then removed. Then we extracted for each image all the prominent regions using the representation and algorithm described earlier in this chapter. The regions which do not correspond to masses were split evenly between training and cross-validation data sets (approximately 2,500 each). In comparison with the 5,000 normal tissue regions, there are only 40 masses (subsequently confirmed as either benign or cancerous after biopsy).

Features

As a result of discussions with a number of radiologists and on the basis of our own experience over the last few years, a number of features were selected for investigation. Ideally, the features would have been developed from considerations of the h_{int} surface representation of a mass; but our work on novelty detection predated its development. Strong evidence that the analysis would have benefited from being formulated in the context of h_{int} is shown in Section 9.4.

BOX 13.3: Quantitative measures of the discriminatory power of a feature

• The F-ratio:

$$\frac{(\mu_1 - \mu_2)^2}{\sigma_1^2 + \sigma_2^2},$$

where μ and σ are the means and standard deviations for the normal tissue and masses. This is sometimes referred to as the ratio of between-class scatter to within-class scatter.

• The Bhattacharyya distance [5]:

$$-\ln \int [p(\mathbf{x} \mid \omega_1)\, p(\mathbf{x} \mid \omega_2)]^{1/2} \; d\mathbf{x},$$

which is a measure of the overlap between the two density functions.

• The number of false positives generated if a threshold is adopted such that the known masses are identified as being novel on the basis of that feature alone. Here, the number of false positives is equated to the number of normal tissue regions which are wrongly classified as being novel.

The features fall into four main categories, which relate to the shape, the texture, the boundary (edge gradients) and the context of the bounded contour of the region. These features are standard in image analysis; here the key step was to rank them according to their ability to discriminate between normal and abnormal tissue. That is, the distribution of values for a highly ranked feature for novel data will not overlap significantly the corresponding distribution for the normal data. We investigated three separate measures of the discriminatory power of the features. The details are provided in Box 13.3. Not surprisingly, there is a high degree of correlation between these measures. The five features that were found to score highly on all three indices were:

1. The standard deviation of the intensities within the region;
2. A number of texture measures, typically the average intensity auto-correlation;
3. The average of the edge gradients around the contour of the region;
4. The ratio of the volume to the area of the contour bounding the region; and
5. A measure of the contrast between the region and the surrounding area.

For all five features, the abnormalities lie to the right of the peak of the distribution (as shown for the sum of the edge gradients in Figure 13.11).

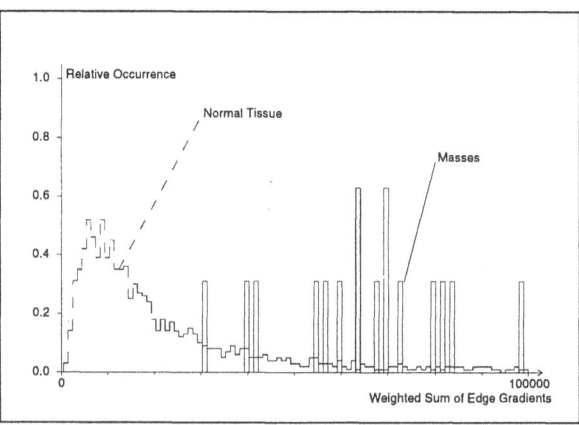

Figure 13.11.   Histograms of weighted sum of edge gradients for both normal and abnormal tissue contours.

BOX 13.4: Using a Parzen window to estimate the probability density function $\hat{p}(\mathbf{x})$

There are as many kernels as there are feature vectors (one per "normal" region in the training database). The estimate of $p(\mathbf{x})$ for spherical kernels is given by:

$$\hat{p}(\mathbf{x}) \; = \; \frac{1}{N\,(2\pi)^{d/2}\,\sigma^d} \sum_{j=1}^{N} \exp\,-\frac{(\mathbf{x} - \mathbf{x}^j)}{2\sigma^2} \qquad (13.2)$$

where $\mathbf{x}^j$ is the feature vector (dimension d) of the jth region and σ is the "width" of each kernel which controls the degree of smoothness of the estimated density function and is usually chosen using cross-validation [1].

Next, we develop a probability density function . Methods for obtaining probability density estimates can be found in the statistical pattern recognition literature[63]. We have explored both Gaussian mixture models and Parzen windows. A mixture model certainly has the flexibility necessary to model general distributions. However, we chose to use Parzen windows because the method requires fewer assumptions than the Gaussian mixture model. Box 13.4 contains the details.

With Parzen windows, the global parameter is set according to an estimate of data density which is an average across all of the input space covered by the cross-validation data. In many medical problems, the distribution of features, even for normal cases, is non-uniform and there are valid regions of input space with low data density. (This is evident from Figure 13.11 as the distribution of values for normal tissue is clearly asymmetric – there are significant numbers of normal data in the tail of the distribution). If a global novelty threshold is used to define the probability density function, feature vectors belonging to such regions will invariably be assessed as being novel, irrespective of how "similar" they might be to the training patterns in that region of input space. This is illustrated in the rather complex Figure 13.12 which shows the values for two of our features for the training data (i.e. normal tissue only). Also shown are the novelty boundaries for two different thresholds. In the first case (corresponding to a probability of 99% of the training data being normal), almost the whole of the normal data is included within the boundary (the outer markings in the figure). However, the fan-shaped distribution of the data is poorly modelled. If the threshold is raised to correspond to a cumulative probability of 95%, the fit improves but normal cases in the region of low data density begin to appear as novel. If the threshold is raised further (the inner closed contour near the origin in the figure - corresponding to a cumulative probability of 80%), the fit around the high-density region is now adequate but there are also far too many false positives.

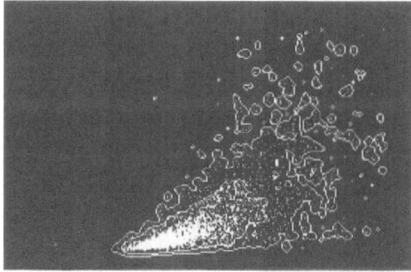

Figure 13.12.   Global Parzen windows equiprobable contours

The solution which we have adopted is to make use of a local novelty threshold which depends on the data density in that region of input space. This requires the input space to be partitioned according to data density and for an estimate of the density function to be calculated independently within each partition, The partitioning of input space can be achieved with one of a number of clustering algorithms, such as K-means[3]. The exact number of clusters, K, is not critical. As shown in Figure 13.13, we have chosen a value of 4 for K; with 3 or 5 clusters, or indeed 8 or 16, the novelty boundaries would not be significantly different. With more clusters, the novelty boundary in the transition region between clusters is smoother but data understanding (in this case, the association of a cluster with a particular type of bounded contour in the original image) rapidly becomes more difficult.

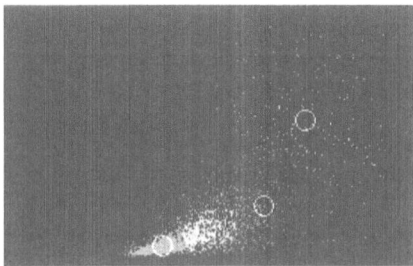

Figure 13.13.   Cluster membership in 2-D for $K = 4$

The novelty boundary obtained with an independent Parzen window estimator for each of the 4 clusters is shown in Figure 13.14 (for a cumulative probability of 99%). The desired result is achieved in the sense that the novelty boundary now encompasses the whole of the low-density data smoothly and also tightly fits the high-density data. The algorithm used to learn a description of normality and to test for novelty can now be summarised as in Box 13.5.

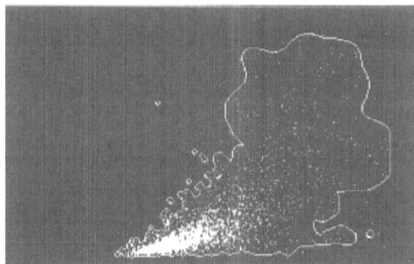

Figure 13.14.   Local Parzen Windows equiprobable contours

Results

We now present some results using the technique from a study in which 24 masses were used to select the five most discriminatory features. Though this was preliminary work, it was considered important, even at this early stage, to test the concept of novelty detection using the approach described

---

BOX 13.5: Algorithm to learn a description of novelty

(1) The curvilinear structures are removed from all images.
(2) The bounding contours of the higher intensity patches are identified and the known real masses excluded. The 5 selected input features are extracted from all the bounding contours and split evenly between the training and cross-validation databases.
(3) A zero-mean, unit variance transform is applied to the features so that each feature is given equal importance.
(4) The K-means algorithm is used for partitioning the 5-D data with $K = 4$ in this case.
(5) A Parzen estimator of the probability density in each of the K regions is computed as in the previous box.
(6) The novelty boundary is set using a cumulative probability value of 95% over all the cross-validation data set.

Test for novelty of a region, given the learned model of normality

(1) The likelihood of a test vector, i.e. the value of the density function for that vector, is calculated as $max\{\hat{p}(\mathbf{x})\}$, where $k = 1, \ldots, K$, with $K = 4$ in this case.
(2) If the test vector is novel (i.e. outside the novelty boundary), the corresponding contour in the original image is noted.

---

above, both with these 24 masses and a further 16 masses which had not been used to select features. In all 40 cases, the mass-like structure was correctly identified as being novel, the probability value being lower than the novelty threshold (except for two very large benign masses for which the segmentation procedure fails).

A significant number of false positives were discovered, corresponding to bounded contours extracted from normal tissue. With most of these, there were 3 or more features at the very edge of the distribution (beyond the 95% cumulative probability). Once this sub-set of feature vectors had been identified, it was possible to return to the bounded contours which had generated them. A typical example is displayed in Figure 13.15 which shows a breast image with two such false positives, regions of normal tissue with abnormal shapes. The problem arises because the segmentation procedure extracts any bounded contour which it finds in the image, regardless of shape. The two contours shown in Figure 13.15 do not correspond to mass-like structures but the statistical properties of the pixels within these elongated or jagged shapes are such as to give rise to abnormally high feature values. The solution to this problem is either to include knowledge about the expected shape of the masses or to use a filtering procedure at its output.

FALSE-POSITIVE CONTOURS

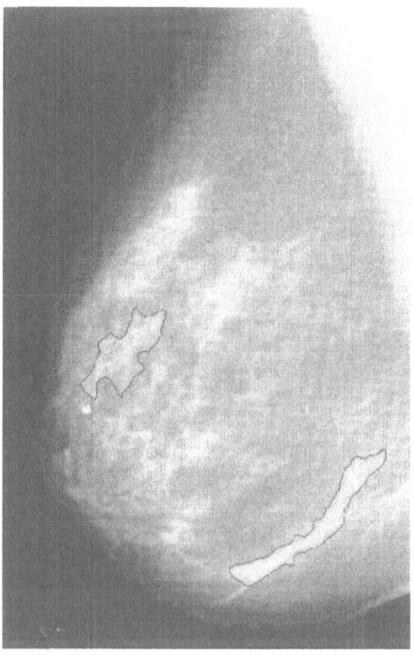

Figure 13.15. Examples of bounded contours from normal tissue wrongly classified as being novel

The novelty detection approach using local Parzen estimators correctly highlights regions of interest in mammograms which need to be drawn to the attention of a human expert. All the masses so far investigated have been identified as novel (except for two failures of the segmentation procedure). The level of false positives has now been reduced to just over one per image on average. A typical result is shown in Figure 13.16: (a) shows the image of a left breast in which a trained radiologist has identified a cancerous mass (which is not obvious to the untrained eye); (b) shows all the bounded contours generated by the segmentation procedure, all of which are assessed as normal except for the mass identified by the radiologist which is classified as being highly novel by the algorithm (and shown in bright white) and another, less novel, contour which may be of some interest to the radiologist. The level of performance of the novelty detection algorithm is already interesting; but clearly further work is needed before it could be deployed clinically.

NOVEL MASSES

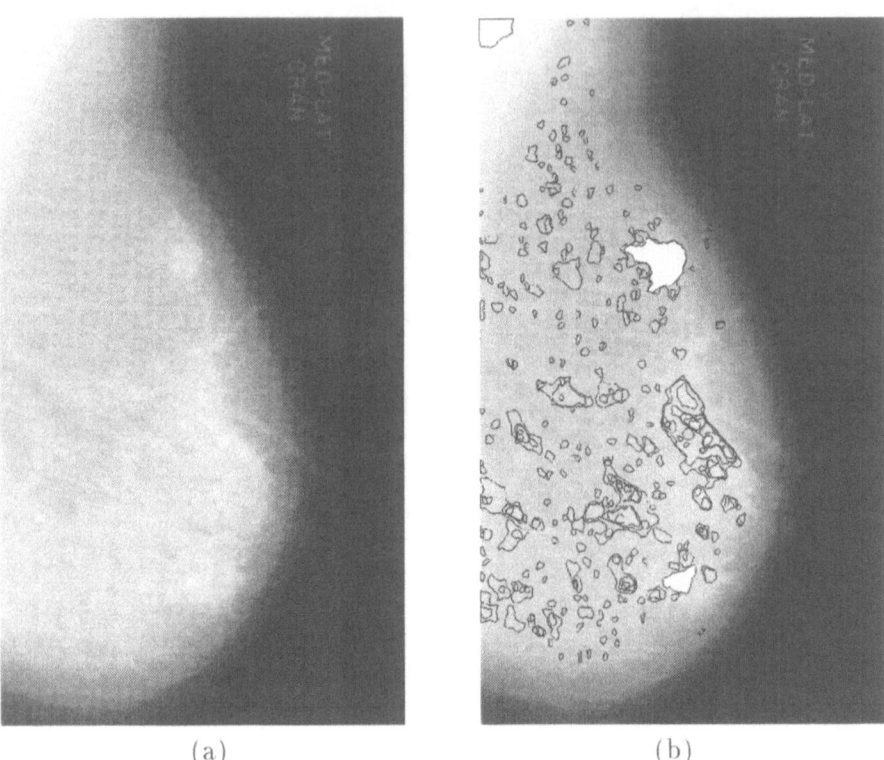

(a)   (b)

Figure 13.16.   (a) Original mammogram   (b) Bounded contours generated by segmentation algorithm, with two contours being detected as novel and shown here in bright and less bright white.

13.8. Summary: Masses

The key to most matching algorithms in image analysis is a good representation of the images to be matched, and the algorithms presented in this chapter are no exception. The representation of nested salient fibroglandular structures facilitates matching both temporal and bilateral pairs of mammograms, while prominent regions facilitate the interpretation of a density as an abnormal mass. In this latter connection, the use of a neural network that learns normality and then searches in the extremes of its notion of normality to find abnormality is fundamental to medical image analysis in screening applications, where, thankfully, the class of interest is massively under-represented in the population.

This chapter concludes our analysis of x-ray mammography. The next chapter recounts our early exploration of a very different image modality: breast MRI.

PART III

Further Breast Image Analysis

CHAPTER 14

BREAST MRI

14.1. Introduction

The techniques developed so far in this monograph reflect current diagnostic and screening practice in mammography in the sense that they are based predominantly on x-ray images. In this chapter we change tack to discuss mammography based on Magnetic Resonance Imaging (MRI). We begin by discussing the need for breast imaging techniques to complement x-ray, and we summarise some of the evidence in support of the diagnostic effectiveness of MRI. Then, beginning in Section 14.2, we describe the work we have carried out in our Laboratory in collaboration with our colleague Paul Hayton, in association with Niall Moore, Pieter Pretorius, and Lionel Tarassenko. The image processing system **xmri** that has been developed from this work has been installed at the John Radcliffe Hospital in Oxford and was the subject of a recent clinical trial[204]. We stress that breast MR is a rapidly developing field with considerable potential. The results described here should be regarded as indicative but preliminary.

As we made clear in Chapter 1, though x-ray mammographic imaging technology, diagnostic practice, and image analysis have made enormous strides over the past decade, there is room for considerable improvement. More than 70–80% biopsies turn out to be benign and 8–25% of cancers are missed [43, 71, 130, 131, 222]. Whereas some radiological findings are characteristic of benign or malignant disease (for example, teacup micro-calcifications or spiculated opacities, respectively), others are quite indeterminate and can represent either benign or malignant disease. Similarly, certain fibrocystic breast diseases have a high risk of leading to cancer, but screening is difficult because these women often present at examination with dense breasts which makes detection of abnormalities difficult.

Although it seems clear that x-ray mammography, as it is currently understood, is likely to remain the principal imaging modality for diagnosing breast disease over the next few years, its shortcomings are that it is a two-dimensional projection of a three-dimensional object, and that it has limited applicability. We discuss these in turn.

X-ray mammography is projective

In order to reduce patient dosage to an acceptable level, the breasts are compressed (tightly) between parallel plates while a mammogram is taken. The most that a single mammogram can show is the integral of non-fat tissue in the direction of the x-ray beam (a representation that we have called h_{int} throughout this monograph). It follows that localisation of a lesion or microcalcification on the basis of an x-ray mammogram is inherently poorer than might be hoped for compared with truly three-dimensional imaging.

Can this shortcoming be overcome? That is, could there be a three--dimensional x-ray image of the breast? An obvious candidate is x-ray computed tomography (CT)([254], Chapters 4, 5); but this is not currently a practical method for breast imaging because of the relatively high radiation dose required. There are possibilities to overcome this restriction and increase the rate of image formation, such as the *Morphomet* system developed by GE Medical Systems at Buc in France. An alternative might be to attempt three-dimensional reconstruction from a small number of views, especially if it were to be combined with the technique described in Chapter 10 to reduce the dosage of an x-ray by removing the anti-scatter grid. This is, in fact, the goal of tomosynthesis [168, 182] which shows promise but which awaits full-field digital mammography. Finally, one might think about adapting the techniques of stereo developed in computer vision [70] in which a three-dimensional representation of the visible world is computed from two, two-dimensional images. This is significant as increasingly both a cranio-caudal and a medio-lateral oblique view are taken. However, as we discussed in Chapter 9 the different compressions of the breasts and the non-rigid deformation of breast tissue renders difficult the three-dimensional reconstruction from those two views and the problem has only recently begun to be studied.

We conclude that though it is possible to imagine routine, low-dose, three-dimensional x-ray imaging of the breast similar to that in CT and MRI a practical version is nowhere near available.

Mammography has limited applicability

Currently, mammographic screening is limited in application to women over 50. Indeed, the benefit of mammographic screening for women rather younger than age 50 has not yet been demonstrated. The major reason is that, as we again noted in Chapter 1, the breast of a woman of child-bearing age consists predominantly of glandular tissue and so the mammogram appears dense. Involution changes increasingly large proportions of the glandular tissue to fat which is translucent. However, it is not only younger women that cause problems for x-ray mammography: scar tissue following a lumpectomy or the changes wrought by hormone replacement therapy can render mammograms ineffective.

Can these shortcomings be overcome? There do not seem to be any novel x-ray energy bands that give sufficient and reliable discrimination between glandular/adipose tissue and cancerous tissue, although dual-energy x-rays have potential. It seems that the only possibility is afforded by advanced image processing: perhaps it will be possible (using h_{int} of course!) to improve dramatically the visibility of cancers in mammograms of dense breasts thereby extending the range of applicability of mammography.

MRI as an alternative to x-ray mammography

The upshot of these two limitations is that there is an urgent need for imaging techniques complementary to x-ray mammography, particularly for younger women, and especially those known epidemiologically to be at risk of developing breast cancer. We discuss two of these, nuclear medicine and 3D ultrasound in the next chapter. However, of the several alternative imaging technologies that have been experimented with, MRI shows the most promise. MRI has certain natural advantages: the breast is imaged in 3-D (as a set of 2-D slices) instead of 2-D; images can be taken of pre-menopausal women; the signal-to-noise ratio is high (compared to ultrasound); the scan itself has no harmful effects on the patient; and image processing has played a key role in the development of MRI throughout the past 20 years. In the rest of this chapter we assume some basic understanding of MRI; see the first few chapters of [207] for further background.

However, the disadvantage of standard MRI is that it does not work nearly as well as x-ray mammography in discriminating between abnormalities and their surrounding glandular tissue. As we shall see, the identification of abnormalities currently requires a contrast agent to be injected into the patient's bloodstream. MRI is also currently much more expensive than x-ray mammography, though this is largely because whole body machines are currently used, in conjunction with a breast coil. Already, smaller, cheaper, body part specific MRI machines are being developed, not least for breast imaging. There is the further disadvantage that there are many more images per patient to be examined. Currently, patients are referred to a MRI centre if they are deemed to be at high risk of breast cancer or if a mammogram screening produces ambiguous results.

Before discussing (contrast-enhanced) breast MR in more detail, we consider the case of microcalcifications as an example of the confusion and controversy that currently surrounds the issue. The detection of microcalcifications has been an intensively-researched problem in mammography because microcalcifications are often the earliest sign of breast cancer, and early detection significantly improves prognosis. MRI mammography has been criticised because it is essentially useless for identifying microcalcifications, for two reasons. First, MRI is inherently poor at detecting calcium (see [112] and the discussion and references in [88]). Second, even if it could detect calcium well, there is currently a considerable disparity between the spatial resolution of MRI and x-ray mammography (1mm cubed voxels as opposed to 50 micron pixels; a linear factor of 20). In fact, these two criticisms may not be so damning as appears at first sight! Indeed, [88] notes that: "Surprisingly, when microcalcifications were the only mammographic sign, contrast enhancement was always seen at dynamic MR imaging in our study", while Kaiser ([138], p.66) stresses the importance of angiogenesis, the increased blood flow which is found surrounding a tumour as a result of the microvessels grown by the tumour in order to promote itself. He argues that: "The inability to detect microcalcifications is no disadvantage, because the existence of tumour angiogenesis seems to be a much more reliable sign of malignancy", and this can be detected by breast MRI. Clearly, there is need for a great deal more research to clear up many such issues! [256] is a good introduction to a number of the controversies surrounding breast MRI.

Development of breast MRI

Kaiser [138] suggests that there have been four key steps in the development of breast MRI over the past fifteen years:

1. MRI examinations using a whole body magnet and normal body coil (i.e. without special surface coils). This was not shown to be diagnostically useful, mainly because of the low signal-to-noise ratios that resulted, the relatively poor spatial resolution, and the slowness of the examination.

2. The development of the special (single) breast coil *circa* 1984 encouraged exploratory breast MRI examinations using standard T1- and T2-weighted spin echo sequences. Stack observes that "tissue characterisation of breast disease with MR imaging and relaxation parameters has not proved reliable [228]. This failure to characterise tumour tissue and differentiate tumour constituents on the basis of inherent magnetic relaxation is generally accepted as being due to overlap in relaxation

values." An additional problem that arises with (early versions of) the standard RF-coil for MR mammography is the substantial corruption of the B1 field (the "bias field"); see [90, 93] and the references therein for techniques to correct for this automatically and retrospectively.

3. Contrast enhancement agents such as salts of gadolinium and dysprosium enable much better differentiation of tissue types since certain MR intensities rise over time by an amount that is characteristic of the type of tissue. In particular, carcinoma and fibroadenomas can be easily distinguished from scar tissue, whereas this is often difficult on the basis of x-ray mammography alone. However, the extent to which they can be distinguished from each other is a matter of considerable debate in the literature, as we discuss in more detail below. Several authors note the analogy between the use of contrast agents in breast MRI and the use of x-ray iodine contrast media in CT.

4. Finally, faster imaging sequences have been developed, generically known as gradient echo sequences, such as fast low-angle shot imaging (FLASH), and fast low angle with steady progression (FISP). Kaiser [138] asserts that "gradient echo sequences are about 5 times more sensitive to gadolinium diethylene triamine pentaacetic acid (Gd-DTPA) than spin echo sequences". In the work described below we have used a gradient echo sequence known as Fast Multi-Planar Spoiled GRASS (FMPSPGR).

Better RF coils, faster, more specific imaging sequences, better understanding of contrast agent take-up and more reliable image processing are all contributing to make breast MRI an increasingly useful clinical tool. One final preliminary remark: in brain MRI, white matter, grey matter, air and cerebrospinal fluid have homogeneous intensity ranges and so abnormalities show up at different intensity levels providing image contrast between abnormalities and their surrounding tissue. Conventional breast MRI can show excellent contrast between densities and surrounding fatty tissues [2, 53, 80]. However, as the above quotation from Stack indicates, research continues to show that it is difficult to differentiate carcinoma from many benign tissue changes [110, 212, 66]. Heywang-Köbrunner [109] summarised research findings by concluding that apart from the diagnosis of fibroadenomas there is no widely accepted role for plain MR imaging of the breast.

For this reason, the use of contrast agents is currently the key, for they provide dynamic information about breast tissue that enables discrimination.

Contrast agents and contrast-enhanced breast MRI

In materials with unpaired electrons (e.g. the elements gadolinium and dysprosium), the electron magnetic dipoles respond to an external magnetic field in much the same way as do the weaker nuclear magnetic dipoles and produce a magnetic resonance signal. Such materials are described as paramagnetic. Although there are other types of contrast agent, those based on paramagnetic compounds, administered by intravenous injection, are the most common. The only contrast agent that has as yet been approved by the Food and Drugs Administration (FDA) for clinical use is Gd-DTPA.

Paramagnetic contrast agent affects the MR signal as a result of the dipolar interaction between the proton nuclear spins of the tissue and the unpaired electrons within the compound. This interaction causes a decrease in the MR relaxation time (T1 weighted) and a corresponding signal increase. This explains why the best results to date on tissue differentiation have used T1 weighted image sequences; in fact, T2 weighted sequences often show little or no contrast enhancement [52]. Experimental results [125, 28] have found a linear relationship between observed MR signal enhancement and contrast agent concentration. When the contrast agent is injected into the bloodstream, the observed signal increase enables examination of the contrast agent concentration for a region of interest (ROI) and consequently the blood flow and leakage of vessels into the extracellular space of the breast tissue. It is this signal enhancement relative to the original pre-contrast value which can be related to blood flow and ultimately used for diagnosis.

Stack [228] notes that "the pathophysiologic mechanism causing the differential effect of contrast material enhancement on tumors and normal tissue is not known. Most malignant tumors larger than 1cm in diameter are highly vascularised at both the growing edge and within the tumor, with flow being roughly proportional to size. Benign lesions, except for fibroadenomas, are generally relatively poorly vascularised. Absence of high blood flow in the latter group probably accounts for the marked difference in the early change in signal intensity between malignant and benign disease." Kaiser [138] further elaborates the same idea: "In general, the signal increase after the injection of Gd-DTPA corresponds only to the vascularisation of a tumour and not to the malignancy itself. The astonishing uniformity of the maximum enhancement in carcinomas can perhaps be explained by the increased vascularity of malignant tumours due to early tumour angiogenesis, which can be checked by the combined use of Gd-DTPA and gradient echo sequences. A malignant tumour of more than 2mm in size requires - in order to be able to support uncontrolled growth - an increased perfusion of alimentary substances and a transport of metabolic products; an increased production of new capillaries from existing vessels is needed." Many other authors have offered similar explanations [109, 139, 112, 199, 213, 88]. This may also explain why, as we noted earlier, contrast-enhanced breast MR can support the detection of carcinomas that present in x-ray mammography only in the form of microcalcification clusters.

Contrast-enhanced MR imaging can be undertaken either as a steady state uptake image, or by assessing the rate of contrast agent uptake. Heywang-Köbrunner [111] showed that estimating the dynamics of intensity change as a result of the update of Gd-DTPA improves the differentiation between benign and malignant lesions in the breast. A sequence of FLASH (Fast Low Angle SHot) or GRASS (GRadient Acquisition in Steady State) images are captured to plot the course of the contrast agent uptake by the tissues. For similar reasons, Dao et al. [52] showed that an analysis of the rise in the contrast-enhanced signal intensity over time could enable reliable differentiation between recurrent carcinoma and postirradiation fibrosis.

It is evident that in order to differentiate tissue types on the basis of their contrast-enhanced dynamics it is necessary that the MR sequence give sufficient temporal sampling of the signal. To demonstrate the importance of this, Stack [228] employed a spin echo sequence with a short repetition time (four images per minute) to differentiate tissue types. At the time, many other published studies used sequences for which acquisition times of 5 minutes were not uncommon. This is important because, as he shows, the major difference between (for example) carcinoma and fibroadenoma occurs in the first minute or so, indeed the values are identical after 4 minutes. He observes that "the enhancement profile of [the] tumour demonstrated a more gradual increase, different from that of the malignant lesions. This may account for the failure of conventional sequences to enable the distinction of malignant and fibroadenomatous lesions on the basis of enhancement". Similarly, Kaiser [138] notes that "the most important criterion of a malignant tumour is a strong initial increase in signal intensity after the injection of Gd-DTPA" in the dynamic (11 slice) FLASH sequence that he used. He also shows that the most significant difference in uptake rate is in the first minute after injection. Research on the rate of contrast-agent takeup is nowadays summarised in the form of enhancement (sometimes called Kaiser) curves. Figure 14.1 shows the type of curve presented by Kaiser [138] which show the different enhancement characteristics for different tissue types. In Kaiser's study, 399 out of 543 MRI examinations in a skewed dataset gave more information than the x-ray result. In 70 of these the

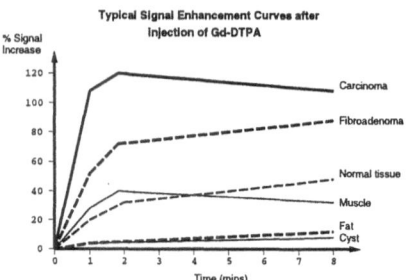

Figure 14.1. Example MR signal enhancement curves after injection of Gd-DPTA.

exact size of the carcinoma could be defined whereas in the mammogram the carcinoma was either undetected or imprecisely defined.

In all of the studies cited above, the lesions were almost always palpable. Some work has been carried out on lesions that are not palpable. This is of significance because non-palpable lesions are generally small, hence earlier in their development, and thus in turn more amenable to treatment. In cases where a mammographic mass has proved negative on biopsy or fine needle aspiration, [163] asserts that contrast enhanced MRI has a role to play in the assessment of suspected recurrent carcinoma. Further to this, [113] used dynamic Gd-DTPA enhanced MRI to assess indeterminate masses. The technique showed good differentiation between normal tissues associated with the architectural distortion and scar tissues resulting from previous surgical intervention that can mimic malignancy on mammography, and the abnormal tissues associated with disease. In addition to giving good results in the classification of known lesions subsequently proved on pathology, the technique proved capable of detecting a 4mm lesion which was not visible on mammography or static Gd-DTPA MRI.

To the best of our knowledge, Gilles et. al. [89] carried out the first study of the accuracy of contrast-enhanced MR imaging in the diagnosis of non-palpable breast tumours. Patients lay prone with their breast suspended in a custom-built holder containing a surface coil of diameter 12.7cm. A spin-echo sequence was used (600msec repeat time with 12msec echo). Images were taken before bolus injection of contrast agent and 47 or 94 seconds after. The simple process of pixel-by-pixel image subtraction was used to detect enhancement and gave encouraging results. However, the effect of image motion due to respiratory or cardiac motions are clearly visible on the results.

14.2. Image processing systems for breast MR

Image formation

An MR image is considered to be a 3D volume of the imaged body part, here (a section of) the breast, though it consists of a set of 2D images of parallel tissue slices that may not be contiguous. In our (typical) case, a volume consists of 16 slices, each approximately 5mm thick and comprising 256×256 pixels, each pixel corresponding to a tissue volume measuring approximately 1mm $\times$ 1mm in the image plane. There is a gap of 3mm between each slice. It follows that the volume imaged measures $256 \times 256 \times 125$mm^3. We use a dedicated double breast coil and the volume imaged covers the whole of both breasts; see Figure 14.5 for a typical slice of a typical (post-contrast) breast MR image.

In contrast-enhanced breast MR it is customary to take one or more pre-contrast T1-weighted image volumes followed by as many image volumes as the machine can generate within a pre-set period, typically 8-10 minutes for the reasons explained above. In our case, two T1-weighted axial FMP-SPGR gradient echo acquisitions are taken, then a further 6-8 acquisitions immediately following the intravenous administration of 0.1mmol.kg^{-1} Gd-DTPA and a 20 ml normal saline flush. Each acquisition takes one minute. The algorithms we have developed average the two pre-contrast volumes as the basis for comparison and the six remaining volumes to estimate contrast enhancement pixel by pixel. The full data set per patient comprises 112 images each occupying 64 KBytes, a total of 7.168 Mbytes per patient, which is a huge amount of information. Considerations such as these are speeding the introduction of Picture Archiving and Communication Systems (PACS) based on hospital-wide local area networks that can transfer text (e.g. patient records) and images of different modalities on demand to a clinician's workstation.

Current systems

An MR image is considered to be a 3D volume of the imaged body part, Every commercial MRI machine has an associated software system; such systems have improved enormously over the past decade both in ease of use and in functionality. They seem, at first glance, to provide the functionality needed for analysing contrast-enhanced breast MR image sequences, since they mostly enable visualisation of the entire data set in cine-mode, have an assortment of filtering algorithms to enhance each image, enable contrast enhancement curves to be plotted for a pixel, or averaged over a region of interest (ROI), and offer image subtraction as an algorithm for difference detection. Behrens et. al. [12] argued that "these tools are often difficult to use, thus error prone, and take a substantial amount of time to be performed" and developed a more friendly user-interface. Few details are provided, particularly of the classification algorithms.

The vast majority of commercial MR software systems have, in fact, far more fundamental limitations than the ease of use of the interface. Pixel differencing is only effective if there is no patient movement, so that the pixel at (x, y) in the ith image slice at time t, which we denote by $I_i^t(x, y)$, corresponds to the same small tissue volume ("voxel") as $I_i^{t+1}(x, y)$, for all i, t, x, y. If there were even slight movement (greater than the size of a pixel), that is, more than 1mm in the plane of the image, at any time over the seven minutes of the data acquisition, brightness values corresponding to different tissue voxels would be used to construct an enhancement curve that does not correspond to the breast physiology and which may be completely misleading. Indeed, we will see later that almost all the false positives in a clinical trial of a prototype imaging system stemmed from tissue motion. In much of current practice, in particular in our own work, patients are positioned prone with the breasts pendulous and confined, but not immobilised, in a double breast coil. We have found it virtually impossible to prevent motion over seven minutes, not least due to breathing and to flexing of the pectoral muscles, and such motion thwarts pixel differencing. Motion estimation is a key requirement for analysing breast MR.

More generally, a poor algorithm for motion estimation will be ineffective at identifying small (non-palpable) lesions, and, even for larger ones, may distort the lesion boundary, or remove evidence of surrounding cancerous processes. From the standpoint of the medical image processing community, there has been very little attempt to register images over time, or to model the predicted rise in intensity due to the uptake of contrast agent. Such an evaluation is necessary in order to achieve better localisation, specificity, aid differentiation of normal vascular structures from tumourous tissue, contribute to diagnosis, and to aid quantitative analysis of suspect regions. It is precisely these problems of intensity rise modelling and registration over time that we have been addressing in our work on breast MR and which is embodied in the **xmri** system.

Motion artifacts

An MR image is considered to be a 3D volume of the imaged body part, There are several causes of motion during breast MR examinations. The patient lies prone, normally with her arms forward as shown in Figure 14.2. The patient's body is supported on the couch, so, assuming the patient is not deliberately trying to move, translation in the Z direction is less likely than motion in the XY plane (which is the axial imaging plane) since it requires considerable effort to move forwards or backwards whilst lying on one's front.

In addition to translations along the Z-axis, rotations about the X-axis are also unlikely. Furthermore, since the slice thickness is of the order of 5mm, the effects of small translations along the Z-axis or small rotations about the X and Y axis will be negligible. This argument was backed when a scan was performed on a volunteer, where the volunteer was asked to deliberately move during the scan (Oil capsules were attached to the patient's breasts so that the true motion was known). Even with the patient making an effort to move, the motion was predominantly in the XY plane.

MRI SET-UP

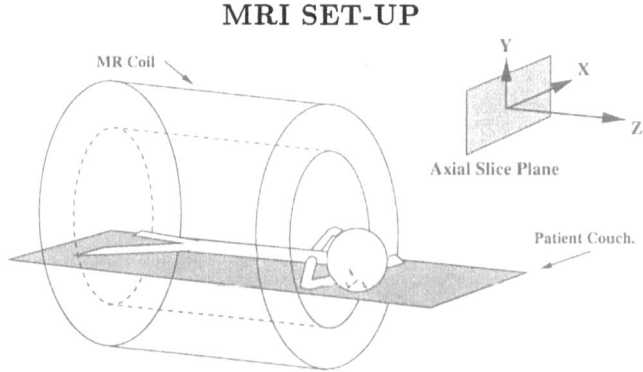

Figure 14.2. The patient lies prone inside the MR machine. The axial slice plane (XY plane) is indicated.

The patient's breasts hang pendulous inside the double breast coil (Figure 14.3). The motion is therefore constrained: the breasts will remain inside the double breast coil. Therefore, an upper bound on the expected translation or displacement of a point can be estimated at about 25mm. For a scan to be diagnostically useful we require that the images be registered to an accuracy of less that 1 pixel (approximately 1mm on average) so that a clinician would see no motion after registration.

The examination lasts 7 minutes, and any tensing or relaxing of the pectoral muscles manifests itself as movement which affects the whole of the breast via the 'Cooper's ligaments' which run throughout the breast. Figure 14.4 shows pre and post-contrast images where the patient has tensed

TYPICAL BREAST MRI IMAGES

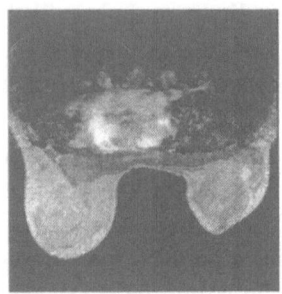 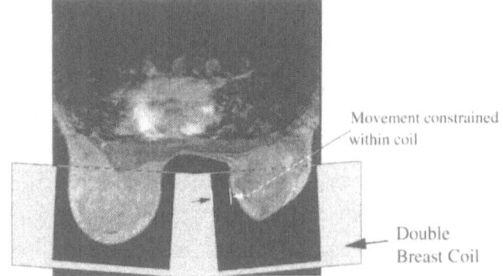

Figure 14.3. A typical MR image of both breasts (left) and a diagrammatic representation of the position of the double breast coil. The breasts are constrained within the double breast coil, so an upper bound on size of motion of the breasts can be estimated.

EFFECTS OF PATIENT MOVEMENT

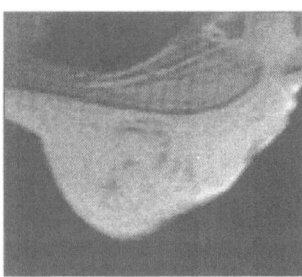 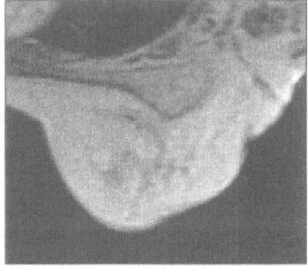

Figure 14.4. Example images showing patient movement due to contraction of the pectoral muscle. The result of applying the registration algorithm to these images will be shown later (Figure 14.20)

her pectoral muscles resulting in a change of shape of the pectoral muscle and movement of the surrounding tissue.

Large movements do occasionally occur when patients are uncomfortable during the scan. Due to the patient lying prone these movements tend to be rotational about the Z-axis.

The next few sections show first (Section 14.7) how the breasts can be effectively segmented from images. Section 14.4 describes the pharmacokinetic model of contrast agent take-up that is key to our image analysis. We then describe two different approaches to motion estimation in Sections 14.6 and 14.5. The pharmacokinetic model is used to identify tissue regions that exhibit strong fast enhancement. Finally, in Section 14.7, we describe a preliminary clinical trial using the **xmri** system to aid diagnosis.

TYPICAL BREAST MRI IMAGE

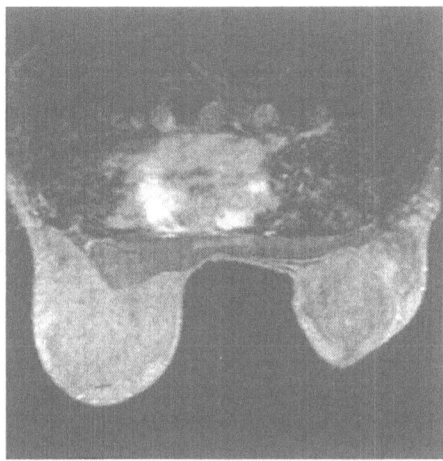

Figure 14.5.   A typical MRI image.

14.3. Breast Segmentation

A first step in the analysis of breast MR images is to segment those areas of the image that correspond to the patient's breasts. The MRI images that we use are taken in the transverse plane and contain large areas that are of no concern to the clinician in the diagnosis of breast cancer, namely the background image of air and the thoracic cavity. Figure 14.5 shows a typical image of a slice of the breasts. As can be seen in Figure 14.5, the image shows the entire thoracic cavity, while the heart is visible posterior to the chest wall with the lungs posterior and lateral to the heart. Note that, as is obvious and as is already evident in Figure 14.5, it is typically the heart that shows the greatest enhancement as the Gd-DTPA courses through it: clearly, a clinician does not want attention drawn by the program to regions of the heart during breast MRI!

The approach we have developed has been to use a two-stage algorithm, first to locate the breast/air boundary and then the chest wall boundary. The former is straightforward: air produces a near-zero MR signal, consequently the boundary of the breast with air is characterised by a sharp rise in MR signal when approaching from the air side. If the geometry of the image is known (it is trivial to identify the geometry automatically by finding the background region), the edge of the breast will be the first significant MR signal encountered when moving through the image from the background towards the breast.

The chest wall is characterised by changes in tissue type and so it may be expected that there will also be corresponding changes in the MR signal at this boundary. However, in this region of the image, there is considerable image noise due to motion of the heart and lungs which are near the chest wall. This makes it difficult to detect the chest wall boundary solely on the basis of local signal changes. Note, though, the location of this boundary relative to the breast edge: if the patient's chest were flat, in the sense of having no breasts, then the chest wall would be a curve lying approximately parallel to the breast edge and located at some distance anterior to the 'flattened' breast edge. This leads to the notion that the chest wall might be located by using the breast edge as a starting point and computationally removing the breasts. We have implemented this idea and it gives very good results.

The morphological closing operator (morphological dilation followed by erosion [101]), applied at increasing scales, closes the breast edge profile until the breasts have been removed. This leaves an initial approximation to the location of the chest wall. Figure 14.6 shows the profiles generated as the breast edge from the image is repeatedly subjected to morphological opening using a circular structuring element where the size is successively increased until it is of the same order as the width of the breast. We call the resulting curve the "MRI breast edge curve", which should not be confused with the breast edge curve used in earlier chapters to estimate breast thickness.

The problem of finding the chest wall boundary is now reduced to finding the most likely boundary that is approximately the same shape as, and located near to, the breast edge curve, and which is characterised by a change in MR signal level. The approach adopted is inspired by the work of Sonka and Zhang [226] and uses a graph search algorithm, a dynamic programming technique, to locate the optimum global boundary that is the same shape as the breast profile. The first stage in the algorithm is to transform the problem into one dimension, by sampling the image orthogonal to the breast edge curve. The chest wall boundary is expected to be parallel and anterior to this curve. We construct a table of edge scores of image points that lie along such parallel curves, where the score measures whether or not the MR intensity gradient is in a direction similar to that of the parallel point on the breast edge curve. If it is, we assign it a high score, since it encourages the interpretation of that parallel curve as being part of the chest wall boundary; if not we assign it a high negative score to reduce the possibility of that interpretation. The algorithm then tries to find the least cost path through the table that is "nearly" parallel to the breast edge curve. Box 14.1 supplies details.

Figure 14.7 shows the search region defined by the breast curve and the

BREAST SEGMENTATION

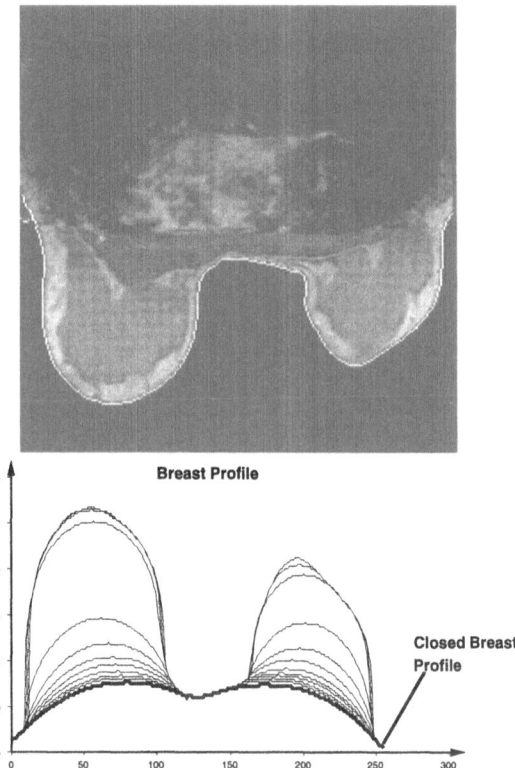

Figure 14.6. MRI image and the profiles showing the result of successively applying the morphological closing operator to the breast edge profile.

optimal chest wall boundary. As with other dynamic programming algorithms it was found that the algorithm was insensitive to the exact values used for the parameters; they can be changed by 10% or more with no significant change to the results. It can be seen that in Figure 14.7, the algorithm finds a good estimate of the chest wall boundary in the presence of noise.

14.4. Pharmacokinetic model for breast MR image analysis

As we have argued throughout this monograph, in order to develop reliable image processing algorithms, in this case for breast MR, or to perform any quantitative analysis, in this case of the dynamic MR signal time course, we require a model of intensity enhancement that is firmly based on the

BREAST SEGMENTATION

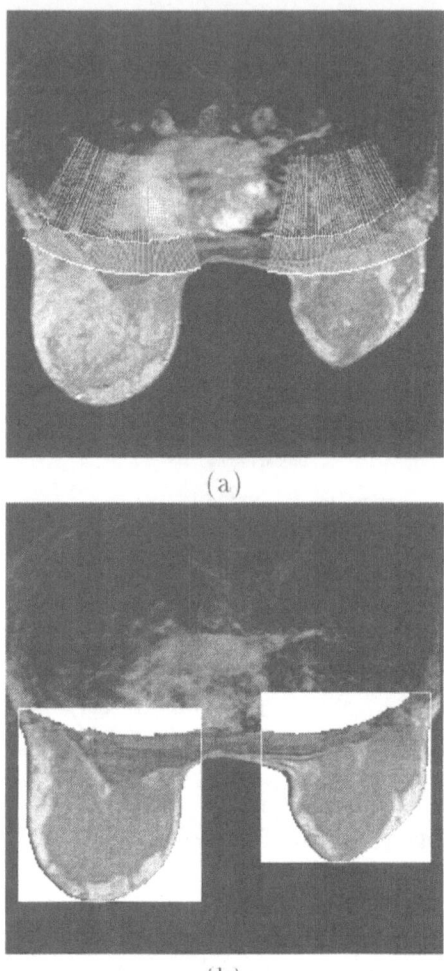

(a)

(b)

Figure 14.7. a) The normals projected from the breast edge curve to define the search region for the optimum global chest wall boundary and the resulting chest wall boundary. b) Final segmentation of the breasts.

physics, in this case of the uptake of Gd-DTPA by tissue. The complexity of the physics underlying MRI prohibit the use of a completely detailed model; nevertheless, we can apply a pharmacokinetic model of the type initially proposed by Tofts and Kermode [244] for measurements on the Blood-Brain Barrier using brain MR. This model has since been adapted to breast MRI [24] [243] and is described in detail by Hoffmann et. al. [125].

BOX 14.1: Algorithm to find the chest wall

Denote the MRI breast edge curve (detected separately in each slice) by
$\mathcal{B} = \{I(x_i, y_i) \mid 0 \leq i \leq n\}$.

(1) *Construct a mapping from image locations parallel and anterior to the breast edge curve to a table T of edge scores.*
Map each point of $\mathcal{B}$ to the point $T(i, 0)$. The chest wall boundary is expected to be parallel and anterior to this curve (corresponding to horizontal paths in the table of edge scores). The pixel locations to map to the table locations $T(i, j) : j > 0$, corresponding to curves parallel to $\mathcal{B}$, are found by sampling orthogonal to the breast edge curve to produce parallel curves of a constant length.

(2) *Define edge scores in the table T*

$$
T(i, j) = \begin{cases}
E_S & \text{if } |Edge| > E_T \;\wedge \\
& |\angle Edge - \angle Breast\ Edge\ Curve| < \pi/6 \\
-A_P & \text{if } |Edge| > E_T \;\wedge \\
& |\angle Edge - \angle Breast\ Edge\ Curve| > \pi/6 \\
0 & \text{otherwise}
\end{cases}
$$

where: $Edge$ is an isotropic estimator of the square of the gradient of the intensity [173], $\angle A$ is the angle of A, E_S is the score for a good edge in the same direction as the breast edge curve, and A_P is the penalty for an edge in the wrong direction. This step of the algorithm assigns a score for each pixel in the table depending on the angular difference between the edge direction and the breast edge curve direction. If there is no strong edge present there is no score.

(3) *Find the optimum curve through the table T in two steps:*

(a) Construct a table $C_{i,j}$ of cumulative scores for paths through the table T using the principle of optimality: if the path computed for the first n points is the optimum path, and the optimum decision is made at the nth point, the resulting path through $n + 1$ will be optimum. More precisely, the cumulative scores at the start of the table are just the edge scores :

$$
\forall_j \;\; C_{0,j} = T_{0,j}
$$

The cumulative scores are then calculated by :

$$
C_{i+1,j} = T_{i+1,j} + \begin{cases}
C_{i,j-1} - M_P & \text{if } C_{i,j-1} - M_P > C_{i,j} \\
C_{i,j+1} - M_P & \text{if } C_{i,j+1} - M_P > C_{i,j} \\
C_{i,j} & \text{otherwise}
\end{cases}
$$

where M_P is a penalty for a movement deviating from the 'ideal' horizontal path through the table (where a horizontal path corresponds to a curve parallel to the breast curve).

(b) From the possible paths computed, choose that with the highest total score. Once the cumulative scores have been computed, the optimum path through the table is given by the highest cumulative score at the end of the table. The actual path can be recovered by storing a table of the choices made by the update rule above. These decisions can then be followed back through the table to obtain the estimate of the chest wall.

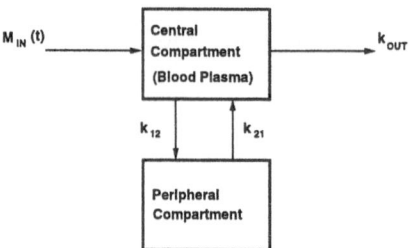

Figure 14.8. Two-compartment pharmacokinetic model of a region of interest. k_{12} and k_{21} are the exchange rates between the two compartments.

We are interested in the signal change due to the contrast agent which is related to the quantity of contrast agent in the extracellular space of the tissue. A so-called two compartmental model is used, in which the blood plasma is approximated as a central compartment and the extracellular space (as small as a voxel) of the tissue as a peripheral compartment, see Figure 14.8.

The model relies on the experimental observation that relative signal increase at a voxel is proportional to contrast agent concentration. The amplitude of an enhancement profile varies according to the tissue-specific parameter T1 [243]. We do not attempt to segment pixels on the basis of enhancement characteristics alone, which would require correcting for different T1 values, but seek only those regions that enhance significantly more than normal tissue; this is exactly what a clinician is doing when examining pre- and post-contrast subtraction images.

We have developed a model of contrast enhancement using a novel mathematical derivation which enables us to analyse the behaviour of the model and to choose the best form of the model to use [105]. Previous work on pharmacokinetic models, referred to in the previous paragraph, simply used an approximation to decouple the equations comprising the model and then solved them using initial conditions. A practical feature of our derivation is that it enables us to examine different, increasingly realistic, models of bolus injection. We find that the different models lead to only slight differences in the temporal course of the intensity rise function.

Two equations can be written for the Gd-DTPA concentrations in each of the two compartments of the model shown in Figure 14.8 based on the overall conservation of contrast medium in each compartment. The quantity of contrast medium is given by $M = C.V$ where C is the concentration and V the volume. The rate of change of contrast medium in a compartment is the difference between the amounts of contrast agent entering and leaving it. For example, the rate of change of contrast medium in the blood plasma

BOX 14.2: Pharmacokinetic model of exchange of contrast agent with a region of interest.

Denote by C_c, C_p, V_c and V_p the concentrations and volumes of the central and peripheral compartments respectively, as shown in Figure 14.8. k_{12} and k_{21} are the exchange rates between the two compartments and k_{out} the rate at which contrast agent leaves the system. Then,

$$V_c \frac{dC_c}{dt} = k_{21} V_p C_p - (k_{12} + k_{out}) V_c C_c + M_{in}$$

$$V_p \frac{dC_p}{dt} = k_{12} V_c C_c - k_{21} V_p C_p$$

Using standard Laplace transform methods [105], the transfer function relating measured concentration of Gd-DTPA, $C_p(s)$, to the input function of Gd-DTPA, $X(s)$ is given by:

$$\frac{C_p(s)}{X(s)} = \frac{A}{(s+a)(s+b)}$$

where $X(s)$ is the Laplace transform of M_{in}/V_c and:

$$a = \frac{k_1 + \sqrt{k_1^2 - 4k_2}}{2} \qquad b = \frac{k_1 - \sqrt{k_1^2 - 4k_2}}{2}$$

where $k_1 = k_{out} + k_{21}$, $k_2 = k_{21}(k_{out} - k_{12})$ and $A = V_c k_{12}/V_p$.

is given by the net of that entering it from the outside $M_{in}(t)$ resulting from the bolus injection, that entering it from the extracellular space of the tissue k_{12}, that leaving it for the extracellular space of the tissue k_{21}, and that leaving the system $k_{out}(t)$. The precise forms of the two differential equations are written in Box 14.2.

As shown, those two equations can be solved to give a function relating the observed concentration $C_p(s)$ over time of Gd-DTPA in the peripheral compartment to the input bolus function. The solution to the equations depends on the initial conditions, which correspond to a model of bolus injection. The contrast agent used for a Pharmacokinetic MRI examination is normally injected as fast as possible. In practice, because the viscosity of contrast agent may cause a vessel to rupture, and because the contrast agent can only pass through the syringe at a finite rate, it is injected rather more slowly and over a period of seconds. In other work Buckley et al, [28], approximate this input function as an impulse, whereas Hoffmann et al [125] use a continuous infusion of contrast agent over time. In Box 14.3 we derive the intensity rise function $C_p(t)$ for several different bolus models:

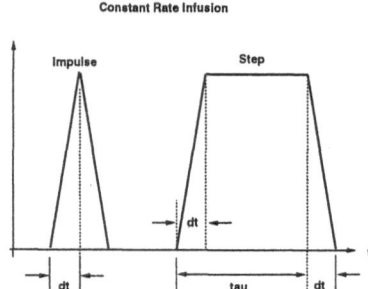

Figure 14.9.   Using ramp inputs for a better approximation to a Bolus and Constant Rate Infusion.

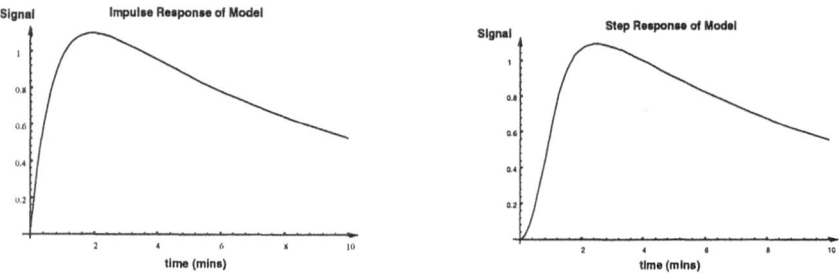

Figure 14.10.   a. Impulse response of the model for parameters $A = 2$, $a = 1.5$, $b = 0.1$. b. Step response of the model for parameters $A = 2$, $a = 1.5$, $b = 0.1$, $\tau = 60s$.

(i) instantaneous injection of the contrast agent; (ii) a steady injection of contrast agent over several seconds; and (iii) a brief ramp-up followed by a constant flow followed by a brief ramp down (Figure 14.9). The latter shows that increasingly elaborate bolus models can easily be inserted into the model. Figure 14.10 shows that the impulse and steady injection bolus models both lead to very similar intensity rise functions.

Notice that in each bolus model, the resulting concentration function is essentially a difference between two exponentials, one of which corresponds to the rise in enhancement, and one of which corresponds to wash out. In each case, the model has three parameters a, b, A that depend on the type of tissue at the particular voxel that is enhancing. More interesting is the inverse problem: given a sequence of intensities of the same tissue voxel (assuming of course that we have estimated and compensated for any breast motion so that it really is the same tissue volume), estimate the model parameters a, b, A and use them to identify regions of the image

BOX 14.3: Derived model functions for three (idealised) bolus injections of Gd-DTPA.

Instantaneous: We can approximate this input function as an impulse, $X(s) = \mathcal{L}(\delta(t)) = 1$, therefore:

$$C(s) = \frac{A}{(s+a)(s+b)}$$

It follows from Box 14.2 that:

$$C(t) = \frac{A}{a-b}(\exp^{-bt} - \exp^{-at})$$

Continuous infusion: In this case, we have

$$X(t) = U - Uu(t - \tau)$$
$$X(s) = \frac{U}{s} - \frac{U}{s}\exp^{-s\tau}$$

where $u(t - \tau)$ is the Heaviside Step Function. It then follows from Box 14.2 that:

$$C(t) = f(t) - f(t - \tau)u(t - \tau)$$
where
$$f(t) \quad - \quad \frac{A}{ab}\left(1 + \frac{b\exp^{-at} - a\exp^{-bt}}{a-b}\right)$$

where A, a and b are reparameterisations of the compartmental variables.

Ramp infusion: The Ramp Input of slope k for the case of the step (or impulse if $\tau = dt$) is given by :

$$X(t) = kt - k(t - dt)u(t - dt)$$
$$\quad -k(t - \tau)u(t - \tau) + k(t - \tau - dt)u(t - \tau - dt)$$
$$X(s) = \frac{1}{s^2}\left(1 - \exp^{-sdt} + \exp^{-s\tau} - \exp^{-s(\tau+dt)}\right)$$

It then follows from Box 14.2 that:

$$C(t) = f(t) - f(t - dt)u(t - dt)$$
$$\quad -f(t - \tau)u(t - \tau) + f(t - \tau - dt)u(t - \tau - dt) \quad \text{where}$$
$$f(t) = \frac{A}{(ab)^2(a-b)}\left((abt - (a+b))(a-b)\right)$$
$$\quad + \left(a^2\exp^{-bt} - b^2\exp^{-at}\right)$$

that are enhancing substantially and rapidly. An algorithm to estimate the model parameters is presented in the next subsection, and can be omitted by readers who are not interested in the technical details: in what follows, we review the results.

Once the model has been fitted at each pixel in a slice of the breast, that is to say to the sequence of (currently) corresponding pixels for this slice across the image sequence, we seek areas of 'high' enhancement. The details of how we do this are given below. The reader might like to look ahead to Figures 14.13, 14.14 and 14.15 which show MRI slices from two different patients with the model parameters fitted and overlaid on the images. The regions are highlighted so that bright areas correspond to regions that exhibit a large and fast relative signal increase. (The brightness key is meant only to give a qualitative indication of enhancement - the best and most reliable way to visualise this information is an open problem.) Areas of high enhancement that have been identified are shown with a box around the segmented region. Figure 14.11 shows the fitted model curves for the pixels with the highest enhancement (model parameter A) in the regions selected (outlined with a double white box) in each of those three figures.

All three slices in Figures 14.13, 14.14 and 14.15 contain tumours which can be easily seen in the model-mapped images. Figures 14.14 and 14.15 are particularly interesting in that the overlaid model parameters, Figures 14.16 and 14.17, for the selected regions (outlined in double white boxes) show that there is higher enhancement at the edges of the tumours than in the centre. This exemplifies the marked peripheral enhancement characteristic of marginal angiogenesis, as discussed earlier in this chapter. Very large tumours may be expected to outgrow their blood supply, resulting in central necrosis. This appears, in fact, to be what has occured for the tumour shown in Figures 14.16 and 14.14, evidence for this interpretation being shown by a close examination of the image surface of the post-contrast image, where the centre of the tumour is at the same, unenhanced level as the surrounding tissue.

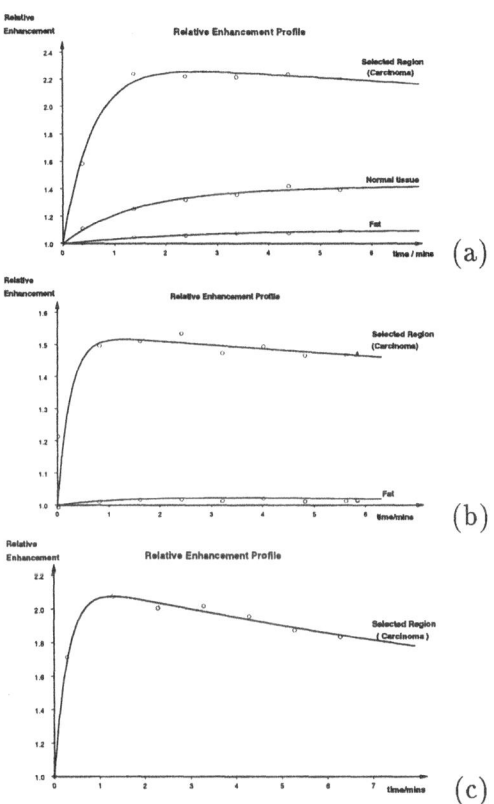

Figure 14.11.   Graphs (a),(b) and (c) show the fitted model curves for the pixels with the highest enhancement (model parameter A) in the regions selected (outlined with a double white box) in Figures 14.13, 14.14 and 14.15 respectively.

> The next subsection can be omitted by readers who
> are less interested in the technical details of fitting
> the contrast enhancement model to a set of recorded
> intensities.

Fitting the model

Since the MR signal increase is proportional to contrast agent concentration[1] $C(t)$, we can deduce the dynamics of $C(t)$ by fitting the model derived in Boxes 14.2, 14.3 to a sequence of intensities in order to estimate the model parameters a, b, A. To reduce the effect of noise, the model is applied not to the original images I_i^t, but to smoothed versions $\overline{I}_i^t$, formed from local averages at each voxel.

The model equation is non-linear in the parameters, so the Levenberg-Marquart algorithm [172] was used iteratively to fit the model. A Simplex Minimisation scheme [181] as used by Buckley et al [28] was also investigated and compared to the Levenberg-Marquart algorithm, but was found to be less accurate, less robust and was slower to converge than the Levenberg-Marquart algorithm.

Due to the non-linearity of the model equation, if standard residuals were used for fitting, data samples at high gradient areas of the model curve would have a larger effect on the fit than data samples at low gradient points. The ideal residual measure is the orthogonal distance from the curve to the data samples, though this is difficult to calculate. In order to minimise this effect, an approximation to the orthogonal distance was estimated based on the Modified Euler method, as follows.

Referring to Figure 14.12, we denote the contrast enhancement function by $f(t)$, the intensity at time point t_i by $I(t_i)$, and the residual at time t_i by $R(t_i)$, that is, $R(t_i) = I(t_i) - f(t_i)$. The time derivative $f'(t)$ of the enhancement function is easily derived from the analytic form chosen for $f(t)$, corresponding to a choice of bolus injection, and enables us to draw a tangent to the curve $f(t)$ at each data point. From the tangent to the curve at time t_1, we can predict t_2

$$t_2 = t_{predict} = t_1 + \frac{R(t_1)}{f'(t_1)}$$

---

[1]We drop the subscript $C_p(t)$ for legibility.

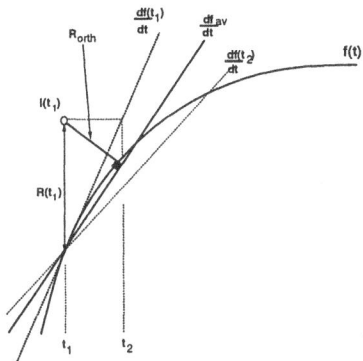

Figure 14.12. The method used to approximate the orthogonal residual to the model curve from a data point used for fitting. This is calculated using the average of the current and predicted gradients of the curve in a similar way to the Modified Euler method.

Using the average of the gradients, $f'(t_1)$, $f'(t_2)$, of the curve at t_1 and at the predicted t_2, we can approximate the orthogonal distance to the curve as

$$R_{orth}(t_1) = R(t_1) \sin \theta$$

where

$$\theta = \frac{\pi}{2} - tan^{-1}(f'_{av})$$

$$f'_{av} = \frac{1}{2} \left\{ f'(t_1) + f'\left(t_1 + \frac{R(t_1)}{f'(t_1)} \right) \right\}$$

In order to prohibit model fits that are unrealistic in the presence of noise, penalty methods [165] were used to restrict the possible values of the model parameters. Penalty methods are implemented by changing the model fitting criteria (see [165] for a full description). Whereas normally we seek to minimise the sum of the squared orthogonal residuals, we now seek to minimise:

$$\mathcal{X}^2 + \sum_{i=1}^{n} c_i P_i(A, a, b) \quad \text{where} \quad P_i(A, a, b) = \max[0, g_i(A, a, b)]$$

$$\text{and} \qquad \mathcal{X}^2 = \sum_{i=1}^{n} R_{orth}^2(i)$$

where there are n bounds to enforce on the parameters. To prevent a negative enhancement such that $A > 0$, $g_1(A, a, b) = -A$.

We have discovered that areas of "high" enhancement can be found effectively by an algorithm that seeks "hills" on the enhancement surface. Key to our approach is the Graduated Non-Convexity (GNC) surface fitting

DISPLAYING MODEL PARAMETERS

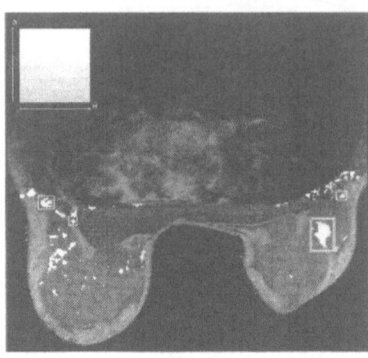 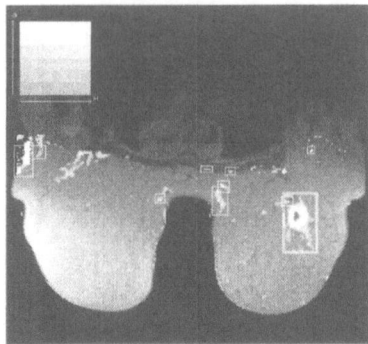

Figure 14.13. Overlaid map of model parameters. The tumour is visible in the left breast.

Figure 14.14. Overlaid map of model parameters. The tumour is visible in the left breast.

algorithm [16]. The goal is to fit a smooth surface to data that is assumed to be noisy. Two smoothness models can be used:

— The *"thin plate"*: where there is a limit to how rapidly the surface can bend; the approximating surface must break and insert a discontinuity if it is to follow data that has a localised high rise, corresponding to a hill with steep sides;

— The *"membrane"*: there are no discontinuities and the approximating surface smoothly follows the noisy data to second order.

In our application, GNC is applied twice to the data, once using the thin plate model and once using the membrane. If the data is noisy but otherwise slowly undulating, these two approximations will be similar, and the membrane approximation is accepted. On the other hand, at a localised region of high enhancement, the thin plate model will insert a discontinuity in order to achieve a closer fit, while the membrane will smoothly follow the sharp rise without a discontinuity. Consequently, the two approximating surfaces diverge and this can be used to detect such regions (accept the thin plate approximation) and to model the surrounding background (accept the surrounding membrane approximation). Further details of the approach can be found in [104].

14.5. Image registration

We noted earlier that unless patient movement is estimated and taken into account, the enhancement curves will be fitted to intensity values that do not correspond to the same tissue volume. Of course, one can attempt to

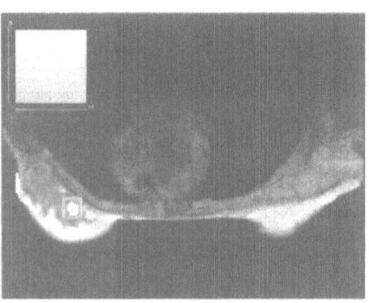

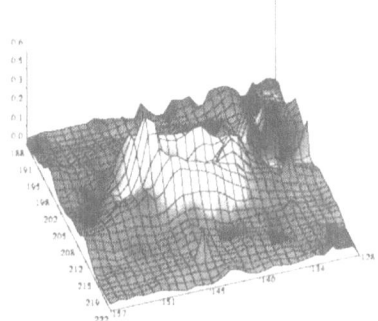

Figure 14.15. Overlaid map of model parameters. The tumour is visible in the right breast.

Figure 14.16. Plot of model parameters (see also Figure 14.17 (b)) for the region selected (outlined with double box) in Figure 14.14.

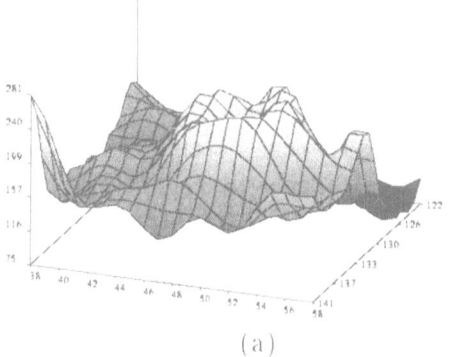

(a)

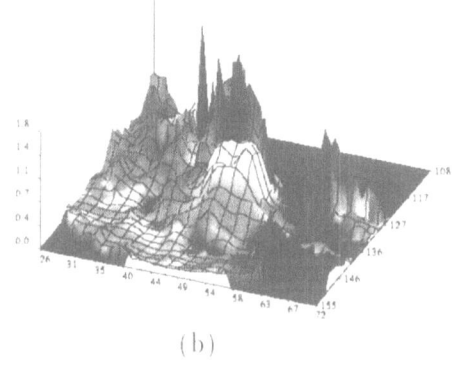

(b)

Figure 14.17. For the image in Figure 14.15 : (a) shows the image surface in the post-contrast image (time = 3 minutes) (b) The variation in model parameters : height represents amount of enhancement A and brightness represents rate of enhancement a.

finesse this problem by fitting enhancement curves to regions of interest (ROIs) that are sufficiently large that the effects of motion are minor. To some extent we already do a little of this by fitting enhancement curves to smoothed intensity data formed by local averaging of intensity values; but the bigger the ROI the less localised can be the information provided to the radiologist. Motion can be due simply to the breathing of the patient, to the patient adjusting her position, or to her flexing her pectoral muscles to get more comfortable during the relatively long (7 minutes) MRI examination. In order to analyse accurately the enhancement of an abnormality, and to delineate the shape of the tumour as precisely as possible, this motion must be estimated and corrected for. From an image analysis standpoint, the hardest motions to correct for are those that are large, sudden, and non-rigid, as typified by flexing of the pectoral muscles. Previous work on correcting for motion in dynamic MRI images, [270], assumes a rigid body displacement and seeks only to align the MRI volumes.

Maintz et al [171] provide a detailed survey of medical image registration techniques. The impracticability of inserting extrinsic registration objects into the breast coil, necessitates the development of "intrinsic" registration techniques that are based on the anatomy of the patient only. Furthermore, the lack of specific landmarks in the breast encourages the development of algorithms based on properties of voxels, that is that use the intensities of the voxels themselves and define a measure of similarity between different images/sub-images. The registration parameters are then optimized to maximise this measure.

As we noted in Section 14.2, in our work we make the simplifying assumption that motion is predominantly in the planes of the image slices, that is, that the ith slice corresponds to an almost identical block of tissue at all times. We may generalise this to volume motion in the future. Consider each separate stack of six images, one per slice of the MRI data set. If there were no movement, then all the pixels would be "lined up", so that enhancement curves could be fitted to each pixel location of the images in the stack. More generally, because of motion at each time step, the local tissue displacement due to motion has to be estimated before the enhancement curves can be fitted. For example, Figure 14.18(c) shows the result of subtracting two successive images from the same stack: the sideways motion means that the asymptomatic, fatty edges of the breast appear most significant when the enhancement curves are fitted! Techniques to estimate such local displacements, or image motion, are called "optic flow", and algorithms abound for estimating the "motion (or flow) field" of an image pair such as I_i^t, I_i^{t+1}. An example of the kind of flow field to be estimated is shown in Figure 14.18(d).

Two very different strategies suggest themselves for registering the image slices and computing the model fits for all pixels in all slices:

1. *Estimate the motion field at each time and each slice, then fit the enhancement curves.* The advantage of this approach is that it can build on existing algorithms for estimating motion fields. The disadvantage is that it does not exploit the constraint that the image sequence corresponds to a breast that is enhancing as a result of contrast agent injection. Motion estimation is key to the quantitative analysis of breast MRI and so we have developed an algorithm which is described in the next section.

2. *Use the enhancement curve model error fits to estimate the motion.* This approach is at the opposite end of the spectrum: it makes very strong use of the type of image change that we expect to see, but uses a relatively dated motion estimation algorithm. The basic idea is

IMAGE REGISTRATION

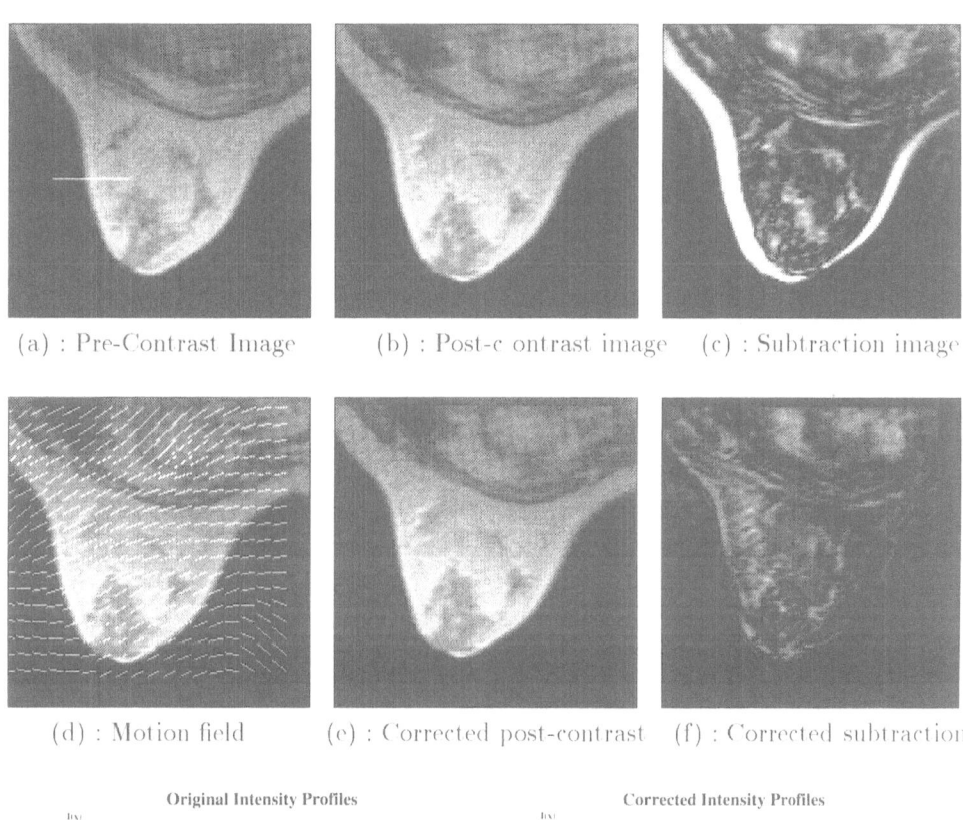

(a) : Pre-Contrast Image   (b) : Post-c ontrast image   (c) : Subtraction image

(d) : Motion field   (e) : Corrected post-contrast   (f) : Corrected subtraction

Figure 14.18. Results of the registration algorithm applied to pre and post-contrast MR images from a patient who moved during the scan. Images (a),(b) and (c) show the pre, post contrast and subtraction images respectively. Image (d) shows the computed motion field. Images (e) and (f) show the corrected image and the corrected subtraction image. The intensity profiles show the variation in intensity along the line shown in image (a). These demonstrate the accuracy of the registration at the left breast edge. The horizontal displacement between the resulting breast edges is less than half a pixel.

that if the images $I_i^0, I_i^1, \ldots, I_i^6$ were perfectly registered, and if the motion field was smooth over time, then the sum of the errors in the fitting process described previously would be minimised. We have also developed a version of the algorithm that explores this idea and it is described in Section 14.6.

Breast motion estimation

The key problem that all motion estimation algorithms have to contend with is local ambiguity in the motion field: remember that the goal is to find, for each slice i and each time t the displacement $u(x, y, t), v(x, y, t)$ such that pixel $I_i^t(x, y)$ corresponds to $I_i^{t+1}(x + u(x, y, t), y + v(x, y, t))$. To estimate the displacement, algorithms typically search image I_i^{t+1} in a neighbourhood centred on (x, y). Occasionally, this neighbourhood will contain a unique point that is so "similar" to (x, y) (in a sense defined by the specific motion estimation algorithm) that the displacement of that point can be estimated directly. However, for many pixels there will be a number of what appear to be equally good choices in this neighbourhood. The solution is to assume a (piecewise) smooth motion field and gradually propagate the displacements from points we are sure about to their neighbours.

Voxel-property based algorithms use the full image content to determine the transformation between two images. They require a measure of similarity to be defined between the images or sub-images. Vemuri [249] proposed an algorithm which uses the sum of squared differences as its measure of similarity. The problem with the method is it assumes that the second order variation of the motion field is constant, that is, that local accelerations are small and that the location of the optimum is known approximately. Neither of these assumptions hold for many breast motions.

Bro-Nielsen [25] used a fluid flow model for the deformation. His work is based on that of Christensen [42] who developed a viscous fluid flow model. This computes a force on the transformation composed of an image force, which alters the transformation such that the images move toward one another, and a viscous fluid force derived from a partial differential equation describing fluid flow. The transformation is adjusted at each iteration in the direction of this force until an equilibrium stopping condition is reached. Thirion [242] performs non-rigid registration using what he terms 'demons' which drive the image transformation based on the difference in image intensity gradients. Bro-Nielsen [25] showed that 'demons' are very similar to the fluid flow algorithm, and can be considered as a special case of that algorithm. These algorithms have given promising results on brain MRI images; but would require considerable adjustment to work on contrast-enhancing breast images.

Viola [250] proposed an algorithm to register images by maximisation of mutual information. Mutual information is a statistical measure that describes how likely it is that one random variable is functionally related to another. The algorithm seeks to optimize the parameters of a transformation (rigid or affine) to maximise the mutual information between the two images. Wells and Viola [258] applied this algorithm to register an MR volume with CT and PET volumes. We use mutual information as a similarity measure in the algorithm we have developed.

Optical flow based methods derive their similarity measure from the *motion constraint equation*, proposed by Horn and Schunck [126] which assumes that brightness is conservative. i.e we expect pixels in two different images which correspond to the same physical point in space to have the same intensity. This does not hold for contrast enhancement. Most existing methods attempt to find an optimal value for the motion at each pixel and then reduce errors by smoothing of the resulting motion field. These errors arise largely because of two factors. The first is flow measurement inaccuracy, arising from the various noise processes which occur throughout the image generation, along with non-modeled changes in the image. The second cause of "error" is the aperture effect [126] which refers to the fact that from the motion constraint equation, only the component of motion in the direction of the local intensity gradient can be estimated directly; the orthogonal motion component must be inferred from measurements elsewhere.

A weakness with published optic flow approaches is that no alternatives to the first estimate of the motion field at a point are considered. Rather, using local similarity measures, a single choice is forced and the algorithm then spends many iterations propagating information from neighbouring points in order to undo the consequences of this initial choice. The procedure has lost/ignored the initial evidence that could have contributed to the final solution. The algorithm we have developed stores all possible flow vectors at each image position, along with their initial relative probabilities. The following two mini-sections develop the motion estimation algorithm by discussing:

1. The similarity measure used
2. Bayesian motion estimation

Similarity measure

Any voxel property based registration algorithm requires a method of determining whether two subimages represent the same anatomical location. For breast MR images this must be considered carefully. MR signal intensities are subject to change between images due to contrast enhancement - this change can be of the order of 100%. Indeed, it is this non-uniform enhancement that is the key to diagnosis. We have experimented with a number of similarity measures based on intensity correlation and mutual information (see below). Hayton [104] reports a number of experiments to choose between a number of similarity measures. These suggest that the difference between them is that correlation measures the error or disagreement between two image locations whereas the mutual information measures compute the supporting evidence or agreement. The registration is computed from areas of agreement, which predominate, and is extended across locals areas of disagreement by interpolation. These localised areas of disagreement are where the contrast is taken up strongly, i.e. the area is potentially suspicious. As a consequence of the contrast uptake, mutual information is more suitable for computing registration of breast MR images. The differences in results using a variety of mutual information measure were found to be negligible.

Mutual information (or relative entropy) is defined in terms of the entropy and joint entropy of the two random variables. The only assumption required, in this case, is that two pixels that have the same intensity in the first image also have the same intensity in the second image. In breast MR images, this is not always true over the whole image - it holds for normal tissue, but places where it does not hold are of diagnostic interest. It is, however, likely to be true on a local scale over most of the image. The similarity measure we used is given in Box 14.4.

Bayesian motion estimation

The initial similarity scores at a given location in the image corresponding to the set of allowed displacements (motions) can be considered as estimates of the prior probabilities of those motions. Bayes' theorem can be used to locally update the estimated probability at each image location of each motion given the current motion field and a suitable model of the motion deformation. Box 14.5 supplies the details of the deformation model that we have used; but the essence is that for each neighbouring location, the maximum probability of similar motions, weighted by a Gaussian, is taken. The probability of the surrounding motions given a particular mo-

---

BOX 14.4: Mutual information and similarity measure

The entropy of a random variable X is defined by:
$$H(X) = -\int p(X)\ln p(X)dx.$$
Joint and conditional entropies $H(Y,X)$ and $H(Y|X)$ relate the predictabilities of two random variables, and are defined respectively as :

$$H(Y,X) = -\int\int p(Y,X)\ln p(Y,X)\ dxdy$$

$$H(Y|X) = -\int\int p(Y|X)\ln p(Y|X)\ dxdy$$

$$H(Y|X) = H(X,Y) - H(X)$$

The mutual information is defined as $M(X,Y) = H(Y) - H(Y|X)$, so that the mutual information can be written as :

$$M(X,Y) = H(X) + H(Y) - H(Y,X)$$

Under a transformation T, for probability density estimates $a(x)$ and $b(x)$, the mutual information becomes :

$$M(a(x), b(T(x))) = H(a(x)) + H(b(T(x))) - H(a(x), b(T(x)))$$

In maximising this measure, transformations are encouraged which project onto the more complex parts of b such that a and b are functionally related. The similarity measure S_x we use is a function, here mutual information f, of the signal intensities at two image locations:

$$S_x(\mu) = f\left(I(x), I(x+\mu)\right) \qquad \text{where} \qquad x = \begin{pmatrix} x \\ y \end{pmatrix} \quad \mu = \begin{pmatrix} u(x,y) \\ v(x,y) \end{pmatrix} \quad (14.1)$$

---

tion as the correct one is estimated as the product of these maxima from each location.

Bayes' theorem can be used to estimate the probability of a motion at a location given the surrounding motions. Box 14.6 supplies the details. After applying Equation 14.4 in Box 14.6 iteratively, the resulting motion field can be computed by taking, as the estimate of the motion at each sampled point in the image, the motion corresponding to the maximum posterior probability. The method has some similarity to the standard Markov Random Field method. The difference is that normally, Markov Random field algorithms estimate a set of discrete labels. Consequently a model is required (often taken to be a Gaussian) of the prior distribution given a particular estimated label. The algorithm is summarized in Box 14.7.

A motion flow field between a pre and post-contrast image pair is a set
of motion estimates at discrete locations in the image. In order to correct
for movement, the motion at every pixel must be evaluated. To do this,
we interpolate the motion from the given discrete set of locations. For this
we use Declerck's approximating B-Spline mesh algorithm [58] which fits a
cubic tensor product B-Spline mesh to the motion field. This has worked
well in practice.

BOX 14.5: Motion deformation

We assume that we only need consider neighbouring motion estimates:

$$P(u_{S\backslash x}|u_x) \equiv P(u_{\delta x}|u_x)$$

Since the probabilities of the different motions at a single location are not
independent, we find that a suitable model for $P(u_{S\backslash x}|u_x)$ is:

$$P(u_{\delta x}|u_x) = \prod_{\delta x} \max_{v \in \mathcal{N}_u} \left(P(v_{x+\delta x}) \exp^{-\left(\frac{(v-u)^2}{2\sigma_u^2}\right)} \right)$$

where $P(v_{x+\delta x})$ is the probability of motion v at $\mathbf{x} + \delta \mathbf{x}$ and $\mathcal{N}_u$ is the set of
motions similar to u (the set of motions such that $|v - u| < \varepsilon$). The model in
Equation 14.5 considers each neighbouring location $\mathbf{x}+\delta\mathbf{x}$. For each neighbouring location, the maximum probability of similar motions $u + \delta u$, weighted by
a Gaussian, is taken. The probability of the surrounding motions given u as
the correct motion is estimated as the product of these maxima from each location. The update algorithm requires multiplications and taking maxima. It is
therefore computationally cheaper to take logarithms of the similarity data so
that all multiplication operators become additions. The model equations then
become :

$$P_{log}(u_{\delta x}|u_x) = \sum_{\delta x} \max_{v \in \mathcal{N}_u} \left(P_{log}(v_{x+\delta x}) - \left(\frac{(v-u)^2}{2\sigma_u^2}\right) \right)$$

Examples

We present results for three typical patients who moved during the MR
scan and show that, using the registration algorithm described above, the
motion can be corrected for to an accuracy of 1mm.

The patient in Figure 14.18 moved by approximately 10mm. The image
sequence was such that the radiologist reported that the scan was "near impossible to interpret". There was nothing clinically significant in the scan,
though this cannot be determined from the subtraction images or enhancement graphs, and was difficult to determine by visual observation alone.

BOX 14.6: Update equation

Bayes' theorem:

$$P(u_x|u_{S\backslash x}) \propto P(u_{S\backslash x}|u_x)P(u_x) \qquad (14.2)$$

where $P(u_x)$ is the prior probability of displacement (motion) u at location $\mathbf{x}$ and $u_{S\backslash x}$ denotes the motion flows of the surrounding locations. The denominator of Bayes Theorem is a normalisation factor, which can be explicitly forced by normalising the estimates of $P(u_x)$ at each iteration by :

$$\sum_u P(u_x) \;\; = \;\; 1 \qquad (14.3)$$

Using the log probabilities as in Box 14.5, the **update equation** becomes :

$$P_{log}(u_x|u_{S\backslash x}) \propto P_{log}(u_{S\backslash x}|u_x) + P_{log}(u_x) \qquad (14.4)$$

BOX 14.7: Bayesian Registration Algorithm

(1) Compute similarity scores at a set of equally spaced sample locations across the image for all possible motions according to Equation 14.1.

(2) Normalise the set of similarities at each location to estimate the prior probabilities $P(u_x)$ using Equation 14.3.

(3) Take natural logarithms of the prior probabilities.

(4) Compute the posterior probability of each motion given its surrounding estimates using the update Equation 14.4

(5) Re-normalise the estimated probabilities. Goto Step (3) unless we've completed the required number of iterations.

(6) Find the motion field by taking, as the estimate of the optic flow at each location, the displacement corresponding to the maximum posterior probability.

The intensity profiles in Figure 14.18 verify that there is no enhancement on the left hand side of the breast which can be seen in the corrected subtraction image and show that the breast edge has been registered to an accuracy of less than half a pixel.

In Figure 14.19, the patient has a tumour which is circled in the subtraction image. The patient has moved approximately 2mm between pre- and post-contrast images. The surface plots show the intensity surfaces of the subtraction images in the region around the tumour with and with-

IMAGE REGISTRATION FOR PATIENT MOVEMENT

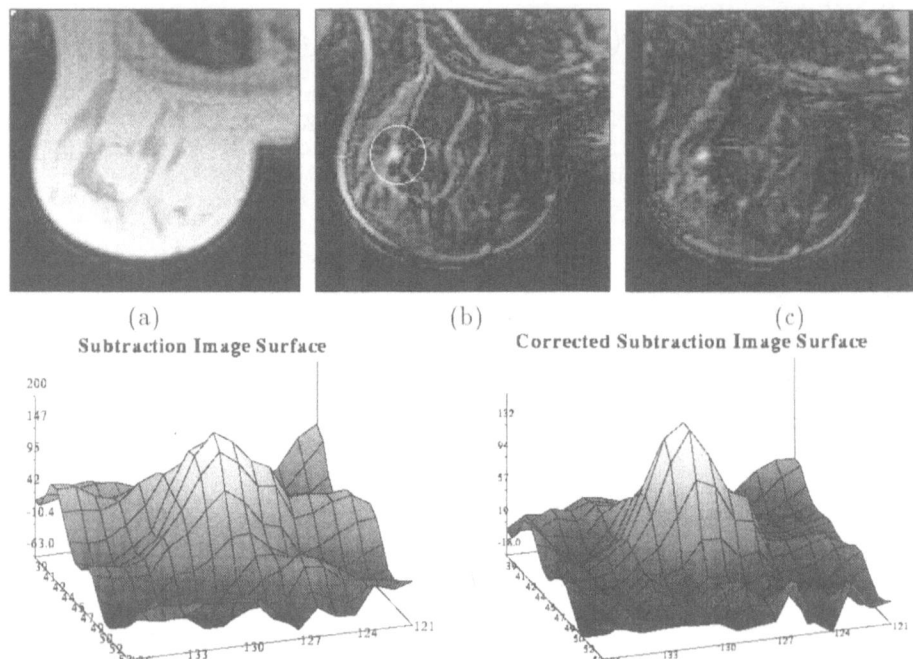

Figure 14.19.   Results of the registration algorithm applied to pre and post-contrast MR images from a patient who moved during the scan. Images (a) and (b) show the pre-contrast and subtraction images respectively. There is a tumour present which is circled in the subtraction image. Image (c) shows the corrected subtraction image. The surface plots show the intensity surfaces from the subtraction images within the region of interest (circled in image (b)).

out motion correction. The peak in the surface corresponds to the tumour and is more strongly peaked in the corrected subtraction surface plot. This implies that even though the motion is very slight, after applying the registration algorithm, the tumour is better localized in the motion corrected image.

In Figure 14.20, the registration algorithm has been used to correct the post-contrast image for a patient who relaxed her pectoral muscles between the pre and post-contrast acquisitions. The movement is extremely non-rigid (the pectoral muscle changes shape and moves approximately 15mm). The patient has a tumour which also moves 7 or 8mm as a result of the movement within the breast. It is interesting to note that in this case, the movement is almost confined within the breast, with the breast edge moving only about 3mm. The registration algorithm correctly identifies the motion

IMAGE REGISTRATION FOR PATIENT MOVEMENT

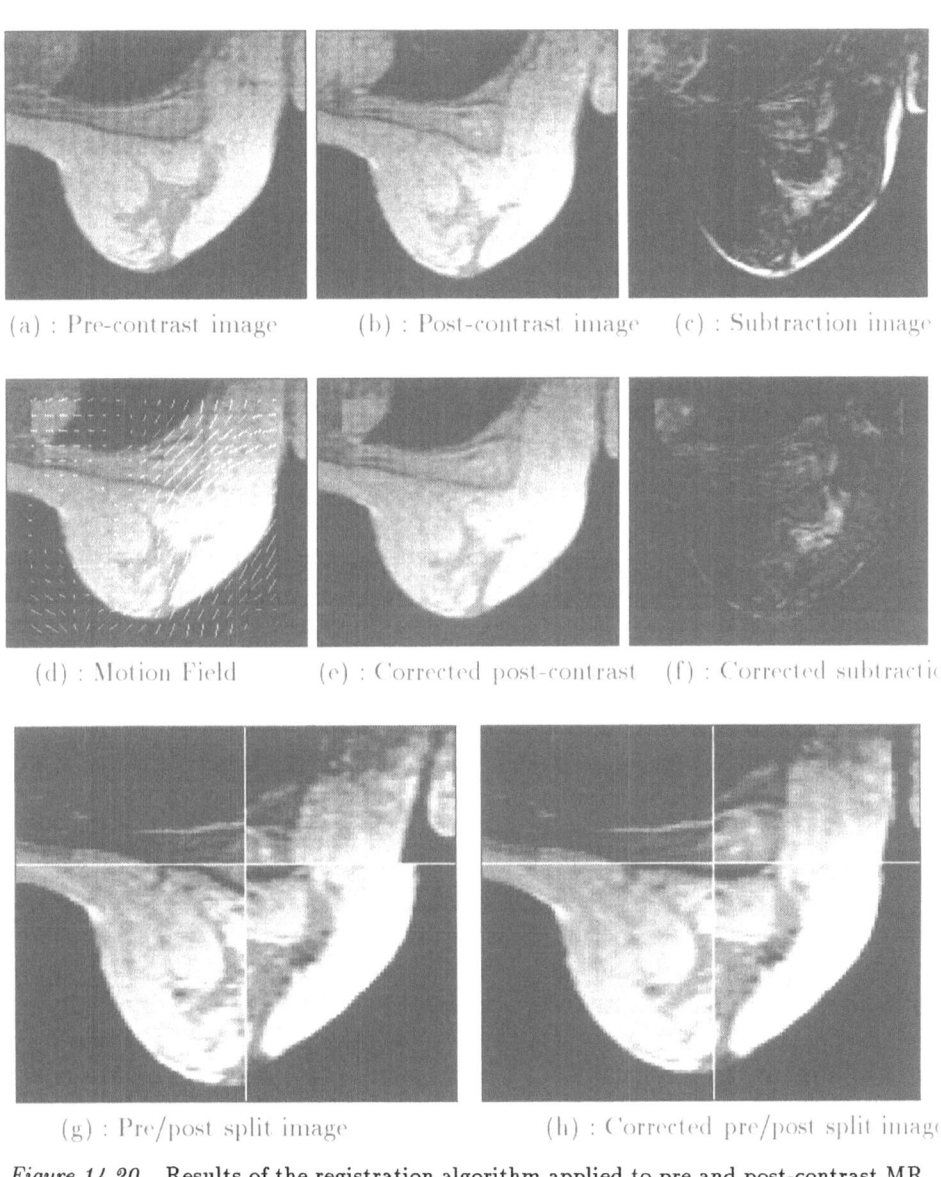

(a) : Pre-contrast image   (b) : Post-contrast image   (c) : Subtraction image

(d) : Motion Field   (e) : Corrected post-contrast   (f) : Corrected subtraction

(g) : Pre/post split image   (h) : Corrected pre/post split image

Figure 14.20. Results of the registration algorithm applied to pre and post-contrast MR images from a patient who moved during the scan. Images (a),(b) and (c) show the pre, post contrast and subtraction images respectively. Image (d) shows the computed motion field. Images (e) and (f) show the corrected image and the corrected subtraction image. Images (g) and (h) are split between pre and post-contrast images. The pre-contrast image is to the top left and bottom right quadrants, the post-contrast image in the bottom left and top right quadrants. Image (g) is split between the original pre and post contrast images; image (h) between the pre and corrected post-contrast images.

field and the tumour in the corrected post-contrast image has been moved
back to the correct position. The largest error in the corrected post-contrast
image is at the right hand edge of the pectoral muscle where there is a 1
pixel error between the edge in the pre and corrected-post contrast image.
The split images are formed by displaying the pre-contrast image in the top
left and bottom right quadrants[2] of the image and the post-contrast image
in the bottom left and top right quadrants. These images show motion
errors at the quadrant boundaries. In the motion corrected split image,
the boundaries of the pectoral muscle and fibroglandular tissue are aligned
demonstrating the algorithm has correctly registered the images.

14.6. Motion from enhancement curve model errors

In this section we explore a complementary idea, namely that the contrast
enhancement model, and the algorithm to fit it to a set of 7 data samples,
can be used also to estimate image motion. More precisely, the idea is that:

*if the images were perfectly registered, the mean square errors of the
model fits would be minimised subject to the motion field being smooth over
the image.*

Box 14.8 shows how this idea is made precise in the form of an algorithm.
The approach was inspired by Horn and Schunck's pioneering work on the
estimation of a motion field [126], with a modification to take account of the
change in intensities across the image due to the contrast agent (see [105]
for details).

In order to develop and test the algorithm, global translations were
imposed on all images in an MRI sequence, and the algorithm run. Since
the algorithm requires smooth derivatives for the gradient of the error fit,
each image in the sequence was smoothed. A scaled implementation of the
algorithm was used since the model field is required to be smooth. This
results in a single vector displacement being computed for a $X \times X$ region,
where X is the scale factor. A single representative model fit was used
for each $X \times X$ region. The algorithm assumes the intensity surface to be
continuous and smooth and requires intensity values at locations between
pixels. Bi-linear interpolation is used to estimate inter-pixel intensities.

Figure 14.21 shows the variation of mean square registration errors and
average model residuals as the algorithm proceeds. Figure 14.22 shows the
computed displacement field and the model residual images with and without correcting for motion using the registration field. The model residual
images (intensities scaled by a factor of 10 for contrast) are computed by:

$$I_{\text{residual}}(x, y) = |I(x, y, t) - M(x, y, t)|$$

[2]The quadrants are delineated by the cross.

BOX 14.8: Algorithm to estimate motion field from enhancement model errors

Denote the displacement at pixel (x, y), at time t, by $u(x, y, t), v(x, y, t)$. If we fix (x, y) we have a set of seven intensity values to which the contrast enhancement model can be fitted to yield a curve $M_{(x,y)}(t) = M_{(x,y)}(t; u, v)$.

(1) For each pixel location (x, y), calculate the model curve $M_{(x,y)}(t)$ for the current displacement estimate $u(x, y, t), v(x, y, t)$.

(2) Estimate the gradient of the model error fit, at each time t:

$$
\begin{aligned}
E_u(t) &= \left| I(x + u + 1, y + v, t) - M_{(x,y)}(t) \right| - \\
&\quad \left| I(x + u - 1, y + v, t) - M_{(x,y)}(t) \right| \\
E_v(t) &= \left| I(x + u, y + v + 1, t) - M_{(x,y)}(t) \right| - \\
&\quad \left| I(x + u, y + v - 1, t) - M_{(x,y)}(t) \right|
\end{aligned}
$$

(3) Update the estimate of the displacement field in each image concurrently

$$
\begin{aligned}
u^{n+1}_{(x,y)} &= \bar{u}^n_{(x,y)} - \frac{\lambda}{1 + \sqrt{(E_u^2 + E_v^2)}} E_u \\
v^{n+1}_{(x,y)} &= \bar{v}^n_{(x,y)} - \frac{\lambda}{1 + \sqrt{(E_u^2 + E_v^2)}} E_v
\end{aligned}
$$

in which mention of t has been suppressed for clarity, and in which $\bar{u}^n_{(x,y)}$ is the average in a neighbourhood of (x, y) of the estimates of $u(x, y, t)$ at time t at iteration n.

(4) **if** the estimate of u or v changed at iteration n at any pixel (x, y) at any time t, **goto** step (1), **else stop.**

---

where I(x,y,t) is the intensity at (x, y) at time t and $M(x, y, t)$ is the model value at time t for pixel (x, y) for the current slice. Obviously, if the model fits were perfect the image I_{residual} would be totally black so these images in the presence of enhancement are somewhat analogous to subtraction images. The post-registration image is evidently much improved over the pre-registration model residual image. Also of interest is the fact that the only area exhibiting large residuals in the post-registration image is the top right corner. This is due to the motion of the heart which produces image artifacts in the MRI phase encoding direction (in this case horizontally). There are no features from the original image visible in the residual image demonstrating that the tissue boundaries are correctly registered.

Figures 14.21, 14.22 and 14.23 demonstrate that the algorithm is working successfully. Figure 14.24 shows the regions that are identified as having significant enhancement with and without application of the registration

algorithm. It should be noted that without registration the calculation of
a significant enhancement limit fails to converge as a result of the non-
exponential distribution of enhancements. For comparison, the limit was set
here manually to be the same for both corrected and uncorrected sequences.
The algorithm has been found to converge successfully in image sequences
which exhibit significant enhancement. This is understandable since, in the
absence of significant enhancement the model residuals are dominated by
noise so the minimisation in poor.

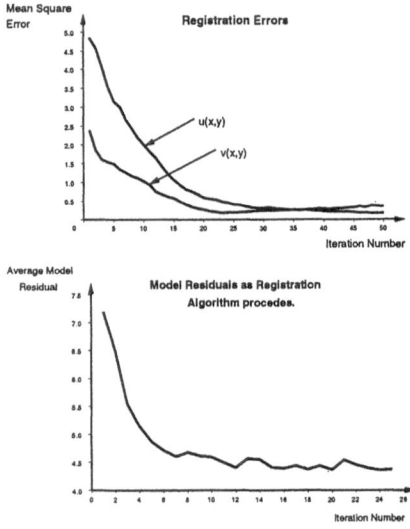

Figure 14.21. Variation of registration errors and model residuals as the registration
algorithm proceeds.

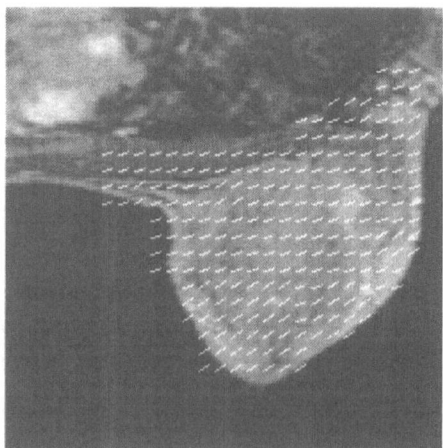

Figure 14.22. Computed displacement field for segmented breast image.

MODEL RESIDUAL IMAGES

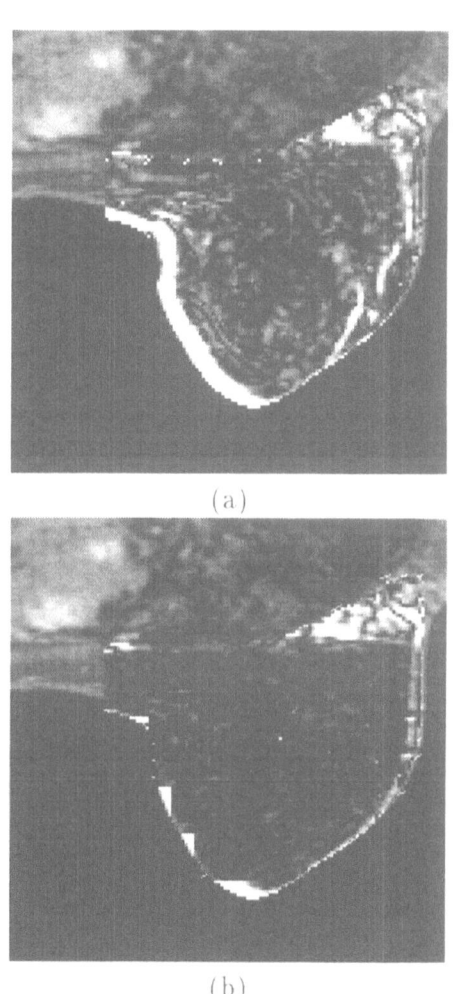

(a)

(b)

Figure 14.23.   Model residual images a) pre-registration. b) post-registration.

SEGMENTATION WITH REGISTRATION

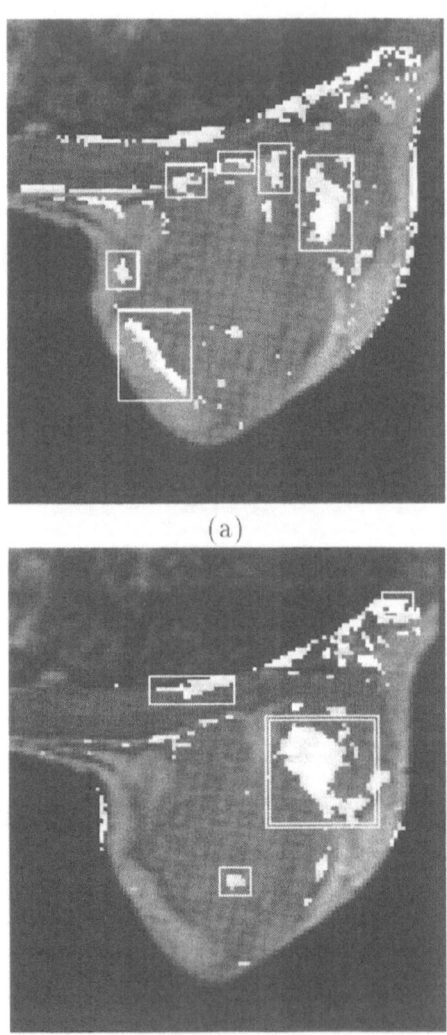

(a)

(b)

Figure 14.24. a) Unregistered segmented regions. b) Segmented regions after applying the registration algorithm. The figure shows an invasive adeno-carcinoma whose localisation is greatly improved after registration.

14.7. Clinical trial

A preliminary clinical evaluation of the model-based analysis algorithm was carried out at the Oxford Magnetic Resonance Imaging Centre (OMRI) by two of our radiologist colleagues Pieter Pretorius and Niall Moore. The aim was to assess the potential of the automated algorithms to identify areas of enhancement, which had previously been identified as suspicious by a radiologist experienced in breast MR examinations.

Methods

Six breast MR examinations were retrospectively selected from examinations performed at OMRI between October 1995 and January 1997. A total of 13 suspicious enhancing lesions were reported prospectively and histological confirmation is available in all six cases. All the examinations were performed on a 1.5T machine (Signa IGE Medical Systems). The patients were positioned prone with the breasts confined in a dedicated double breast coil. The dynamic imaging sequence consisted of 2 sets of pre-contrast T1-weighted axial FMPSPGR acquisitions (16 slices per set covering the whole of both breasts) then a further 6 acquisitions immediately following the intravenous administration of 0.1mmol.kg^{-1} Gd-DTPA and 20ml normal saline flush.

The examinations had been reported by one of the radiologists after image transfer to the IGE independent console. Image analysis involved viewing the dynamic sequences as an animation sequence. Areas of enhancement were further examined using ROI analysis to determine the amplitude and temporal profile of enhancement. This was presented as a signal time course. The model-based analysis was carried out on the dynamic series of each examination on a graphics workstation. All areas of enhancement greater than 40% identified by the program were evaluated by the other radiologist and were assigned to one of three categories: 1) True enhancement corresponding to lesion mentioned in the radiologist's report, 2) True enhancement not mentioned in the report, and 3) Artifactual enhancement due to movement of the breast.

Results

The program identified a total of 66 areas of enhancement from all of the slices of the six examinations. Of the 13 lesions identified by the radiologist in the initial reports, 12 were identified by the model and represented 21 foci of enhancement. An additional 24 foci of true enhancement were identified for which no histological data exists. Using the radiologist's report as gold standard, the results translate to a sensitivity of 92%. 21 foci of enhancement could clearly be attributed to movement resulting in misregistration, 18 of these foci occurred in a single case. Table 14.1 summarises the experimental results.

Discussion

The pharmacokinetic model shows great promise as a tool to help radiologists search out areas of enhancement in breast images. To be clinically useful, it would need to prove itself as a sensitive and time efficient way of finding areas of enhancement which could then be further evaluated by the radiologist. The cognitive processes employed by a radiologist when determining the significance of an area of enhancement include consideration not only of the enhancement characteristics but also of morphological criteria and information gained from other imaging modalities and clinical findings as discussed in Chapter 15. By contrast, the model was designed to identify areas purely on the grounds of enhancement characteristics. All areas of enhancement not due to movement were therefore considered to be true positives even if they had been discounted by the radiologist. The large number of foci identified by the model was strongly influenced by the conservatively chosen threshold (40%).

In this assessment, the good sensitivity was counteracted by a high number of false positives due to movement, especially in case 2. Unless this is remedied, it would leave the radiologist with the very time consuming task of eliminating a large number of false positives during his/her evaluation. The clinical trial was, in fact, carried out before the motion estimation algorithm described in Section 14.5 was developed. As this book goes to print, a substantial clinical trial is underway.

14.8. Summary: Breast MRI

Contrast-enhanced breast MRI offers an increasingly important complementary imaging modality to x-ray mammography. A pharmacokinetic model of contrast agent take-up by different kinds of breast tissue, combined with a technique for estimating breast motion, enables abnormally enhancing regions to be drawn to the attention of the radiologist. Other imaging modalities are being developed, most notably 3D ultrasound and nuclear medicine, and though we are only now beginning work on these, we sketch progress by others in the next chapter.

Histological diagnosis	Number of lesions and foci of enhancement detected by		Additional foci of enhancement not mentioned in report	False Positives results
	Radiologist	Model		
1. Infiltrating ductal carcinoma	3	3(6)	14	1
2. Infiltrating ductal carcinoma	3	2(3)	4	18
3. Infiltrating ductal carcinoma	2	2(4)	0	0
4. Fibroadenoma	1	1(1)	5	1
5. Fibroadenoma	1	1(1)	0	0
6. Infiltrating ductal carcinoma	3	3(6)	1	1
Totals	13	12(21)	24	21

TABLE 14.1. Breakdown of results for each of the 6 cases. For the foci of enhancement detected by the model, $a(b)$ means that of the enhancing regions noted by the radiologist, a of them were detected by the model as b separate regions (a single tumour may be visible in several slices at more than one location).

CHAPTER 15

OTHER MODALITIES AND FUTURE PROSPECTS

15.1. Introduction

This monograph is a contribution to the rapidly evolving field of mammography, a field that has evolved over the past two decades into a sophisticated technical medical speciality. Progress has been based on the interplay between emerging and improving techniques for breast imaging, massive advances in computing power and usability allied to substantial improvements in image processing, and, above all, a surge in our understanding of the relationship between breast images and breast disease.

The book has been as much about a model-based approach to image processing as it has been the description of a particular set of technical advances. We have argued that in order to be reliable and predictable, mammographic image processing must be based on a physical model of how the image is formed. For the case of x-ray mammography, this involved developing a model of the way that x-rays pass through breast tissue of different types, are absorbed, and scattered before exposing the film. In like manner, in the case of MR breast imaging, we showed how a pharmacokinetic model of the uptake of contrast agent by tissue could be used to register and segment suspicious regions. We have also stressed throughout the monograph the importance of image processing scientists and engineers working in close cooperation with clinicians, since it is the clinicians who identify the problems, and it is the engineers' and scientists' job to help the clinicians solve those problems.

By virtue of our close interaction with clinicians, the problems that we have tackled in the monograph are real and relevant, and because our approach is firmly rooted in physics-based models, we believe that the results and techniques we have presented will not become outdated as soon, as is often the case in applications of computing. Nevertheless, the subject is evolving rapidly and there remain many open problems. In this final chapter we briefly mention a number of directions in which we expect to see major progress over the next few years, and which we would expect as a consequence to include in any future editions of the book!

We begin in Section 15.2 with a discussion of all-digital mammography, then discuss in Section 15.3 a number of recent developments in image-guided (minimally invasive) surgery, which has, to date, primarily relied on x-ray stereotaxis and ultrasound. We then turn our attention to two of the most promising alternative imaging technologies for mammography, namely nuclear medicine in Section 15.4 and ultrasound in Section 15.5. The combination, or fusion, of data of different sorts is increasingly important, since in medical image processing, as in all other demanding applications of image processing, it is clear that no single imaging modality suffices for all cases, and, equally, since many hospitals call for a number of different modalities in their diagnostic procedures. Finally, the past two decades has also seen major developments in automated reasoning systems, particularly those based on uncertain information. A clinician takes account of non-image based data, such as patient history, age, appearance, and symptoms to help interpret images, and uses both to inform diagnoses. Section 15.6 sketches some relevant work in developing such artificial intelligence systems.

15.2. Digital mammography

The film-screen technology used in conventional mammography, which we described in Part I, is the last remaining non-digital imaging modality used in radiology. X-ray film was the origin of radiology, and remains central to its operation in clinical mammography. Radiology rooms are often organised around a central film processing station. There are, however, a number of limitations to film screen mammography[263]:

- Long-term storage is costly in space and in maintaining image quality, while image transmission between clinicians is inevitably slow.
- There is a compromise between contrast and latitude, that is the film is only useful where the rate of change of film density with the logarithm of relative exposure is high. In practice, this means that increasing the contrast decreases the useful range of log relative exposures.
- The film granularity limits spatial resolution.

It seems certain that this last bastion of analogue image acquisition will fall, sooner rather than later. The increasing use of computers to present, access and process images, the equally increasing availability of Picture Archiving and Communication Systems (PACS) based on high bandwidth computer networks that facilitate the rapid electronic transfer of images between distant sites, and the efficiency and cost advantages of storing images electronically rather than on film, all argue cogently for digital mammographic images. Currently, digital mammographic images are first produced on film, then digitised by a laser scanner, though Dance [254] notes (p.67-8) that "any information that is recorded on film at very low or high density will be degraded because of the form of the film characteristic". To minimise film usage (since it is intrinsically not re-usable), a large variety of sizes of film have to be kept in stock. In contrast, digital images can be of any size, appropriate to the application, and image analysis algorithms can accept digital images of any size. In an all-digital system, image capture and display are decoupled: this reduces the need for repeat exposures, particularly if there is reliable software enhancement of the type we have described in Part II of this monograph. Furthermore, there is the potential for rapid review of any image in the database. An image can be stored and then any portion can be displayed at any resolution or in any way relevant to the application: storage and display are completely decoupled. Indeed, Dr. Faina Shtern [221] of the National Cancer Institute (NCI), Bethesda, Maryland reports that the "NCI convened a consensus conference that reached the following conclusion: 'while there is room for continued development with conventional methods ... [novel technologies including digital mammography] ... represent the most fertile territory for the ... diagnosis of minimal breast cancer' ".

All these issues encourage all-digital image capture, without an intermediate film stage. However, film-based radiology (including the film-screen) has evolved over the past century to meet developing clinical needs. Radiologists are familiar with film, for all its inadequacies. A change to all-digital mammography, will inevitably take time, notwithstanding the advantages enumerated in the previous paragraph, unless and until the resulting digital images are at least as effective for diagnosis (or are perceived to be as effective), and are at least as easy to use as film, or offer quantifiable productivity benefits.

The advantages of all-digital mammography have been recognised for some time. The fact that all-digital systems have not yet replaced film-screen analogue technology partly reflects the cost of changing equipment, partly the need to secure FDA approval, but mostly because it has proved difficult to attain the performance levels of film-screen systems, in at least one of:

- Image quality (including low noise, device sensitivity),
- Spatial resolution,
- Image acquisition time.

We discuss these briefly in turn.

Image quality

The design of an all-digital system involves minimising the radiation exposure to the patient, while maximising the contrast efficiency. This is often equated to the device having a high detective quantum efficiency (DQE), which is defined as the square of the quotient of the signal-to-noise ratio (SNR) of the pattern of photons presented to the detector and the SNR of the pattern of photons absorbed by it. This turns out to be the key parameter that determines the size of objects that can be detected, for example microcalcifications. High DQE at low spatial frequencies most affects the SNR of an image and the quantum statistics of the imaging device, consequently the size of objects that can be detected.

As we noted in Chapters 2 and 7, the dynamic range is large in mammography [170], since there are large variations in breast tissue. High dynamic range poses considerable challenges for full-field mammography device design [241] but these are rapidly being overcome.

Spatial resolution

Conventional film has a very high spatial resolution, estimated by [210] as 5% modulatation transfer at a spatial frequency of 20 line pairs per millimetre. This suggests that a digital sampling aperture of twice this resolution, that is 25 microns, is needed in order for all-digital mammography to have a similar spatial resolution. When one considers that a typical mammogram film measures 10 inches by 8 inches (25.4×20.3cm) a spatial resolution of 25 microns implies images comprising $10,160 \times 8,120$ (82.5 million) pixels. Assuming only 12 bits of intensity resolution per pixel, this requires a staggering 123Mbytes of storage per mammogram!

Is such high spatial resolution needed? This continues to be the subject of debate, which, in the case of mammography, tends to centre on detecting and classifying microcalcifications. Of course, the smaller that microcalcifications can be detected and classified, the better the prognosis, so that the size of what is "needed" by radiologists depends on what can be achieved technologically! Nevertheless, but with this in mind, let us suppose that one wishes to classify microcalcifications as small as 100-200 microns. We noted in Chapter 11 that the shape of microcalcification is important for their classification; this seems, at first glance, to imply that a sampling aperture of at least 100 microns, and possibly 50 or 25 microns, is necessary. Halving the sampling resolution divides the number of pixels by 4, so that the 25.4×20.3cm mammogram referred to in the previous paragraph would generate 20 million pixels if it were sampled at 50 microns, but "only" 5 million if sampled at 100 microns.

Chan et. al. [39] digitised a mammographic film F with a sampling aperture of 100 microns to produce an image I, then used a laser film writer to output the image I onto a film F', also at 100 microns. They showed that a radiologist made considerably more errors in diagnosing microcalcifications from F' than for F: 0.4 true positive fraction (TPF) as opposed to 0.7 for a false positive fraction (FPF) of 0.1. Interestingly, they also showed that if I were "enhanced" by unsharp-masking to form I' prior to writing

F' then a higher TPF resulted for a FPF greater than 0.1, though it was still significantly worse than for the original film. We conjecture that the unsharp-masking process significantly reduced digitiser and printer blur.

Karssemeijer et. al. [142] demonstrated the importance of concentrating on relatively small windows of mammograms that appear to contain microcalcifications. They digitised such a window at 100 microns, then displayed it on a computer screen magnified four-fold (after interpolation to reduce digitisation blocking appearance). The magnified window was then shown to a radiologist, who was asked to classify the microcalcifications as benign or malignant. In contrast to [39], Karssemeijer found that a sampling resolution of 100 microns did not adversely affect diagnosis. Radiologists seem to process an image coarse-to-fine, using a magnifying glass where necessary, further evidence that it is not necessary to digitise all parts of an image to the same extent. Roehrig [210] built on this work by performing a threshold detection experiment with microcalcification phantoms, which were used in [142]. He used two all-digital systems: one had a relatively high spatial resolution of 50 microns, but a relatively poor DQE of 0.2; the other had rather poorer spatial resolution at 85 microns but a higher DQE of 0.6. He found that the latter gave far better discrimination for the microcalcification phantoms.

The implication is that in order to achieve diagnostic accuracy equal to that of film, it is not necessarily the case that all-digital systems need to match film in all respects. There remain, however, many gaps in our knowledge.

Image acquisition time

A film-screen system exposes all parts of the film at once: the image acquisition time is determined largely by the film speed, and is typically less than a second. We noted above that a digital image is likely to comprise between 5 and 82 million pixels. Providing a single active surface with that many elements is currently prohibitively expensive, and so, many prototype all-digital designs build the image up gradually by scanning a digitising device over the area of interest. The acquisition time is then the product of the number of scan sites and the acquisition time per site, the latter being approximately the same as for a conventional analogue film-screen system. For example, Tesic [240] developed a line scanning system in which a linear array of 1024 photodiodes was scanned across a screen. The x-ray beam was collimated through a linear strip before passing through the breast, and then again after emerging at the scintillator. An advantage of the device is the greatly reduced scatter. The exposure time was about 10 seconds, and this is not only a disadvantage for the patient (particularly in mammography, where the breast is compressed), but also for the x-ray tube, whose useful working life is decreased, not to mention the poor image quality due to patient motion. Nowadays, devices exploit the increased packing density and response times of semiconductor devices: CCD chips that cost several hundred dollars fifteen years ago now cost less than ten. For example, a commercial descendant [241] of [240] features a prototype CCD device with a very low dark current, 24 micron pixels, and has 1100×330 pixels per CCD. An alternative design [161] features an array of thin film transistors as its active devices; but no figures are given for the numbers of pixels per device.

In conclusion, several all-digital imaging systems are currently being developed commercially to meet the required spatial resolution, dynamic range, DQE, and low noise requirements; though there remains some discussion over exactly what specifications are necessary to at least compete with film. Some of the devices are already at the stage of clinical trial. We repeat the point that we made at the end of Chapter 1: the advent of all-digital systems will necessitate a revision to Part I of this monograph; but we remain confident that the output will be the h_{int} representation of interesting tissue, and that Part II will remain largely intact.

15.3. Image guided, minimally invasive breast surgery

Until about twenty years ago, the primary therapy for a diagnosed breast cancer was to perform a mastectomy. This has been replaced, particularly for early detected breast cancer, by a policy of breast conservation, based on a combination of increasingly targeted lumpectomies, chemotherapy, and radiation therapy. Breast conservation has been demonstrated to be safe in a number of prospective randomised trials, which find no significant differences, either in disease-free interval, or in overall survival rate, in patients who are treated with breast conservation rather than mastectomy[74]. As is noted in [147], conservative breast surgery not only produces a more acceptable cosmetic appearance than mastectomy, but preserves the patient's body image and enables greater freedom of dress.

Conservative treatment of breast cancer exemplifies the growing interest in minimal invasive surgery/therapy (MIS). The main advantages of MIS are several:

- There tend to be fewer complications, because the treatment involves less trauma to the patient, less anaesthesia is necessary, and there is less risk of intra-operative infection since there is less exposure of organs.
- It costs the health service considerably less, since the length of time that a patient needs to stay in hospital to recover from surgery can be

reduced from weeks to days. Indeed, in some cases, one-day outpatient treatment is possible.

MIS depends critically on accurate, reliable information about the location, nature, and extent of tumours. The full extent of disease must be determined prior to therapy in order to ensure that additional multifocal disease is not missed. Image analysis plays a key role in MIS, so much so that it is often referred to as image-guided, minimal invasive surgery (IGS). IGS implies team work, since it inevitably breaches the traditional boundaries of radiology and surgery and engineering. In the future, mammographic image analysis, such as discussed in this monograph, will play an increasingly important role in the management of breast cancer, that is, in its integrated diagnosis and treatment. In the remainder of this section we sketch developments in two inter-related aspects of breast IGS:

- Image-guided core biopsy;
- Image-guided minimal invasive therapy

Image-guided core biopsy

We recall from Chapter 14 that currently more than 70–80% biopsies turn out to be benign. A number of approaches are being developed to address this problem, in particular image-guided core biopsy. Chare ([77], p.3) describes the *triple assessment* approach to the assessment of breast disease, an approach that is central to the diagnosis and management of breast disease in the UK [85, 92]. Triple assessment involves a team comprising a surgeon, radiologist, and a cytopathologist, who gather and grade (for example, on a five point scale from normal to malignant) clinical, radiological, and cytological evidence respectively. Further information may be sought of each type until a consensus emerges for the management course to follow. Typically, the radiological evidence comprises a mammogram with or without an ultrasound scan of any apparent abnormality. Cytological evidence is normally provided by fine needle aspiration cytology (FNAC), which is "capable of diagnosing over 90% of palpable cancers when performed by an experienced operator and reported by an experienced cytopathologist" ([77], p.4).

With the advent of breast screening, there was a large increase in the number of mammographically-detected non-palpable lesions. Image-guided FNAC with stereotaxis was introduced in Sweden in 1977. More recently, ultrasound guidance has been introduced. However, FNAC has a small but significant false positive and negative rate, particularly with small lesions. Typically, the triple assessment of patients for whom FNAC failed to establish a diagnosis have in the past been subjected to an open surgical biopsy. The UK Breast Screening Programme, based on earlier Swedish experiences, was set up using FNAC and predicted a pre-operative diagnostic rate of over 70%. In order to minimise the number of unnecessary biopsies, core needle biopsy (CNB) is increasingly advocated, with the aim of increasing the pre-operative diagnostic rate to over 90%. It is reported ([77], p.188) that the number of open biopsies has reduced by 62% with the introduction of image-guided CNB.

CNB using biopsy guns has been available for palpable disease for about ten years. CNB requires that a location be specified in the breast: that is a point and direction are specified on the surface of the breast together with a depth to which the needle should penetrate. We noted in Chapter 14 that it is not possible to compute three dimensional positions of lesions from a single mammogram. One approach is to use ultrasound to guide CNB; this is an attractive option for several reasons, not least the availability of (two dimensional) ultrasound in most specialist breast clinics. For those lesions that are visible using it, ultrasound guided CNB has produced diagnostic accuracy rates approaching those obtained using prone table stereotactic digital systems. For those lesions that are not visible by ultrasound, stereotactic localisation is usually used. The breast is compressed, then two images are taken, each at 15° either side of the direction of compression, and a standard binocular stereovision algorithm used to determine the depth of a lesion. A development is the dedicated prone table ([77], chapter 8), which avoids a number of problems (patient movement, inaccuracy, ...) of standard stereotaxis at the cost of providing the capital equipment and dedicated space for breast biopsy. The procedure typically takes 40 minutes.

Future developments stemming from image analysis might include more precise information for the triple assessment, and improved techniques for rapid localisation in 3D of lesions [121].

Image-guided minimally invasive therapy

We noted above that the desire for breast conservation has led to more targeted lumpectomies, as well as increasing use of chemotherapy and radiotherapy. Other minimal invasive techniques are being developed for cancer therapy, and, once more, image analysis has a key role to play, not least in assessing the success of a procedure. Of these, interstitial laser photocoagulation (ILP) is perhaps the most clinically advanced. Bown [21] notes that "as collaboration develops between clinicians and scientists, and our understanding of the interaction between laser light with living tissue evolves, so it becomes possible to see the wide range of conditions that might be amenable to laser therapy in the future." Currently, there is no evidence of the cumulative toxicity problems that arise with radiotherapy and chemotherapy. The most promising developments in laser therapy are based on laser beams that penetrate tissue relatively deeply, particularly those in the near infrared part of the spectrum (800-1500nm). In ILP, the laser light is delivered through an optic fibre that is inserted directly into the target organ. The power is reduced to less than 5 W, but is maintained for several minutes. As Bown [21] notes, "essentially, the diseased tissue is gently cooked". There is no vapourisation, and dead tissues remain in place.

As regards breast cancer therapy, ILP aims to destroy tumours where they arise in the breast; but without leaving a scar or any cosmetic deformity. An early experiment is reported in [178]. Contrast-enhanced MR images were taken before and after ILP to assess whether the area that had been treated with ILP had indeed been necrotised, as a non-enhancing region in the post-resection MR image that had enhanced on the pre-image. The ILP procedure was monitored throughout using real-time ultrasound. Since all patients undergoing the experimental procedure were scheduled for surgical resection, histopathological "ground truth" was subsequently available. The correlation between MR and histopathology for laser burn diameter and residual tumour were both high. Though considerable development is needed before the ILP technique can replace surgical resection, it shows considerable promise, and poses challenging problems for image analysis in assessment and localisation.

Other minimal invasive therapeutic techniques that are under develop ment include focussed ultrasound and radio-frequency heating; but to date there do not seem to have been any published clinical results using them.

15.4. Nuclear medicine

In nuclear medicine, radionuclide-labelled agents, known as radiopharmaceuticals, are injected into the body and are taken up selectively by tissue, for example in the breast. Progress in nuclear medicine has consisted of: (i) a range of increasingly pathology-sensitive and pathology-specific radiopharmaceuticals; (ii) a succession of improvements to imaging devices based on gamma camera devices, notably for planar scintigraphy, single-photon emission tomography (SPET) and PET; (iii) more targeted clinical trials; and (iv) improvements in computer power and image/signal filtering. We discuss these briefly in turn.

Before doing so, we note that, as in the case of x-ray imaging, injecting a radionuclide into living tissue is bound to be cause for concern. However, as [254] (p.258) observe: "in most cases, the concentration of radiopharmaceutical (or radiotracer) is subpharmacological, usually of the order of nanomolar, and at this concentration imparts no measurable effect". They further observe that (p.181): "one of the primary advantages associated with the use of radionuclides in medicine is the large signal (in this case the emitted radiation) obtained from a relatively small mass of radionuclide employed".

Radiopharmaceuticals

An example of a radiopharmaceutical that has been of particular interest in detecting breast cancer is the tracer sestaMIBI labelled with the radionuclide Technetium $^{99}Tc^m$. SestaMIBI was originally developed for myocardial perfusion studies and accumulates particularly in cells with a high energy metabolism such as neoplastic cells. After administration, the radiopharmaceutical begins to decay and emit γ rays or other particles. $^{99}Tc^m$ has a half life of 6.02 hours and decays to ^{99}Tc by emitting a 140 keV γ ray. As we describe below, γ rays of this energy can be imaged effectively by a gamma camera. Radiopharmaceuticals labelled with $^{99}Tc^m$ have been used in over 90% of nuclear medicine studies of breast cancer to date, though there has been a fascination with developing alternatives. Indeed, there is feeling that this fascination with new radiopharmaceuticals has retarded the careful assessment of the clinical potential of the more promising among them [67, 19].

A related though different approach is afforded by positron-emission tomography (PET), which is based on the use of radiohalogens such as fluorodeoxyglucose (FDG). An example of the functional information provided by PET applied to breast cancer is the labelling of steroid hormones with positron-emitting radionuclides. It is important to realise that besides imaging as such, PET can provide functional information such as vascularisation, whose importance we stressed in Chapter 14. We make further reference to this below, and in the next section.

Imaging devices

The key step in the development of nuclear medicine was the invention, and successive refinements, of the gamma camera. Chapter 6 of [254] is a superb account of the physics of radioisotope imaging. In nuclear medicine, ionising radiation can arrive at a detector over a relatively wide solid angle, so it is customary to place a collimator, in its simplest form an array of parallel cylindrical holes drilled in a sheet of lead, between the radiating organ and the detector. This is analogous to the use of anti-scatter grids in x-ray mammography, which we discussed at length in Chapter 10. Typically the detector is a single large area (typically 50cm diameter) thin (6-12mm) scintillating crystal of Thallium-activated Sodium Iodide NaI(Tl), which absorbs γ rays in the energy band 50-500 keV (which includes the 140 keV energy of $^{99}Tc^m$-emitted γ rays) and in turn radiates blue-green light (410 nm). To a good approximation, light photon radiance is proportional to γ irradiation, so intensity is a good measure of radionuclide concentration in the direction normal to the collimator surface. The trend to make the scintillating crystal thinner and thinner impacts the choice of radionuclide, and this, together with its convenient half life, has led to the widespread adoption of $^{99}Tc^m$.

The light emitting from the scintillating crystal is conducted via light guides into a hexagonal array of photomultiplier tubes that cover the crystal surface area from which emerges the electronic signal that can be converted to digital form and which is used to form the stored image. Currently, nuclear medicine images have relatively poor spatial resolution (often 64 pixels square) and have poor quality, mostly because of the poor photomultiplier efficiency that degrades the image signal-to-noise.

The most basic form of the gamma camera is the planar camera that produces a static 2D image. This technique is known as static planar scintigraphy, and it has been the basis of most work to date on breast nuclear medicine. Rapid advances in computer power and cheaper memory have enabled the development of dynamic planar scintigraphy; but it has, not surprisingly, been most targeted at the heart, lungs, and kidneys. Exactly analogous to x-ray mammography, a fundamental limitation of planar scintigraphy is that it cannot differentiate between a single non-overlapped, intensely radiating region and the superposition of two lesser-radiating regions.

Emission-computed tomography overcomes this limitation by generating a genuinely three-dimensional map of tissue activity by combining multiple cross-sectional images. Since, for many applications, the half life is relatively long, it is possible to generate multiple cross sections either by moving a single planar detector along a trajectory that encircles the organ of interest. Alternatively, though more expensively, detectors can be replicated for example in a circle surrounding the subject. It is customary to distinguish single-photon emission tomography (SPET), in which single γ rays are emitted, and PET in which radionuclides are used that emit positrons (e^+) which quickly annihilate in tissue, generating a pair of anti-parallel γ rays each of 511 keV.

Generally, PET tends to give better sensitivity and specificity than either planar scintigraphy or SPET, and the radiation dose tends to be lower. However, PET is currently quite expensive and so it is only available at a few major centres.

Clinical data

Fortunately, there has recently appeared an excellent and comprehensive review of nuclear medicine techniques for the detection of breast cancer, to which the interested reader is referred [19]. Here we sample some of what seem to be the most promising findings. Piccolo et. al. [198] studied the uptake of the radiopharmaceutical $^{99}Tc^m$-methylene diphosphate (MDP) in a biased group consisting of 200 women suspected of having carcinoma of the breast. X-ray mammograms were available in each case, and from the mammograms, 120 indicated neoplasm, 27 were judged highly suspicious, and the judgement was inconclusive in the remaining 53. Postoperative histology revealed that there was in fact neoplasm in 172 cases, and benign breast disease in the remaining 28. Planar scintigraphy images were obtained both anteriorly and posteriorly at three times post injection: 4 minutes, 10-20 minutes, and 2 hours. Of these, it was concluded that the first and last gave no useful information. However, in the images acquired after 10-20 minutes, a photoabundant focal region was visible in 158 of the 172 women that had breast cancer. The focal region was surprisingly bright, with a contrast of approximately 4. Once again, we note that these excellent results are attributable to the rich vascularisation due to angiogenesis. Unfortunately, lesions less than 0.7cm in diameter could not be detected.

Among others, Khalkali and his colleagues have conducted a series of trials with $^{99}Tc^m$-sestaMIBI that have produced some highly encouraging results. In one of these studies [148] 147 patients had 153 lesions (102 of which were subsequently confirmed by biopsy, the remaining 51 by fine-needle aspiration) of which 110 were palpable. The examination was performed with the patient prone, and planar scintigraphy images were taken anterior and lateral oblique 5 and 60 minutes after intravenous injection of $^{99}Tc^m$-sestaMIBI. The sensitivity was 92.1%, specificity 89.2%, positive predictive value 81.0% and negative predictive value 95.8%. The authors suggest that this demonstrates that planar scintigraphy using $^{99}Tc^m$-sestaMIBI has a valuable role to play in reducing the number of biopsies performed. These promising results lead Khalkali and his colleagues to conduct a multi-centre trial (42 sites) with similarly encouraging results. There has been some preliminary work comparing the radiopharmaceuticals $^{99}Tc^m$-MDP and $^{99}Tc^m$-sestaMIBI, but the results are currently hard to evaluate.

Finally, we sample one of the growing number of applications of PET to detect breast cancer. Utech et. al. [246] used whole-body PET to study 124 patients that had recently been diagnosed as having breast cancer. In particular, they determined the average differential take-up ratio of ^{18}F-

fluorodeoxyglucose (FDG) in the axillary lymph nodes. This is, of course, one of the keys to determining the likelihood that metastasis has already started. The PET images enabled all 44 positive axillary lymph nodes to be detected, and no false negatives resulted. This could be a most important development since it may be that axillary lymph node dissection might not be necessary in patients that show no take up of FDG on PET. The possibility of replacing axillary lymph node dissection by PET is currently a hot topic of research, as is the possible detection and localisation of sentinel nodes.

Assessment of nuclear medicine

x-ray mammograms, and even to contrast-enhanced breast MRI, nuclear medicine images are currently of poor spatial resolution and have poor signal-to-noise. Moreover the images are relatively slow to obtain (typically 10-20 minutes). Finally, as we noted above, PET is currently quite expensive and so it is only available at a few major centres and is highly unlikely to provide a basis for screening. The reader may well wonder whether breast nuclear medicine has a real clinical role! The answer is almost certainly "yes", and increasingly so. First, PET and gamma cameras are rapidly improving in quality and reducing in cost. Several commercial systems already have a spatial resolution of 128 pixels square, and the signal to noise is improving as new photomultiplier tubes are developed. More importantly, even current radiopharmaceuticals have demonstrated encouraging pathology specificity and have proven value in replacing surgical procedures that currently have significant morbidity, not least dissection of axillary lymph nodes.

There have also been encouraging developments in image processing of PET and gamma camera images. First, the statistical parameter map technique has shown great promise for functional MRI (which is also functional and which also has poor spatial resolution and signal to noise), and has been applied to enhance and match PET images. Techniques have been developed to register (functional) PET images of the brain with (anatomical) MRI images that have far greater resolution. However, the vast majority of the work reported to date on PET image processing has been applied to the brain, for which MR images have high contrast boundaries. The extension of such techniques to the breast remains largely open.

15.5. Ultrasound

Overview

In his excellent survey of ultrasound of the breast, Fornage [78] notes that breast diseases are routinely evaluated by physical examination and mammography, with sonography being recognised currently as the best adjunct to mammography. He concludes that although it is useful to compare and contrast their relative merits for diagnosis and for interventional guidance, "breast sonography and mammography are complementary not competing procedures". Indeed, given a nonpalpable lesion which is hard to match up between sonography and mammography, sonography can be performed through a window in a modified mammographic compression plate, with the coordinates of the lesion as found in the mammogram marked on the skin. In this way, the information from the two imaging modalities can usefully be combined.

Bamber and Tristam [6] give an excellent introduction to the physics of medical ultrasound, including the engineering principles of imaging, scanning modes, and beam formation. Most medical ultrasound applications use frequencies in the range 5-10 MHz, and sense in pulse-echo (reflective) mode to give an image of reflectivity, also called a B-mode image. Since the average speed of sound in soft tissue is about 1500 metres per second, typical wavelengths in medical imaging range from 0.3mm at 5 MHz to 0.15mm at 10 MHz. Ultrasound is reflected and refracted at interfaces between media of different acoustic impedance. The intensity of an ultrasound pulse/wave decreases exponentially, the attenuation coefficient being the sum of contributions from scatter (10-30%) and attenuation (70-90%). The attenuation is, to a good approximation, linearly proportional to the frequency of the ultrasound. At 5 MHz, the attenuation of breast tissue is about 8 dB per centimetre, while that of bone/calcification is about ten times as large, and that of cyst liquid is about one tenth of normal breast tissue. The greater the acoustic impedance difference between tissues, the greater is the B-mode reflection caused by that tissue boundary. Thus, for example, cysts as small as 3-4mm can be detected very reliably by high-frequency sonography. A typical cyst is anechoic, well circumscribed, and associated with distal sound beam enhancement. There are exceptions, for example cysts that are calcified, for which the high attenuation of the calcium coating of the cyst prevents reflections from deeper tissues. This gives the appearance of a "shadow" in the ultrasound image.

Fibroadenomas are the most common solid benign tumours in breasts of young women and may also develop in post-menopausal women taking HRT. The vast majority of fibroadenomas are hypoechoic, and the margin is usually, though not always, regular, that is, smooth. Carcinomas less than 1cm in diameter are now routinely identified on sonograms. The most common breast cancer is the infiltrating ductal carcinoma: this appears as a focal hypoechoic mass but with irregular borders and which distorts the architecture of the breast. During palpation, real-time sonography demonstrates the tumour's incompressibility and its strong adherence to the surrounding tissues. About 10-15 % of breast carcinomas appear as well-circumscribed nodules on mammograms. Although the sonographic patterns of benign and malignant lesions will always overlap, the improved resolution of modern high-frequency transducers allows increasingly better discrimination between such lesions. Though the above is encouraging progress in ultrasonography of the breast, Fornage notes that "the capability of sonography to detect nonpalpable carcinomas not seen on mammograms has not been acknowledged in the United States, where sonography is still considered an ancillary, operator dependent procedure only useful for differentiating solid from cystic palpable masses".

Fornage concludes that the advantages of sonography over mammography include:

+ Commercially-available ultrasound scanners produce images in real-time;
+ Because ultrasound measures the depth to acoustic impedance boundaries, it is possible to localize lesions quite accurately in three-dimension;
+ At the intensities and frequencies that are used in clinical practice, ultrasound poses no significant health hazards;
+ An ultrasound breast image is normally produced with the woman lying flat on her back while a linear probe is scanned across the breast. This means that it is possible to evaluate small breasts;
+ It is also possible to examine radiologically dense breasts, particularly those of young women. It is also possible to image breasts with implants, lesions near the periphery of the breast, and regional lymph nodes;
+ It is possible to diagnose fluid collections and to visualize directly dilated ducts;
+ It is possible to palpate a lesion under real-time ultrasound monitoring (we return to this below); and
+ An ultrasound examination is less painful for a woman than a mammogram. It is also less time consuming and costly than MRI as well as being not at all claustrophobic.

Fornage further suggests that the disadvantages of sonography relative to mammography include:

- Ultrasound intrinsically has a low signal-to-noise ratio and image quality is further challenged by speckle, clutter, and other sources of noise. In fact, image quality largely depends on the operator's experience; it is difficult to interpret films taken by someone else.
- It cannot be used to visualise (small) microcalcifications and small cancers (currently smaller than 0.7mm though this is changing as technology advances);
- Ultrasound probes have a narrow field of view and it is also difficult to reproduce a given sonogram on serial examinations;

We may summarise the current situation with respect to ultrasonographic image analysis as follows: there has been considerable progress but it still has insufficient sensitivity and specificity to discriminate benign from malignant lesions. In analogy with the work on breast MRI that we presented in Chapter 14 and on nuclear medicine in section 15.4 of this chapter, attention has shifted to investigating whether ultrasound can be used to differentiate between benign and malignant lesions on the basis of their vascularisation.

Dynamics

Cosgrove et. al. [47] note that malignant tumours larger than a few millimetres in diameter usually stimulate the growth of new blood vessels by secreting angiogenesis factor. The result is a multiplicity and disordered pattern of small vessels surrounding a tumour that spread by linking to other nearby vessels (creating shunts). This neoangionesis corresponds to a substantial increase in blood flow around a tumour. Techniques for measuring flow with ultrasound are based on variants to estimating Doppler frequency shifts caused by sensing a moving target [257].

Bamber and Tristam ([6], p.327) develop a simple model in which Doppler frequency shift is proportional to the probing frequency (typically 5 MHz) and to the component of flow in the axial (ie transmitted pulse) direction, and inversely proportional to the speed of ultrasound in tissue. They note that it is necessary to know both the speed and the direction of motion of flow in order to measure the velocity of flow. Since it is difficult to estimate either accurately, the precise determination of flow velocity is difficult. In general, there are many moving scatterers, each producing a different frequency shift. This leads naturally to a Doppler shift spectrum and to Fourier analysis of it, generating either the basic spectra (as a function of frequency and time) or power.

Ultrasound devices are either continuous wave (CW) or pulsed. A CW system is the easiest to construct; but it intrinsically has no resolution in the depth direction. Pulsed systems, originally inspired by pulsed radar systems, can overcome this, but the frequencies outside a pre-determined passband are aliased, and this forces a range-velocity compromise ([6], p.357). If a vessel is well-defined, then the angle θ can be determined, hence the velocity vector v. Combination of echo imaging with pulsed Doppler is commonly called a "duplex" scanner. In colour flow (CF), the computed flow information in a user-selectable window is superimposed, in colour coded form, on the normal grey scale image. Actually, as Ferrara and DeAngelis [72] point out in their excellent review of colour flow mapping, in some applications, particularly in cardiology, the relatively long acquisition times needed for computing colour flow can make it difficult to register the greyscale image and the colour flow data. This is not a major problem for breast ultrasound.

Early reports of the application of colour flow to breast cancer diagnosis [47] were extremely encouraging. Cosgrove et. al. [47] found that 20 of 21 untreated carcinomas showed flow detected by CF, and in nine of these it was considered moderate or high, indeed was "subjectively striking". In contrast, most benign masses showed no detectable flow. The same team later [48] reported a larger series in which they found 88% of malignant lesions and 5% benign lesions showing colour flow. Other authors have reported highly varied results on both the sensitivity and specificity of colour flow for differential diagnosis. An explanation is offered by [128], who note the somewhat paradoxical situation that "as the sensitivity of color Doppler US has increased for depicting low flow volumes and smaller flow velocities, vessels in benign lesions have also become detectable". They argue that this necessitates the development of quantitative measures of flow, and they propose two such: the mean colour value (MCV) (of the coloured pixels) and the colour pixel density (CPD) (the proportion of pixels in the colour flow window that are in fact coloured). They found that the best results were obtained with a machine setting that was optimal for low velocities, and they report the sensitivity in helping to identify carcinomas was 64% for CPD and 92% for MCV. Conversely the specificity was 91% for CPD and 78% for MCV. Oddly, combining the results did not seem to help.

Colour flow imaging is based on pulsed Doppler. However, Carson and colleagues[33] have reported a study in which spectral measurements of flow calculated from CW ultrasound were "observed to be more sensitive to the tumour vasculature" for almost all of the 11 measurements. One such was the estimated relative power in all portions of the observed power spectrum, as is expected for the chaotic flow characteristic of angiogenesis. The somewhat confused state of Doppler-based diagnosis of breast cancer is added to by recent explorations of power Doppler imaging (PDI). For example, [14] note that "because PDI is more sensitive to flow than colour Doppler" they conjectured that it would show even better specificity and sensitivity than CF. In fact, they found that more benign than malignant lesions showed significant PDI flow, and that two thirds of the malignant masses showed less than 10 % PDI flow.

It is not clear how to resolve the various debates and inconsistent results reported in the literature. Perhaps it is a reflection of the difference between the complexity of the underlying pathology and the relative simplicity of the morphological and flow parameters used to date to represent that pathology. Further, Huber[128] suggest that the values that are computed depend on the specific site where the Doppler signal is acquired (tumour centre, periphery, or a neighbouring vessel). Similarly, Weidner's [255] study of angiogenesis showed that areas of substantial new vascularisation could occur almost anywhere in an invasive tumour, that microvessels are sparse in sclerotic areas, and that regions of necrosis within tumours (that appear hypoechoic) are most likely to be avascular. Perhaps more sophisticated representations of three-dimensional morphology and flow could resolve these issues.

Many techniques have been developed for acquiring three-dimensional volumes of ultrasound data. In most cases, they have involved sampling a set of parallel ultrasound slices by immobilising the breast, for example using a modified breast compression device, and using an instrumented linear positioning device to move the ultrasound head relative to the breast [108], [33], [177]. An alternative approach is to track the position and orientation of an ultrasound probe as the clinician makes freehand motions holding it. More recently, three-dimensional phased array ultrasound machines have become commercially available. It is clear that the acquisition, processing, and display of three-dimensional ultrasound data will be an area that will advance rapidly over the next few years, and that it will give fresh insight into the development and diagnosis of breast cancer, not least by enabling the computation of three-dimensional morphology and the three-dimensional flow field surrounding a tumour.

Though neovascularisation is characteristic of malignancy, it is often difficult to detect because the Doppler signals are too small. Contrast agents have been developed for ultrasound[217]. Kedar[145] et al. report experiments with a microbubble contrast agent and found shunts in all cancers but not in any benign lesion. Furthermore, diagnostic confidence increased with the use of the contrast agent. The use of a contrast agent also offers a new set of dynamic features, such as the time to reach maximum intensity, and the subsequent decay time, to help in differential diagnosis.

	No.	easily deforms	intermediate	incompressible
Cancer	37	0%	14%	86%
Cyst	15	80%	20%	0%
Fibroadenoma	18	44%	17%	39%

TABLE 15.1. Compressibility

	No.	mobile	intermediate	fixed
Cancer	37	11%	16%	72%
Cyst	15	7%	7%	87%
Fibroadenoma	18	67%	28%	6%

TABLE 15.2. Mobility

Tissue composition

Though this section has so far concentrated on diagnosis of breast cancer using ultrasound, we conclude by mentioning two other potentially extremely valuable applications in breast disease. First, largely because of its real-time, three-dimensional nature, ultrasound has rapidly gained in popularity for guidance of needle biopsy and other minimal invasive procedures. Fornage[78] reviews the topic, though there have, as we noted in Section 15.3 of this Chapter, been many more recent developments. Second, ultrasound can give valuable information about tissue elasticity. Ueno et. al.[245] note that "by palpation, it is known that cancers show poor mobility and high consistency while benign masses are easily moved and softer. We usually observe the changes in tumour shape and its fixation to surrounding tissues by manual compression under conditions of real-time imaging". They reported the results shown in Tables 15.1 and 15.2 for 70 cases.

Thus, masses that deform easily and are mobile are usually fibroadenomas, while carcinomas are fixed and incompressible. We note the similarity between this work and the idea of differential compression mammography that we described in Chapter 9. Subsequent work by Chen and colleagues [40] substantially develops this idea. A two-dimensional correlation-based algorithm tracked tissue displacements arising from palpation, here taken to mean a translation of the imaging transducer accompanied by a rotation about an axis that corresponds to the linear array. Three kinds of motion were observed: a shear motion of adjacent tissue above the mass; a slight drag of adjacent tissue in the direction of palpation; and an *en bloc* displacement of the mass and adjacent parenchyma. The quantitative measures resulting from the tissue flow fields were consistent with the the earlier qualitative results of [245].

Breast ultrasound continues to develop rapidly and has enormous potential for diagnosis, image guided surgery, and for contributing to the theoretical foundation of cancer development.

15.6. Decision aids

This monograph has described progress in the computer processing of mammographic images, primarily x-rays, but also MRI, nuclear medicine, and ultrasound. Techniques such as those we have described, together with the tumbling cost of computing and imaging equipment, and the rapid spread of computer networks within and between clinical sites, have made available to the clinician a staggering, and rapidly growing, number of images to support clinical decision making. In fact, the growing superabundance of images has generated its own challenge: how to enable clinicians to make effective use of this flood of information. The problem is exacerbated by growing demands on the already busy clinician's time: more patients have to be managed, more decisions have to be made, and more information of diverse sorts is available to support those decisions. Furthermore, not only are decisions made within a team framework such as the triple assessment regime discussed in Section 15.3, further adding to the information pool that underpins any particular decision; but digital image transmission enables clinicians at remote sites to collaborate in decision making. Increasingly stringent clinical regulations and spiralling malpractice insurance costs underline the need to be able to demonstrate that the most authoritative and relevant information was taken into account in decisions relating to patient management. This increasing challenge, and the imperative to confront that challenge, are driving the development of computer-based decision aids. Taylor [237] presents a literature review of computational decision aids.

Clinicians are required to make a wide variety of decisions:

- Whether or not there is a clinically significant finding;
- Whether or not it is necessary to call for further investigations in order to establish (to the clinician's satisfaction) that there is such a finding;
- How to classify or interpret such a finding, leading to a tentative diagnosis;
- How to stage a disease;

– Which treatments to initiate, at which stages, and how to assess the patient's responses to each such.

In making these decisions, a clinician (or team of clinicians) has to mobilise knowledge of a variety of sorts: that specific to this particular patient (family history, age, general condition, etc.), those that are of general applicability (disease types, treatment regimes, etc.), and those that pertain to the protocols for patient management that are in force at the clinician's site. Much of this knowledge can conveniently be expressed textually (e.g. patient record and family history), while some relates directly to images (e.g. the appearance of spiculated lesions or ductal microcalcifications in mammograms). In order to develop a computerised clinical decision aid, the following questions have to be addressed:

– How is the knowledge of each of the various different types represented?
– How is it determined which of the mass of stored knowledge is relevant to the management of any particular patient?
– How are several pieces of information relevant to managing a patient combined in a way that corresponds to clinical reasoning or decision making?
– How, in subsequently changed circumstances (e.g. a follow up image or lack of response to a particular treatment), can the decision making that led to the original diagnosis, prognosis, or treatment be revised without having to start from scratch?
– Since information about a patient, or about the causality or dependence of one piece of information about another, is often uncertain, how can uncertainty be represented and manipulated appropriately?
– Since disease processes are extremely variable and complex, it is often impossible to make precise predictions about a treatment (e.g. rate and amount of response); how can qualitative information about patient management be represented and mobilised?
– How can the knowledge and decision aids be used to develop a tutor that can help starting clinicians learn more effectively?

These are the central questions addressed in artificial intelligence [214, 202] and so it is no surprise that steps toward the development of clinical decision aids are reported in journals such as *Artificial Intelligence* and *Artificial Intelligence in Medicine*. For example, a range of symbolic processing techniques, including semantic networks and frames, have been developed for representing knowledge, particularly that which can be expressed conveniently as text. These techniques facilitate, for example, automatic inheritance and generalisation, so that a request for information about Paget's disease would automatically invoke more general facts about malignant lesions. Such knowledge representation techniques have associated search engines that filter which information seems most relevant in any particular case. Simpler approaches have been developed that are often effective in reasonably narrow applications: these include expert systems, in which knowledge is represented as facts and in which relevance is determined by an algorithm that pattern matches stored facts against those specific to the management of this particular patient. A number of efficient techniques have been developed for belief revision, in which the dependencies of an inferred fact on those from which it was deduced are stored. This enables any particular fact to be modified and the reasoning revised just for those other facts that depended upon it.

A range of approaches to modelling and propagating uncertainty have been developed. Most familiar are those based on Bayesian decision making. Others include the Dempster-Shafer rule that distinguishes between belief and uncertainty, and fuzzy logic. Qualitative reasoning approaches eschew precise numerical values for variables, restricting attention to the sign of a variable (plus, zero, or minus) and the sign of its derivative. Surprisingly, robust systems have been developed to reason about the working of some quite complex non-linear mechanisms such as heat transfer engines, clocks, and sensor-guided robot vehicles.

Although there has been encouraging work on developing computer systems that can support decision making, most of it is restricted to manipulating textual information; to date, hardly any has enabled the mixing of text and images in the way that a real radiologist would. One exception to this is the work of Taylor, Fox, and Todd-Pokropek [239], who propose a model for integrating image processing into a decision aid developed previously by Fox et al. [127]. Fox's symbolic "defeasible" decision procedure consists of four elements:

- *Generic decision rules*: a set of logical rules that govern the processes of proposing "candidates" (i.e. possible solutions), constructing arguments for and against the candidates, and establishing the existence of the evidence required by those arguments;
- *Task specific knowledge*: a set of facts that indicates which classes of the entities described in the domain-level knowledge can serve as candidates and as arguments in the different sorts of decisions that are of interest;
- *Domain-level knowledge*: a set of facts that describe the domain in which the decision is to be made;
- *Case specific knowledge*: a set of facts describing what is known about this particular case.

The task specific knowledge instantiates the generic decision rules in order to identify candidates and arguments, by matching the domain level knowledge to the case specific facts. The arguments for and against a particular decision focus attention on what information is needed to sharpen the decision that is eventually taken: the diagnosis could be X or Y; if it were X you would expect signs S1 and S2, whereas if it were Y you would expect signs S1 and S3; S1 is clearly present but it is hard to say which of S2 and S3 are; test T is a good way to decide this; ... This logic of argumentation has been applied to general medicine and to oncology, based entirely on thousands of facts expressed as text. The prototype decision aid developed by [239] attempts to combine mammographic image processing with Fox's reasoning system. The initial focus has been on reasoning about microcalcifications. Unfortunately, although the architecture of the system is of considerable promise, the "Achilles heel" is the inadequate performance of the image processing routines: the poor sensitivity and specificity undermine the reasoning.

Though computer decision aids of the type developed by [239] are at an early stage, it is clear that they will continue to be developed and that their performance will improve to the point where they are used clinically. Certainly, the need for them will become ever more pressing.

15.7. Summary

We have limited the discussion in this final chapter to a selection of the issues that promise much for the advancement of breast cancer diagnosis and therapy over the next few years. We began by summarising what we consider to be the main ideas we promoted in the body of the text. Promising developments in digital mammography were followed by a glimpse of the exciting developments under way in minimally invasive therapy. We considered two imaging modalities that are currently the subject of intensive research: nuclear medicine and ultrasound. Both of them give information about the dynamics of tumour behaviour, as does MRI mammography. Additionally, ultrasound promises to give important information about tissue composition. Finally, we noted that the ideas of artificial intelligence are leading to systems that can combine information from images and from patient records to make a smart assistant for the clinician.

This selection of topics is just that: a choice. We could have included sections on the digital hospital, the impact of the internet, on image analysis applied to cytopathology, and on the exciting prospect of combining image analysis with developments in molecular medicine in order to detect and quantify the effectiveness of new drug therapies.

Mammography has emerged over the past two decades as an established technique in the fight against breast cancer, enabling clinicians to frame diagnoses earlier and more reliably, and enabling researchers to gain new insights into the disease process. Yet, as the work discussed in this monograph, particularly that in this final chapter, indicates, there remains massive room for improvement. The subject is evolving quickly and research agendas are in preparation internationally on topics such as:

- Novel imaging modalities, typified by 3D ultrasound, that do not involve ionising radiation;
- Functional imaging aimed at *in vivo* cellular and molecular biological tissue characterisation;
- 3D and 4D image analysis, building on ideas such as those described in this monograph, for robust quantitative analysis and for enhanced display of radiological information;
- Telemammography and related information management for facilitating consultations with distant experts;
- Full field digital x-ray mammography, with corresponding developments in mammography workstation design;
- Techniques for guiding minimal invasive mammographic surgery;
- The development of artificial intelligence techniques to assist a team of clinicians manage patient care.

At a time of rapid development on so many fronts it is always tempting to wait one more year before publishing a monograph. However, we believe that the approach to mammographic image analysis that we have developed, organised in the case of x-ray mammography around the h_{int} representation and in the case of MR mammography around the pharmacokinetic model of contrast agent take-up, has reached a point that it provides a novel and interesting perspective on what is a fiendishly difficult problem. Developments on the many problems referred to above, and discussed in more details in this final chapter, will have to wait for the next edition!

Hopefully, the ideas that we discussed in the body of this monograph, together with the developments in areas such as we have sketched in this chapter, will contribute to the over-riding clinical and social goal: a massive reduction in breast cancer mortality and support the development of drug and minimal invasive therapies that effectively cure the disease before it can metastasize.

RECEIVER OPERATING CHARACTERISTIC (ROC) CURVES

The detection techniques described in this monograph, whether performed by human or by computer, are required to choose between two conditions (*positive* and *negative*) for each given image or patient. To assess performance, it is necessary to develop a measure of the diagnostic accuracy of the technique, and ROC curves have been developed as one of a number of such measures. In the simplest case, ROC measures assume that ground truth exists as one of two states *malignant* or *benign* and that this state is known in each case, typically, in the context of this monograph, in the form of histological data. Given such ground truth, the pronouncement made for each patient can be allocated to one of four sets:

- *True positive* (TP): those that are correctly pronounced positive (malignant),
- *False positive* (FP), those that are incorrectly pronounced to be malignant,
- *True negative* (TN), those that are correctly pronounced to be benign, and
- *False negative* (FN), those that are incorrectly pronounced to be benign.

The total set M of outcomes that are in fact malignant comprise those in the sets TP and FN, since if a case is falsely labelled benign, it must, in the two state case, be malignant. Similarly, the total set B of those that are in fact benign comprises the sets TN and FP. Several measures are defined, each of which is expressed as a ratio, to analyse observer performance:

- *Sensitivity*: the ratio $\frac{TP}{M}$, sometimes also called the *true positive fraction*.
- *Specificity*: the ratio $\frac{TN}{B}$. Closely related is the *false positive fraction*, defined as 1-specificity:

$$\text{false positive fraction} = 1 - \frac{TN}{TN + FP} = \frac{FP}{B}.$$

— *Diagnostic accuracy*: the ratio of the number of correct assessments divided by the total number of assessments, that is

$$\frac{TP + TN}{M + B}$$

— *Positive predictive value*: the ratio $\frac{TP}{TP+FP}$

— *Negative predictive value*: the ratio $\frac{TN}{TN+FN}$

As we noted in Chapter 13 it is normally (fortunately) the case that the incidence of malignancies detected in a screening population of apparently healthy women is low. The aim of screening is to detect the set of women with malignancies, and, since one does not want to miss any, this implies that the set FN, consisting of those that are in fact malignant but which are missed, should ideally be empty. It would then be the case that TP would be identical to M, so that sensitivity would be 1.0. One way to increase the likelihood of this is to declare all women who are not correctly judged to be benign, that is, those for whom there is doubt, to be malignant. Inevitably, this would involve declaring a substantial number of women malignant when they are in fact benign, that is it would almost certainly increase the number of FPs. Consequently, though the sensitivity would be 1.0, the specificity would be low. In practice, such a policy is unacceptable since it would involve substantial number of women in further examinations, and while this might not have serious consequences, it clearly is costly and extremely upsetting to those women who are recalled unnecessarily. The moral is that the measures are not absolute and independent, and so one should not seek to maximise one (e.g. sensitivity) without considering others (e.g. specificity).

Receiver operating characteristic (ROC) curves have been developed from such considerations. There is an extensive literature on ROC curves and related measures, and here we present only the basic idea. The ROC is a graph of the false positive fraction (1.0-specificity) vs the true positive fraction (i.e. sensitivity), the points on the curve being obtained by repeating the test, ideally with different data, but possibly also using the same data presented in a randomised fashion on a number of different occasions (it is known that in many cases intra-observer variability is high; but, in this monograph, we are most interested in the case where we seek to develop a measure of an algorithm's performance which factors out, as far as possible, observer variation). The idea is that an algorithm, an individual radiologist, or indeed an entire screening team ([209], p.190) would have an associated ROC curve, which might change (hopefully improve) over time as a result of "learning".

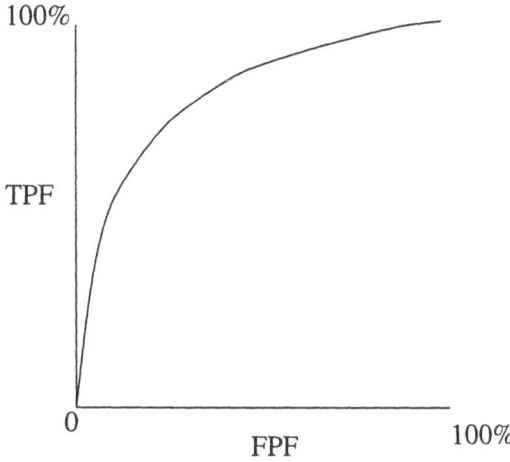

Figure A.1.   An ROC example.

A typical example of a ROC curve is shown in Figure A.1. Ideally, an ROC curve should have the following properties:

- *Informative*: the diagonal straight line connecting $(0,0)$ to $(1,1)$ can be considered as completely uninformative, since at all points on the curve, the fraction of false positives is equal to the fraction of false negatives. Consequently, an ROC curve should lie wholly above this diagonal.
- *Monotonic*: as the fraction of false positives increases, so should the number of true positives. That is, one would not expect to detect a smaller fraction of true positives as the fraction of false positives is allowed to increase.
- *Sharp rise from* $(0,0)$: tolerating even a small fraction of false positives should suffice, in the case of an expert, to get a very high fraction of the true positives. A consequence of this and monotonicity is that the rate of increase in the fraction of true positives should slow down with increasing false positive fraction. Generally, an ROC curve should exhibit a "knee". In the ideal limit, one might aspire to a curve that has a knee that is almost right-angled, that is, the ROC curve would become identical to the line $(0,1)$ to $(1,1)$.

How might different ROC curves be compared? If one curve R_1 were wholly above and to the left of another R_2, we might say that the observer/technique corresponding to R_1 is better than that corresponding to R_2. In general, however, the two ROC curves might cross. For example, one observer might have a greater bias toward sensitivity, another to specificity. For this reason, the integral below the curve is often used as a basis for comparison.

A number of refinements of this simple model have been proposed, including Location ROC (LROC), free-response ROC (FROC), and the alternative free-response ROC (AFROC). The reader is referred to the medical statistics literature for more details.

REFERENCES

1. L. V. Ackerman and E. E. Gose. Breast lesion classification by computer and xeroradiograph. *Cancer*, 30:1025–1035, 1972.
2. A. H. Adams, J. R. Brookeman, and M. B. Merickel. Breast lesion discrimination using statistical analysis and shape measures on magnetic resonance imagery. *Computerised Medical Imaging and Graphics*, 15:339–349, 1991.
3. F. Aghdasi, R. K. Ward, and B. Palcic. Restoration of mammographic images in the presence of signal-dependent noise. In K. W. Bowyer and S. Astley, editors, *State of the Art in Digital Mammographic Image Analysis*, volume 9 of *Series in Machine Perception and Artificial Intelligence*, pages 42 – 63. World Scientific, 1994.
4. V. F. Andolina, S. L. Lille, and K. M. Willison. *Mammographic Imaging: A Practical Guide*. J. B. Lippincott Company, 1992.
5. B. A. Arnold, H. Eisenberg, and B. E. Bjarngard. Measurement of reciprocity law failure in green-sensitive x-ray films. *Radiology*, 126:493 – 498, 1978.
6. J. C. Bamber and M. Tristam. Diagnostic ultrasound. In S. Webb, editor, *The Physics Of Medical Imaging*, Medical Science Series. Institute of Physics Publishing, Bristol and Philadelphia, 1988.
7. G. T. Barnes. Radiographic mottle : A comprehensive theory. *Medical Physics*, 9(5):656 – 667, 1986.
8. G. T. Barnes and I. Brezovich. The intensity of scattered radiation in mammography. *Radiology*, 126:243 –247, 1978.
9. H. Barrett and W. Swindell. *Radiological Imaging*. Academic Press, 1981.
10. S. I. Barry and G. K. Aldis. Comparison of models for flow induced deformation of soft biological tissue. *Journal of Biomechanics*, 23:647 – 654, 1990.
11. M. Baum. Breast cancer : The facts, 1981.
12. U. Behrens, J. Teubner, C. J. G. Eversatz, M. Walz, H. Juergens, and H. Peitgen. Computer assisted dynamic evaluation of contrast-enhanced breast MRI. In H. U. Lemke, M. W. Vannier, K. Inamura, and A. G. Farman, editors, *CAR'96 Computer Assisted Radiology*, Excerpta Medica, International Congress Series 1124, pages 362–367. Elsevier, June 1996.
13. R. Birch, M. Marshall, and G. M. Ardam. Catalogue of spectral data for diagnostic x-rays. HPA Scientific Report Series 30, Hospital Physics Association, London, 1979.
14. R. L. Birdwell, D. M. Ikeda, S. S. Jeffrey, and R. B. Jeffrey Jr. Preliminary experience with power Doppler imaging of solid breast masses. *Amer. J. Roentgenology*, 169:703–707, 1997.
15. C. M. Bishop. *Neural Networks for Pattern Recognition*. Oxford University Press, 1995.
16. A. Blake and A. Zisserman. *Visual Reconstruction*. Series in Artifical Intelligence. M.I.T. Press, 1987.
17. H. Blume, S. Daly, and E. Muka. Presentation of medical images on CRT displays. *SPIE Vol 1897: Image Capture, Formatting and Display*, pages 215 – 231, 1993.
18. H. Blume, H. Roehrig, M. Browne, and T. Ji. Comparison of the physical performance of high resolution CRT displays and films recorded by laser image printers and displayed on light-boxes and the need for a display standard. *SPIE Vol 1232:*

Medical Imaging IV: Image Capture and Display, pages 97 – 113, 1990.

19. E. Bombardieri, F. Crippa, L. Maffioli, and M. Greco. Nuclear medicine techniques for the study of breast cancer. *Euro. J. Nuc. Med.*, 24:809–824, 1997.

20. F. Bookstein. Principal warps: thin-plate splines and the decomposition of deformations. *IEEE Trans. Patt. Anal. and Mach. Intell.*, 11:567 – 585, 1989.

21. S. G. Bown. Laser techniques for cancer therapy. In J. Newsom-Davis and D. J. Weatherall, editors, *Health Policy and Technological Innovation*. Chapman and Hall (Royal Society Technical Meeting Proceedings), London, 1994.

22. K. Bowyer, M. Sallam, G. Hubiak, and L. Clarke. Screening mammogram images for abnormalities developing over time. In *IEEE Nuclear Science Symposium and Medical Imaging Conference*, pages 1270–1272, 1992.

23. D. S. Brettle, J. Thompson, G. J. S. Parkin, and A. R. Cowen. Dual compression mammography using computed radiography. *British J. Radiology*, pages 761 – 763, 1995.

24. G. Brix, W. Semmler, L. R. Schad, G. Layer, and W. Lorenz. Pharmacokinetic parameters in CNS Gd-DTPA enhanced MR imaging. *J. Comp. Assisted Tomog.*, 15:621–628, 1991.

25. M. Bro-Nielsen. *Medical Image Registration and Surgery Simulation*. PhD thesis, Dept of Mathematical Modelling, Technical University of Denmark, 1996.

26. D. Brzakovic, N. Vujovic, V. Neskovic, P. Brzakovic, and B. Fogarty. Mammogram analysis by comparison with previous screenings. In A. Gale, S. Astley, D. Dance, and A. Cairns, editors, *2nd International Workshop on Digital Mammography*, Excerpta Medica International Congress Series 1069, pages 131–139, York, England, 10–12 July 1994. Elsevier Science B.V.

27. F. Buchmann. Extrafocal radiation. *Medica Mundi*, 39:94 – 97, 1994.

28. D. Buckley, R. Kerslake, S. Blackband, and A. Horsman. Quantitative analysis of multi-slice Gd-DTPA enhanced dynamic MR images using a automated simplex minimization procedure. *Magnetic Resonance in Medicine*, 32:646–651, 1994.

29. A. Burch and J. Law. A method for estimating compressed breast thickness during mammography. *British J. Radiology*, 68:394 – 399, 1995.

30. B. Burkhardt, P. Schnur, J. Tufield, and P. Dempsey. Objective clinical assessment of fibrous capsular contrature. *Plastic and Reconstructive Surgery*, 69:794, 1982.

31. C. B. Caldwell and M. J. Yaffe. Development of an anthropomorphic breast phantom. *Medical Physics*, 17(2):273 – 280, 1990.

32. G. A. Carlsson, D. R. Dance, and J. Persliden. Grids in mammography: Optimization of the information content relative to radiation risk. Technical Report ULi-RAD-R-059, Linkoping University, Department of Radiation Physics, 1989.

33. P. L. Carson, D. D. Adler, J. B. Fowlkes, K. Harnist, and J. Rubin. Enhanced color flow imaging of breast cancer vasculature: continuous wave Doppler and three-dimensional display. *J. Ultrasound Med.*, 11:377–385, 1992.

34. J. Caseldine, R. Blamey, E. J. Roebuck, and C. Elston. *Breast Disease for Radiographers*. Wright, 1988.

35. N. J. Cerneaz. *Model-based analysis of mammograms*. PhD thesis, Engineering Science, Oxford University, Parks Road, Oxford, OX1 3PJ, UK, 1994.

36. N. J. Cerneaz and M. Brady. Finding curvilinear structures in mammograms. In N. Ayache, editor, *First International Conference on Computer Vision, Virtual Reality and Robotics in Medicine, CVRMed'95*, Lecture Notes in Computer Science, pages 372 – 382, Nice, France, April 1995. Springer-Verlag.

37. H. P. Chan, K. Doi, C. Galhotra, C. J. Vyborny, H. MacMahon, and P. M. Jokich. Image feature analysis and computer-aided diagnosis in digital radiography: I. automated detection of microcalcifications in mammograms. *Medical Physics*, 14(4):538–548, 1987.

38. H. P. Chan, K. Doi, K. L. Lam, C. J. Vyborny, and R. A. Schmidt. Computer-aided detection of microcalcifications in mammograms: methodology and preliminary clinical study. *Investigative Radiology*, 23(9):664 – 671, 1988.

39. H. P. Chan, K. Doi, H. MacMahon, C. Metz, E. Sickles, and C. Vyborny. Digital mammography - ROC studies of the effects of pixel size and unsharp-mask filtering on the detection of subtle microcalcifications. *Investigative Radiology*, 22:581 – 589, 1987.

40. E. J. Chen, R. S. Adler, P. L. Carson, W. K. Jenkins, and W. D. O'Brien Jr. Ultrasound tissue displacement imaging with application to breast cancer. *Ultrasound in Med. and Biol.*, 21:1153–1162, 1995.

41. Y. Chitre, A. P. Dhawan, and M. Moskowitz. Classification of mammographic microcalcifications using image structure and cluster features. In A. Gale, S. M. Astley, D. Dance, and A. Cairns, editors, *2nd International Workshop on Digital Mammography*, Excerpta Medica International Congress Series 1069, pages 31–40, York, England, 10–12 July 1994. Elsevier Science B.V.

42. G.E. Christensen, R.D. Rabbitt, and M.I. Miller. 3D brain mapping using a deformable neuroanatomy. *Physics in Medicine and Biology*, 39:609–618, 1994.

43. S. Ciatto, L. Cataliotti, and V. Distante. Non-palpable lesions detected with mammography: 512 consecutive cases. *Radiology*, 165:99–102, 1987.

44. E. Claridge. Characterisation of mammographic lesions. In A. Gale, S.M. Astley, D.R. Dance, and A.Y. Cairns, editors, *2nd International Workshop on Digital Mammography*, Excerpta Medica International Congress Series 1069, pages 241 – 250, York, England, 10–12 July 1994. Elsevier Science B.V.

45. D. J. Clark, I. R. Chambers, K. Faulkner, J. Rayson, P. M. Hacking, and J. Milton. Pressure measurements during automatic breast compression in mammography. *J. Biomedical Engineering*, 12:444 – 446, 1990.

46. R. C. Cory and S. S. Linden. The mammographic density of breast cancer. *Amer. J. Roentgenology*, 160:418 – 418, 1993.

47. D. O. Cosgrove, J. C. Bamber, J. B. Davey, J. A. McKinna, and H. D. Sinnett. Color Doppler signals from breast tumours. *Radiology*, 176:175–180, 1990.

48. D. O. Cosgrove, R. P. Kedar, J. C. Bamber, and et. al. Breast diseases: color Doppler US in differential diagnosis. *Radiology*, 189:99–104, 1993.

49. D. R. Dance. An introduction to the physics of mammography. In K Faulkner, editor, *Physics in Diagnostic Radiology*, pages 1 – 11. Institute of Physical Sciences in Medicine, York, UK, 1990.

50. D. R. Dance and G. J. Day. Computation of scatter in mammography by Monte Carlo methods. *Physics in Medicine and Biology*, 29:237 – 247, 1984.

51. D. R. Dance, J. Persliden, and G. A. Carlsson. Calculation of dose and contrast for two mammographic grids. *Physics in Medicine and Biology*, 37:235 – 248, 1992.

52. T. H. Dao, A. Rahmouni, F. Campana, M. Laurent, B. Asselain, and A. Fourquet. Tumor recurrence versus fibrosis in the irradiated breast: differentiation with dynamic gadolinium-enhanced MR imaging. *Radiology*, 187:751–755, 1993.

53. N. Dash. Magnetic resonance imaging in the diagnosis of breast disease. *Amer. J. Roentgenology*, 146:119–125, 1986.

54. D. H. Davies. Digital mammography - the comparative evaluation of film digitizers. *British J. Radiology*, 66:930 – 933, 1993.

55. D. H. Davies, D. R. Dance, and C. H. Jones. Automatic detection of microcalcifications in digital mammograms using local area thresholding techniques. *SPIE Medical Imaging III: Image Processing*, 1092:153 – 161, 1989.

56. G. J. Day and D. R. Dance. X-ray transmission formula for antiscatter grids. *Physics in Medicine and Biology*, 28:1429 – 1433, 1983.

57. P. B. Dean. Overview of breast cancer screening. In K. Doi, M. L. Giger, R. M. Nishikawa, and R. A. Schmidt, editors, *3rd International Workshop on Digital Mammography*, Excerpta Medica International Congress Series 1119, pages 19–26, Chicago, USA, June 1996. Elsevier Science B.V.

58. J. Declerck, G. Subsol, J-P. Thirion, and N. Ayache. Automatic retrieval of anatomical structures in 3D medical images. Technical Report 2485, INRIA, Sophia Antipolis, France, 1995.

59. L. Desponds, C. Depeursinge, M. Grecescu, C. Hessler, A. Samiri, and J. F. Valley. Image quality index for screen-film mammography. *Physics in Medicine and Biology*, 36:19 – 33, 1991.

60. M. H. Dilhuydy. *Anomalies Mammographiques Infracliniques*. Fondation Bergonie, Bordeaux, France, 1994.

61. M. H. Dilhuydy. *Imagerie du Cancer du Sein*. Fondation Bergonie, Bordeaux, France, 1996.

62. J. M. Dinten, J. M. Volle, and M. Darboux. Quantitative interpretation of mammograms based on a physical model of the image formation process. In N. Karssemeijer, editor, *4th International Workshop on Digital Mammography*, pages 267 – 274, Nijmegen, Netherlands, 1998. Kluwer Academic Publishers.

63. R. O. Duda and P. E. Hart. *Pattern Classification and Scene Analysis*. Wiley, 1973.

64. J. M. Egan. A constitutive model for the mechanical behaviour of soft connective tissues. *Journal of Biomechanics*, 20:681 – 692, 1987.

65. G. W. Eklund. Mammographic compression: science or art? *Radiology*, 181:339 – 341, 1991.

66. S. J. el Yousef, R. H. Duchesneau, R. J. Alfidi, J. R. Haaga, P. J. Bryan, and J. P. Lipuma. Magnetic resonance imaging of the breast. *Radiology*, 150:761–766, 1984.

67. P. J. Ell. Keeping abreast of time. *Euro. J. Nuc. Med.*, 22:967–969, 1995.

68. J. Esteve, A. Kricker, J. Ferlay, and D. M. Parkin. Facts and figures of cancer in the European Community. Technical report, International Agency for Research on Cancer, Lyon, France, 1993.

69. A. Fandos-Morera, M. Prats-Esteve, J. M. Tura-Soteras, and A. Traveria-Cros. Breast tumours: composition of microcalcifications. *Radiology*, 169:325–327, 1988.

70. O.D. Faugeras. *Three-Dimensional Computer Vision: A Geometric Viewpoint*. MIT Press, 1993.

71. S. Feig. Breast masses: mammographic and sonographic evaluation. *Radiol. Clin. North Am.*, 30:67–92, 1992.

72. K. Ferrara and G. DeAngelis. Color flow mapping. *Ultrasound in Med. and Biol.*, 23:321–346, 1997.

73. I. Fife. The physical dimensions of compressed breasts. *British J. Radiology*, 64:73 – 74, 1991.

74. B. Fisher, C. Redmond, R. Poisson, and et. al. Eight-year result of a randomized clinical trial comparing total mastectomy and lumpectomy with or without irradiation in the treatment of breast cancer. *New England Journal of Medicine*, 320:822–828, 1989.

75. M. M. Fleck. Spectre: an improved phantom edge finder. In *Proceedings of the 5th Alvey Vision Conference*, pages 127–132, University of Reading, UK, 25–28 September 1989.

76. M. M. Fleck. Multiple widths yield reliable finite differences. *IEEE Trans. Patt. Anal. and Mach. Intell.*, 14(4):412–429, April 1992.

77. Chris Flowers, editor. *Image Guided Core Biopsy of the Breast - A Practical Approach*. Greenwich Medical Media (distributed by Oxford University Press), 1998.

78. B. D. Fornage. Ultrasound of the breast. *Ultrasound Quarterly*, 11(1):1–39, 1993.

79. P. Forrest. *Breast Cancer Screening. Report to the Health Ministers of England, Wales, Scotland and Northern Ireland*. HMSO, London, UK, 1986.

80. E. T. Fossel, G. Brodsky, J. L. DeLayre, and R. E. Wilson. Nuclear magnetic resonance for the differentiation of benign and malignant breast tissues and auxillary lymph nodes. *Annals of Surgery*, 198:541–545, 1983.

81. E. E. Frederick, M. R. Squillante, L. J. Cirignano, R. W. Hahn, and G. Entine. Accurate automatic exposure controller for mammography: Design and performance. *Radiology*, 178:393 – 396, 1991.

82. I. M. Freundlich, T. B. Hunter, G. W. Seeley, C. J. D'Orsi, and N. L. Sadowsky.

Computer-assisted analysis of mammographic clustered calcifications. *Clinical Radiology*, 40:296 – 298, 1989.

83. M. Le Gal, J.-C. Durand, M. Laurent, and D. Pellier. Conduite a tenir devant une mammographie revelatrice de microcalcifications groupées sans tumeur palpable. *La Nouvelle Presse Medicale*, 5:1621–1627, 1973.

84. M. Le Gal, L. Ollivier, B. Asselain, and et. al. Mammographic features of 455 invasive carcinomas. *Radiology*, 185:705–708, 1992.

85. M. Galea and R. W. Blamey. Diagnosis by team work: an approach to conservation. *British Medical Bulletin*, 47:295–304, 1991.

86. S. Geman and D. Geman. Stochastic relaxation, Gibbs distribution, and the Bayesian restoration of images. *IEEE Trans. Patt. Anal. and Mach. Intell.*, 6(6):721–741, 1984.

87. G. E. Giakoumakis and D. M. Miliotis. Light angular distribution of fluorescent screens excited by x-rays. *Physics in Medicine and Biology*, 30(1):21 – 29, 1985.

88. R. Gilles, J. M. Guinebretière, L. Shapiro, and et. al. Assessment of breast cancer recurrences with contrast enhanced subtraction MR imaging: preliminary results in 26 patients. *Radiology*, 188:473–478, 1993.

89. R. Gilles, B. Mesurolle, A. Tardivon, J. M. Guinebretière, J. Masselot, and D. Vanel. Aspects cliniques et mammographiques des rechutes locales des cancers du sein. *Rev. Im. Med.*, 5(12):761–765, 1993.

90. S. Gilles, M. Brady, J.-P. Thirion, and N. Ayache. Bias field correction of breast MR images. In Karl Heinz Hoehne and Ron Kikinis, editors, *Visualisation in Biomedical Computation (VBC'96)*, Lecture notes in computer science 1131, pages 153–158, Hamburg, September 1996. Springer Verlag.

91. R. C. Gonzalez and P. Wintz. *Digital Image Processing*. Addison-Wesley, 2nd edition, 1987.

92. Guidelines for surgeons in the management of symptomatic breast disease in the United Kingdom. *Eur. J. Surg. Oncol.*, 21:1–13, 1995.

93. R. Guillemaud and M. Brady. Enhancement of MR images. In Karl Heinz Hoehne and Ron Kikinis, editors, *Visualisation in Biomedical Computation (VBC'96)*, Lecture notes in computer science 1131, pages 107–116, Hamburg, September 1996. Springer Verlag.

94. R. Guissin and M. Brady. Iso-intensity contours for edge detection. Technical Report OUEL 1935/92, Department of Engineering Science, Oxford University, Parks Road, Oxford, OX1 3PJ, UK, 1992.

95. L. Gylbert. Applanation tonometry for the evaluation of breast compressibility. *Scandinavian Journal of Plastic and Reconstructive Surgery*, 23:223, 1989.

96. L. Gylbert and A. Berggren. Constant compression caliper for objective measurement of breast capsullar contracture. *Scandinavian Journal of Plastic and Reconstructive Surgery*, 23:137 – 142, 1989.

97. C. C. Haagensen. *Disease of the Breast*. W.B.Saunders Company, 1986.

98. G. R. Hammerstein, D. W. Miller, D. R. White, M. E. Masterson, H. Q. Woodard, and J. S. Laughlin. Absorbed radiation dose in mammography. *Radiology*, 130:485 – 491, 1979.

99. W. Hand, J. L. Semmlow, L. V. Ackerman, and F. S. Alcorn. Computer screening of xeromammograms: a technique for defining suspicious areas of the breast. *Computers and Biomedical Research*, 12:445–460, 1979.

100. R. M. Haralick and L. G. Shapiro. *Computer and Robot Vision*, volume 1. Addison-Wesley Publishing, Reading, Mass., 1992.

101. R. M. Haralick, S.Sternberg, and X.Zhuang. Image analysis using mathematical morpholgy. *IEEE Trans. Patt. Anal. and Mach. Intell.*, 9:532 – 550, 1987.

102. A. G. Haus, R. W. Cowart, G. D. Dodd, and J. Bencomo. A method of evaluating and minimizing geometric unsharpness for mammographic x-ray units. *Radiology*, 128:775 – 778, 1978.

103. A. G. Haus, C. E. Metz, K. Doi, and J. Bernstein. Determination of x-ray spectra

incident on and transmitted through breast tissue. *Radiology*, 124:511 – 513, 1977.

104. P. Hayton. *Analysis of contrast enhanced breast MR images*. PhD thesis, Engineering Science, Oxford University, Parks Road, Oxford, OX1 3PJ, UK, 1998.

105. P. Hayton, M. Brady, L. Tarassenko, and N. R. Moore. Analysis of dynamic MR breast images using a model of contrast enhancement. *Medical Image Analysis*, 1(3):1–18, 1996.

106. G. E. Healey and R. Kondepudy. Radiometric CCD camera calibration and noise estimation. *IEEE Trans. Patt. Anal. and Mach. Intell.*, 16:267 – 276, 1994.

107. M. A. Helvie, H. P. Chan, D. D. Adler, and P. G. Boyd. Breast thickness in routine mammograms - effect on image quality and radiation dose. *Amer. J. Roentgenology*, pages 1371 – 1374, 1994.

108. A. Hernandez, O. Basset, I. Dautraix, and I. E. Magnin. Acquisition and stereoscopic visualization of three-dimensional ultrasonic breast data. *IEEE Trans. Ultrasonics, Ferroelectrics, and Frequency Control*, 43:576–580, 1996.

109. S. H. Heywang-Köebrunner. Nonmammographic breast imaging techniques. *Current Opinions in Radiology*, 4:146–154, 1992.

110. S. H. Heywang-Köebrunner, R. Basserman, G. Fenzi, W. Nathrath, D. Hahn, R. Beck, I. Krische, and W. Eiermann. MRI of the breast histopathological correlation. *Euro. J. Radiology*, 7:175–182, 1987.

111. S. H. Heywang-Köebrunner, T. Hilbertz, R. Beck, and et. al. Gd-DTPA enhanced MR imaging of the breast in patients with postoperative scarring and silicon implants. *J. Comp. Assisted Tomog.*, 14:348–356, 1990.

112. S. H. Heywang-Köebrunner, A. Wolf, E. Pruss, and et. al. MR imaging of the breast with Gd-DTPA: use and limitations. *Radiology*, 171:95–103, 1989.

113. P. F. Hickman, N. R. Moore, and B. J. Shepstone. The indeterminate breast mass: assessment using contrast enhanced magnetic resonance imagery. *British J. Radiology*, 67:14–20, 1994.

114. R. P. Highnam. *Model-based enhancement of mammographic images*. PhD thesis, Computing Laboratory, Oxford University, Parks Road, Oxford, OX1 3PJ, UK, 1992.

115. R. P. Highnam and M. Brady. Model-based enhancement of far infra-red images. *IEEE Trans. Patt. Anal. and Mach. Intell.*, 19:410 – 415, 1997.

116. R. P. Highnam, M. Brady, and B. J. Shepstone. Computing the scatter component of mammographic images. *IEEE Trans. Med. Imaging*, 13:301 – 313, June 1994.

117. R. P. Highnam, M. Brady, and B. J. Shepstone. A representation for mammographic image processing. *Medical Image Analysis*, 1:1 – 19, 1996.

118. R. P. Highnam, M. Brady, and B. J. Shepstone. The h_{int} representation and calcifications. In *Medical Image Understanding and Analysis 97*, pages 121 – 124, Oxford, UK, 1997. BMVA.

119. R. P. Highnam, M. Brady, and B. J. Shepstone. Mammographic image analysis. *Euro. J. Radiology*, 24:20 – 32, 1997.

120. R. P. Highnam, M. Brady, and B. J. Shepstone. Estimation of breast thickness in mammography. *British J. Radiology*, pages 646 – 653, June 1998.

121. R. P. Highnam, Y. Kita, M. Brady, B. J. Shepstone, and R. E. English. Determing correspondence between views. In N. Karssemeijer, editor, *4th International Workshop on Digital Mammography*, pages 111 – 118, Nijmegen, Netherlands, 1998. Kluwer Academic Publishers.

122. R. P. Highnam, B. J. Shepstone, and M. Brady. Mammograms at different compression plate widths for the detection of breast cancer. In *Radiology and Oncology 91, Work in Progress*, page 3. British Institute of Radiology, 1991.

123. R. P. Highnam, B. J. Shepstone, and M. Brady. Mammograms at different compressions for the detection of breast cancer. In *Symposium Mammographicum, Imperial College, London*, 1992.

124. R. P. Highnam, B. J. Shepstone, and M. Brady. Mammograms at different compressions for the detection of breast cancer. *British J. Radiology*, 1996.

125. U. Hoffmann, G. Brix, M. V. Knopp, T. Heß, and W. J. Lorenz. Pharmacokinetic mapping of the breast: A new method for dynamic MR mammography. *Magnetic Resonance in Medicine*, 33:506–514, 1995.

126. B. K. P. Horn and B. G. Schunck. Determining optical flow. *Artificial Intelligence*, 17:185–203, 1981.

127. J. Huang, J. Fox, C. Gordon, and A. Jackson-Smale. Symbolic decision support in medical care. *Artificial Intelligence in Medicine*, 5:415–430, 1993.

128. S. Huber, S. Delorme, M. V. Knopp, H. Junkermann, I. Zuna, D. von Fournier, and G. van Kaick. Breast tumours: computer assisted quantitative assessment with color Doppler US. *Radiology*, 192:797–801, 1994.

129. I. W. Hutt, S. M. Astley, and C. R. M. Boggis. Prompting as an aid to diagnosis in mammography. In A. Gale, S. M. Astley, D. Dance, and A. Y. Cairns, editors, *2nd International Workshop on Digital Mammography*, Excerpta Medica International Congress Series 1069, pages 388 – 389, York, England, 10–12 July 1994. Elsevier Science B.V.

130. D. Ikeda and I. Anderson. Ductal carcinoma in situ: atypical mammographic appearances. *Radiology*, 172:661–666, 1989.

131. V. Jackson, K. Dines, L. Bassett, R. Gold, and H. Reynolds. Diagnostic importance of the radiographic density of noncalcified breast masses: analysis of 91 lesions. *Amer. J. Roentgenology*, 157:25–28, 1991.

132. V. P. Jackson, A. M. Lex, and D. J. Smith. Patient discomfort during screen-film mammography. *Radiology*, 168:421 – 423, 1988.

133. C. E. Jamison, R. D. Marangoni, and A. A. Glaser. Viscoelastic properties of soft tissue by discrete model characterization. *Journal of Biomechanics*, 1:33 – 46, 1968.

134. R. Jennings, R. Eastgate, M. Siedband, and D. Ergan. Optimal x-ray spectra for screen-film mammography. *Medical Physics*, 8:629 – 639, 1981.

135. T. Ji, H. Roehrig, H. Blume, and J. Guillen. Optimizing the display function of display devices. *SPIE Vol 1653: Image Capture, Formatting and Display*, pages 126 – 139, 1992.

136. P. C. Johns and M. J. Yaffe. Coherent scatter in diagnostic radiation. *Medical Physics*, 10:40 – 50, 1983.

137. P. C. Johns and M. J. Yaffe. X-ray characterisation of normal and neoplastic breast tissue. *Physics in Medicine and Biology*, 32:675 – 695, 1987.

138. W. A. Kaiser. Dynamic magnetic resonance breast imaging using a double breast coil: an important step towards routine examination of the breast. *Frontiers in European Radiology*, 7:39–68, 1990.

139. W. A. Kaiser and E. Zeitler. MR imaging of the breast: fast imaging sequences with and without Gd-DTPA. *Radiology*, 170:681–686, 1989.

140. N. Karssemeijer. Stochastic model for automated detection of calcifications in digital mammograms. *Image and Vision Computing*, 10(6):369 – 375, 1992.

141. N. Karssemeijer. Adaptive noise equalization and recognition of microcalcification clusters in mammograms. *Int. J. of Pattern Recog. and Artif. Intell.*, 7:1357 – 1376, 1993.

142. N. Karssemeijer, J. T. M. Frieling, and J. H. C. L. Hendricks. Spatial resolution in digital mammography. *Investigative Radiology*, 29:413–419, 1993.

143. N. Karssemeijer and G. M. te Brake. Detection of stellate distortions in mammograms. *IEEE Trans. Med. Imaging*, 15:611 – 619, 1996.

144. N. Karssemeijer and L. van Erning. Iso-precision scaling of digitized mammograms to facilitate image analysis. In *SPIE Medical Imaging V : Image Processing*, volume 1445, pages 166 – 177, 1991.

145. R. P. Kedar, D. Cosgrove, V. R. McCready, J. C. Bamber, and E. R. Carter. Microbubble contrast agent for color Doppler US: effect on breast masses. *Radiology*, 198:679–686, 1996.

146. W. P. Kegelmeyer and M. C. Allmen. Dense feature maps for the detection of

microcalcifications. In A. Gale, S. M. Astley, D. Dance, and A. Cairns, editors, *2nd International Workshop on Digital Mammography*, Excerpta Medica International Congress Series 1069, pages 3–13, York, England, 10–12 July 1994. Elsevier Science B.V.

147. G. M. Keibert, J. C.J.M. de Haes, and C. J. H. van der Velde. The impact of breast conserving treatment and mastectomy on the quality of life of early breast cancer patients: a review. *J. Clin. Oncol.*, 9:1059–1070, 1991.

148. I. Khalkali, J. A. Cutrone, I. G. Mena, L. E. Diggles, R. J. Venegas, H. I. Vargas, B. L. Jackson, S. Khalkali, J. F. Moss, and S. R. Klein. Scintimammography: the complementary role of $^{99}Tc^m$-Sestamibi prone breast imaging for the diagnosis of breast carcinoma. *Radiology*, 196:421–426, 1995.

149. C. Kimme, B. O'Loughlin, and J. Sklansky. Automatic detection of suspicious abnormalities in breast radiographs. In T. L. Kunii A. Klinger, K. S. Fu, editor, *Data Structures, Computer Graphics and Pattern Recognition*, pages 427 – 447. Academic Press, New York, 1977.

150. C. Kimme-Smith, L. W. Bassett, R. H. Gold, and S. Chow. Increased radiation dose in mammography due to prolonged exposure, delayed processing, and increased film darkening. *Radiology*, 178:387 – 391, 1991.

151. Y. Kita, R. P. Highnam, and M. Brady. Correspondence between two different views of x-ray mammograms using simulation of breast deformation. In *Computer Vision and Pattern Recognition Conference*, Santa Barbara, California, USA, June 1998. Computer Society Press.

152. D. J. Klein, H. P. Chan, E. P. Muntz, K. Doi, K. Lee, P. Chopelas, H. Bernstein, and J. Lee. Experimental and theoretical energy and angular dependencies of scattered radiation in the mammography energy range. *Medical Physics*, 10:664 – 668, 1983.

153. S. L. Kok-Wiles. *Comparing mammogram pairs in the detection of mammographic lesions*. PhD thesis, Engineering Science, Oxford University, Parks Road, Oxford, OX1 3PJ, UK, 1998.

154. S. L. Kok-Wiles, M. Brady, and R. P. Highnam. Comparing mammogram pairs for the detection of lesions. In N. Karssemeijer, editor, *4th International Workshop on Digital Mammography*, pages 103 – 108, Nijmegen, Netherlands, 1998. Kluwer Academic Publishers.

155. S. Kumar and D. Goldgof. Recovery of global non-rigid motion - a model based approach without point correspondences. In *Proc. CVPR '96*, pages 18–20, San Francisco, June 1996. IEEE Press.

156. K. Lam and H. P. Chan. Effects of beam equalization on mammographic imaging. *Medical Physics*, 17:242 – 249, 1990.

157. J-L. Lamarque. An Atlas of the Breast, 1988.

158. M. Lanyi. *Diagnosis and Differential Diagnosis of Microcalcifications*. Springer-Verlag, 1987.

159. T. Lau and W. F. Bischof. On techniques for detecting circumscribed masses in mammograms. *Computers and Biomedical Research*, 24:273–295, 1991.

160. J. Law. The influence of focal spot size on image resolution and test phantom scores in mammography. *British J. Radiology*, 66:441 – 446, 1993.

161. D. L. Lee, L. K. Cheung, L. S. Jeromim, and E. Palecki. Imaging performance of a direct digital radiographic detector using selenium and a thin-film transistor array. In H.U. Lemke, M. W. Vannier, K. Inamura, and A. G. Farman, editors, *Computer Assisted Radiology: CAR 96*, International Congress Series 1124, pages 41–46, Paris, June 1996. Elsevier Excerpta Medica.

162. F. Lefebvre, H. Benali, R. Gilles, and R. D. Paola. A simulation model of clustered breast microcalcifications. *Medical Physics*, 21(12):1865–1874, 1994.

163. H. G. Lewis-Jones, G. H. Whitehouse, and S. J. Leinster. The role of magnetic resonance imaging in the assessment of local recurrent breast carcinoma. *Clinical Radiology*, 43:197–204, 1991.

164. T. Lindeberg. Detecting salient blob-like image structures and their scales with a scale-space primal sketch. *The International Journal of Computer Vision*, 11:283–318, 1993.

165. D.G. Luenberger. *Introduction to Linear and Non-Linear Programming*. Addison-Wesley, 1973.

166. S. D. Magalhaes, J. Eichler, and O. Goncalves. Calculation on x-ray scattering of 17.4kev radiation and image degradation in mammography. *Nuclear Instruments and Methods in Physics Research B*, 95:87 – 90, 1995.

167. I. Magnin, M. Alaoui, and A. Bremond. Automatic microcalcifications pattern recognition from x-ray mammograms. In *SPIE: Science and Engineering in Medical Imaging*, volume 1137, pages 170–175, 1989.

168. A. D. Maidment, M. Albert, E. F. Conant, and S. A. Feig. Three dimensional visualisation of breast cancer. In N. Karssemeijer, editor, *4th International Workshop on Digital Mammography*, pages 57 – 60. Kluwer Academic Publishing, Nijmegen, Netherlands, 1998.

169. A. D. Maidment and M. J. Yaffe. Analysis of signal propagation in optically coupled detectors for digital mammography: I. phosphor screens. *Physics in Medicine and Biology*, pages 877 – 889, 1995.

170. A. D. Maidment, M. J. Yaffe, D. B. Plewes, G. E. Mawdsley, I. C. Soutar, and B. G. Starkowski. Imaging performance of a prototype scanned-slot digital mammography system. *SPIE*, 1896:93–103, 1993.

171. J. B. A. Maintz and M. A. Viergever. A survey of medical image registration. *Medical Image Analysis*, 2(1):1–36, 1998.

172. D. W. Marquart. An algorithm for least squares estimation of non-linear parameters. *Journal of the Society of Applied Mathematics*, 11:431–441, 1963.

173. J. Merron and M. Brady. Isotropic gradient estimation. In *Proc. IEEE Conf. on Computer Vision and Pattern Recognition*, volume 2, pages 652–659, San Francisco, June 1996. IEEE Computer Society Press.

174. P. Miller and S. Astley. Automated detection of mammographic asymmetry using anatomical features. *Int. J. Pattern Recog. and Artif. Intell.*, 7:1461–1476, 1993.

175. B. S. Monsees. Evaluation of breast microcalcifications. *Radiol. Clin. North Am.*, 33(3):1109–1121, 1995.

176. J. R. Moore. Applanation tonometry of breasts. *Plastic and Reconstructive Surgery*, 63:9, 1979.

177. A. Moskalik, P. L. Carson, C. R. Meyer, J. B. Fowlkes, J. M. Rubin, and M. A. Roubidoux. Registration of three-dimensional compound ultrasound scans of the breast for refraction and motion correction. *Ultrasound in Med. and Biol.*, 21:769–778, 1995.

178. H. Mumtaz, M. A. Hall-Craggs, and et. al. Laser therapy for breast cancer: MR imaging and histopathological correlation. *Radiology*, 200:651–658, 1996.

179. E. P. Muntz, T. Fewell, R. Jennings, and H. Bernstein. On the significance of very small angle scattered radiation to radiographic imaging at low energies. *Medical Physics*, 10:819 – 823, 1983.

180. S. Naimuddin, B. Hasegawa, and C. Mistretta. Scatter-glare correction using a convolution algorithm with variable weighting. *Medical Physics*, 14:330 – 334, 1987.

181. J. A. Nelder and R. Mead. A simplex method for function minimisation. *Computer Journal*, 7:308–313, 1965.

182. L. T. Niklason, B. T. Christian, L. E. Niklason, D. B. Kopans, P. J. Slanetz, D. E. Castleberry, B. H. Opsahl-Ong, C. E. Landberg, and B. Giambattista. Digital breast tomosynthesis: potentially a new method for breast cancer screening. In N. Karssemeijer, editor, *4th International Workshop on Digital Mammography*, pages 51 – 56. Kluwer Academic Publishing, Nijmegen, Netherlands, 1998.

183. R. M. Nishikawa, M. L. Giger, C. J. Vyborny, and R. A. Schmidt. Computer-aided detection of clustered microcalcifications: an improved method for grouping

detected signals. *Medical Physics*, 20(6):1661–1666, 1993.

184. R. M. Nishikawa, Y. Jiang, M. L. Giger, and et. al. Performance of automated cad schemes for the detection and classification of clustered microcalcifications. In A. Gale, S. M. Astley, D. Dance, and A. Y. Cairns, editors, *2nd International Workshop on Digital Mammography*, Excerpta Medica International Congress Series 1069, pages 13–20, York, England, 10–12 July 1994. Elsevier Science B.V.

185. R. M. Nishikawa and M. J. Yaffe. Signal-to-noise properties of mammographic film-screen systems. *Medical Physics*, 12:32 – 39, 1985.

186. J. A. Noble. *Descriptions of image surfaces*. PhD thesis, Engineering Science, Oxford University, Parks Road, Oxford, OX1 3PJ, UK, 1989.

187. R. Novak. *Transformation of the female breast during compression at mammography with special reference to the importance for localization of a lesion*. PhD thesis, Department of Diagnostic Radiology at Lakarhuset and Karolinska Sjukhuset, Sweden, 1989. Acta Radiologica Supplement 371.

188. C. W. Oomens, D. H. van Campen, and H. J. Grootenboer. A mixture approach to the mechanics of skin. *Journal of Biomechanics*, 20:877 – 885, 1987.

189. M. M. Osman and E. M. Afify. Thermal modeling of the normal woman's breast. *Journal of Biomechanical Engineering*, pages 123 – 130, 1984.

190. M. M. Osman and E. M. Afify. Thermal modeling of the malignant woman's breast. *Journal of Biomechanical Engineering*, pages 269 – 276, 1988.

191. J. Parker, D. R. Dance, and D. H. Davies. Classification of ductal carcinoma in-situ by image-analysis of calcifications from digital mammograms. *British J. Radiology*, 68:150–159, 1995.

192. K. J. Parker, S. R. Huang, R. A. Musulin, and R. M. Lerner. Tissue response to mechanical vibrations for sonoelasticity imaging. *Ultrasound in Med. and Biol.*, 16:241 – 246, 1990.

193. T. C. Parr, S. M. Astley, C. J. Taylor, and C. R. Boggis. Model-based classification of linear structures in digital mammograms. In *3rd International Workshop on Digital Mammography*, Excerpta Medica International Congress Series 1119, Chicago, USA, 9-12th June 1996. Elsevier Science.

194. J. Patnick, editor. *NHS Breast Screening Programme Review 1996*. NHS Breast Screening Programme, Old Fulwood Road, Sheffield, England, 1996.

195. E. A. Patrick, M. Moskowitz, V. T. Mansukhani, and E. I. Gruenstein. Expert learning system network for diagnosis of breast calcifications. *Investigative Radiology*, 26:534–539, 1991.

196. D. R. Pennes and M. J. Horner. Disappearing breast masses caused by compression during mammography. *Radiology*, 165:327, 1987.

197. M. E. Peters, D. R. Voegeli, and K. A. Scanlan. *Breast Imaging*. Churchill Livingstone (London, New York, Melbourne), 1989.

198. S. Piccolo, S. Lastoria, C. Mainolfi, P. Muto, L. Bazzicalupo, and M. Salvatore. Breast scintigraphy with $^{99}Tc^m$-methylene diphosphate scintimammography to image primary breast cancer. *J. Nuc. Med.*, 35:718–724, 1995.

199. W. Pierce, S. Harms, D. Flamig, R. Griffey, and et. al. Three-dimensional Gd-enhanced MR imaging of the breast: pulse sequence with fat suppression and magnetisation transfer contrast. *Radiology*, 181:757–763, 1991.

200. P.Maragos. Tutorial on advances in morphological image processing and analysis. *Optical Engineering*, 26:623 – 632, 1987.

201. M. Poissonnier, R. P. Highnam, M. Brady, B. J. Shepstone, and R. E. English. Integration of low-level processing to facilitate microcalcification detection. In N. Karssemeijer, editor, *4th International Workshop on Digital Mammography*, pages 185 – 188, Nijmegen, Netherlands, 1998. Kluwer Academic Publishers.

202. D. Poole, A. Mackworth, and R. Goebel. *Computational Intelligence: A Logical Approach*. Oxford University Press, Oxford, 1997.

203. C. A. Poynton. Gamma and its disguises. *Journal of the Society of Motion Picture and Television Engineers*, 102:1099 – 1108, 1993.

204. P. Pretorius, P. Hayton, N. R. Moore, and M. Brady. A clinical assessment of the use of a model of contrast enhancement for analysis of dynamic MR breast images. In *Medical Image Understanding and Analysis 97*, pages 57 – 60, Oxford, UK, 1997. BMVA.

205. F. W. Prior, D. S. Channin, S. H. King, M. Schaller, R. Koch, W. Sperner, and R. Kenney. High resolution digital mammography using DIMA and CR: Preliminary results. In A. Gale, S. M. Astley, D. Dance, and A. Y. Cairns, editors, *2nd International Workshop on Digital Mammography*, Excerpta Medica International Congress Series 1069, pages 143 – 151, York, England, 10–12 July 1994. Elsevier Science B.V.

206. P.Wells, editor. *Scientific Basis of Medical Imaging*. Churchill Livingstone, 1982.

207. P. Rinck. *Magnetic Resonance in Medicine*. Blackwell Scientific Publications, 1993.

208. D. Roberts and N. Smith. *Radiographic Imaging*. Churchill Livingstone, 1988.

209. E. J. Roebuck. *Clinical Radiology of the Breast*. Heinemann Medical Books (Oxford), 1990.

210. H. Roehrig, E. A. Krupinski, and W. J. Dallas. Necessary spatial resolution in digital mammography. In H.U. Lemke, M. W. Vannier, K. Inamura, and A. G. Farman, editors, *Computer Assisted Radiology: CAR 96*, International Congress Series 1124, pages 53–59, Paris, June 1996. Elsevier Excerpta Medica.

211. A. Rosenfeld and A. C. Kak. *Digital Picture Processing : Volumes 1, 2*. Academic Press, 1982.

212. R. J. Ross, J. S. Thompson, K. Kim, and R. A. Bailey. Nuclear magnetic resonance imaging and evaluation of human breast tissue: preliminary clinical trials. *Radiology*, 143:195–205, 1982.

213. D. Rubens, S. Totterman, A. Chacko, K. Kothari, W. Loganyoung, J. Szumowski, J.H. Simon, and E. Zachariah. Gadopentetate dimeglumine enhanced chemical shift MR imaging of the breast. *Amer. J. Roentgenology*, 157:267–270, 1991.

214. S. Russell and P. Norvig. *Artificial Intelligence: A Modern Approach*. Prentice Hall, Englewood Cliffs, NJ, 1995.

215. T. J. Ryan and S. P. Curri. Cutaneous adipose tissue. *Clinics in Dermatology*, 7, 1989.

216. M. Sallam and K. Bowyer. Registering time sequences of mammograms using a two-dimensional image unwrapping technique. In A. Gale, S. M. Astley, D. Dance, and A. Y. Cairns, editors, *2nd International Workshop on Digital Mammography*, Excerpta Medica International Congress Series 1069, pages 121–130, York, England, 10–12 July 1994. Elsevier Science B.V.

217. R. Schlief. Ultrasound contrast agents. *Radiology*, 3:198–207, 1991.

218. J. Seibert and J. Boone. X-ray scatter removal by deconvolution. *Medical Physics*, 15:567 – 575, 1988.

219. L. Shen, R. M. Rangayyan, and J. E. Leo Desautels. Detection and classification of mammographic calcifications. *Int. J. Pattern Recog. and Artif. Intell.*, 7(6):1403–1416, 1993.

220. P. Shrivastava. Model to analyse radiographic factors in mammography. *Medical Physics*, 7:222, 1980.

221. F. Shtern. Novel digital technologies for improved control of breast cancer. In H.U. Lemke, M. W. Vannier, K. Inamura, and A. G. Farman, editors, *Computer Assisted Radiology: CAR 96*, International Congress Series 1124, pages 357–361, Paris, June 1996. Elsevier Excerpta Medica.

222. E. A. Sickles. Mammographic features of 300 consecutive nonpalpable breast cancers. *Amer. J. Roentgenology*, 146:661–663, 1986.

223. E. A. Sickles. Management of probably benign breast lesions. *Radiol. Clin. North Am.*, 33(3):1123–1130, 1995.

224. W. Simpson, F. Neilson, and P. J. Kelly. Descriptive terms for mammographic abnormalities: observer variability in application. *Clinical Radiology*, 51:709–713, 1996.

225. J. H. Smith, S. M. Astley, A. P. Hufton, and C. R. M. Boggis. Quantification of breast parenchyma in digitized mammograms. In *Medical Image Analysis and Understanding 97*, pages 137 – 140, Oxford, UK, 1997. BMVA.

226. M. Sonka, X. Zhang, M. Siebes, M. S. Bissing, S. C. DeJong, S. M. Collins, and C. R. McKay. Segmentation of intravascular ultrasound images: a knowledge-based approach. *IEEE Trans. Med. Imaging*, 14:719 – 732, 1995.

227. T. T. Soong and W. N. Huang. A stochastic model for biological tissue elasticity in simple elongation. *Journal of Biomechanics*, 6:451 – 458, 1973.

228. J. P. Stack, O. M. Redmond, M. B. Codd, P. A. Dervan, and J. T. Ennis. Breast disease: tissue characterisation with Gd-DTPA enhancement profiles. *Radiology*, 174:491–494, 1990.

229. E. A. Stamakis, A. Y. Cairns, and I. W. Ricketts. A novel approach to aligning mammograms. In A. Gale, S. M. Astley, D. Dance, and A. Y. Cairns, editors, *2nd International Workshop on Digital Mammography*, Excerpta Medica International Congress Series 1069, pages 355–364, York, England, 10–12 July 1994. Elsevier Science B.V.

230. L. Stanton, J. Day, T. Villafana, C. Miller, and D. Lightfoot. Screen-film mammographic technique for breast cancer screening. *Radiology*, 163:471 – 479, 1987.

231. J. Suckling, D. R. Dance, D. J. Lewis, and S. G. Blacker. Parenchymal delineation by human and computer observers. In A. Gale, S.M. Astley, D.R. Dance, and A.Y. Cairns, editors, *2nd International Workshop on Digital Mammography*, Excerpta Medica International Congress Series 1069, pages 315 – 324, York, England, 10–12 July 1994. Elsevier Science B.V.

232. D. C. Sullivan, C. A. Beam, S. M. Goodman, and D. L. Watt. Measurement of force applied during mammography. *Radiology*, 181:355 – 357, 1991.

233. L. Tabar and P. B. Dean. *Teaching Atlas of Mammography (2nd ed.)*. Thieme Inc., New York, 1985.

234. L. Tarassenko. *A guide to neural computing applications*. Arnold, London, 1998.

235. L. Tarassenko, P. Hayton, N. J. Cerneaz, and M. Brady. Novelty detection for the identification of masses in mammograms. In *Fourth Int. Conf. Artif. Neural Networks*, pages 442 – 447, Cambridge, UK, June 1995. Institute of Electrical Engineers.

236. P. Taylor, R. Owens, and D. Ingram. Multi-scale pattern classification using phase congruency. In K. Doi, M. L. Giger, R. M. Nishikawa, and R. A. Schmidt, editors, *3rd International Workshop on Digital Mammography*, Excerpta Medica International Congress Series 1119, pages 405 – 410, Chicago, USA, 9-12th June 1996. Elsevier Science.

237. P. M. Taylor. Invited review: computer aids for decision-making in diagnostic radiology - a literature review. *British J. Radiology*, 68:945–957, 1995.

238. P. M. Taylor. *Computer assisted decision making for image understanding in medicine*. PhD thesis, University of London (University College), 1998.

239. P. M. Taylor, J. Fox, and A. Todd-Pokropek. A model for integrating image processing into decision aids for diagnostic radiology. *Artificial Intelligence in Medicine*, 9:205–225, 1997.

240. M. M. Tesic, R. A. Mattson, G. T. Barnes, R. A. Sones, and J. B. Stickney. Digital radiology of the chest: design features and considerations for a prototype unit. *Radiology*, 148:259–264, 1983.

241. M. M. Tesic and M. F. Piccaro. Digital mammography system design and performance. In H.U. Lemke, M. W. Vannier, K. Inamura, and A. G. Farman, editors, *Computer Assisted Radiology: CAR 96*, International Congress Series 1124, pages 47–52, Paris, June 1996. Elsevier Excerpta Medica.

242. J-P. Thirion. Fast non-rigid matching of 3D medical images. Technical Report 2547, INRIA, Sophia Antipolis, France, May 1995.

243. P. Tofts, B. Berkowitz, and M. Schnall. Quantitative analysis of dynamic Gd-DTPA enhancement in breast tumours using a permeability model. *Magnetic Resonance*

in Medicine, 33:564–568, 1995.

244. P. Tofts and A. Kermode. Measurement of the blood-brain barrier and leakage space using dynamic MR imaging 1. fundamental concepts. *Magnetic Resonance in Medicine*, 17:357–367, 1991.

245. E. Ueno, E. Tohno, S. Soeda, Y. Asaoka, K. Itoh, J. C. Bamber, M. Blaszczyk, J. Davey, and J. A. McKinna. Dynamic tests in real-time breast echography. *Ultrasound in Med. and Biol. (Supp 1)*, 14:53 – 57, 1988.

246. C. I. Utech, C. S. Young, and P. F. Winter. Prospective evaluation of fluorine-18 fluorodeoxyglucose positron emission tomography in breast cancer for staging of the axilla related to surgery and immunocytochemistry. *Euro. J. Nuc. Med.*, 23:1588–1593, 1996.

247. L. Valatx, I. E. Magnin, and A. Brémond. Automatic microcalcifications and opacities detection in digitised mammograms using a multiscale approach. In A. Gale, S.M. Astley, D.R. Dance, and A.Y. Cairns, editors, *2nd International Workshop on Digital Mammography*, Excerpta Medica International Congress Series 1069, pages 51–57, York, England, 10–12 July 1994. Elsevier Science B.V.

248. D. Vanel. *Imaging Strategies In Oncology*. Martin Dunitz Ltd, London, 1993.

249. B.C. Vemuri, H. Shuangying, D. Sahni, C. Leonard, C. Mohr, R. Gilmore, and J. Fitzsimmons. An effecient motion estimator with application to medical image registration. *Medical Image Analysis*, 2(1):79–98, 1998.

250. P. Viola and W. Wells. Alignment by maximization of mutual information. In *ICCV*, pages 16–23. IEEE Computer Society Press, June 1995.

251. N. Vujovic, P. Bakic, and D. Bzrakovic. Detection of potentially cancerous signs by mammogram follow up. In K. Doi, M. L. Giger, R. M. Nishikawa, and R. A. Schmidt, editors, *3rd International Workshop on Digital Mammography*, Excerpta Medica International Congress Series 1119, pages 421 – 424, Chicago, USA, 9-12th June 1996. Elsevier Science B.V.

252. D. J. Watmough and K. M. Quan. Breast compression to increase the sensitivity of light-scanning for the detection of carcinoma; potential hazard? *Journal of Biomedical Engineering*, pages 173 – 174, 1992.

253. D. J. Watmough and K. M. Quan. X-ray mammography and breast compression. *The Lancet*, 340:122, 1992.

254. S. Webb, editor. *The Physics of Medical Imaging*. Medical Science Series. Institute of Physics Publishing, Bristol and Philadelphia, 1988.

255. N. Weidner, J. P. Semple, W. R. Welch, and J. Folkman. Tumour angiogenesis and metastasis: correlation in invasive breast carcinoma. *New England J. Medicine*, 324:1–8, 1991.

256. J. C. Weinreb and G. Newstead. Controversies in breast MRI. *Magnetic Resonance Quarterly*, 10(2):67–83, 1994.

257. P. N. T. Wells, M. Halliwell, R. Skidmore, A. J. Webb, and J. P. Woodcock. Tumour detection by ultrasonic Doppler flow signals. *Ultrasonics*, 15:231–232, 1977.

258. W. M. Wells III, P. Viola, H. Atsumi, S. Nakajima, and R. Kikinis. Multi-model volume registration by maximization of mutual information. *Medical Image Analysis*, 1(1):35–51, 1996.

259. F. Winsberg, M. Elkin, J. Macy, V. Bordaz, and W. Weymouth. Detection of radiographic abnormalities in mammograms by means of optical scanning and computer analysis. *Radiology*, 89:211 – 215, 1967.

260. C. B. Woodman, A. G.Threlfall, C. R. M. Boggis, and P. Prior. Is the three year breast screening interval too long? Occurrence of interval cancers in NHS breast screening programme's north western region. *British Medical Journal*, 310:224–226, 1995.

261. X. Wu, G. T. Barnes, and D. M. Tucker. Spectral dependence of glandular tissue dose in screen-film mammography. *Radiology*, 179:143 – 148, 1991.

262. Z-Y. Xie and M. Brady. Fractal dimension image for texture segmentation. In *Proceedings of 2nd International Conference on Automation, Robotics and Computer*

Vision, volume 1, pages CV–4.3.1 to CV–4.3.5, 1992.

263. M. J. Yaffe. Development of full-field digital mammography. In N. Karssemeijer, editor, *4th International Workshop on Digital Mammography*, pages 3 – 10, Nijmegen, Netherlands, 1998. Kluwer Academic Publishers.

264. J. M. Yancey, G. F. McNeely, and R. E. Kinard. Breast traction mammography. *Amer. J. Roentgenology*, 156:1321, 1991.

265. F-F. Yin, M. L. Giger, K. Doi, C. E. Metz, and C. J. Vyborny. Computerized detection of masses in digital mammograms: Analysis of bilateral subtraction images. *Medical Physics*, 18:955 – 963, 1991.

266. J. L. Young, C. L. Percy, and A. J. Asire. *Surveillance, Epidemiology, End Results: Incidence and Mortality Data 1973-1977*. US Department of Health and Human Services (NIH) 81-2330, Government Printing Office, 1981.

267. W. Zhang, K. Doi, M. L. Giger, W. Yuzheng, and et. al. Computerized detection of clustered microcalcifications in digital mammograms using a shift-invariant artificial neural network. *Medical Physics*, 21(4):517–524, 1994.

268. B. Zheng, W. Qian, and L. P. Clarke. Digital mammography: mixed feature neural network with spectral entropy decision for detection of microcalcifications. *IEEE Trans. Med. Imaging*, 15(5):589–597, 1996.

269. X. Zhou and R. Gordon. Geometric unwrapping of digital subtraction mammography. In *Proc. Vision Interface '88*, pages 25–30, 1988.

270. C. Zuo, A. Jiang, B. Buff, T. Mahon, and T. Wong. Automatic motion correction for breast MR imaging. *Radiology*, 193(3), 1996.

INDEX